CIRCULATION, NEUROBIOLOGY AND BEHAVIOR

DEVELOPMENTS IN NEUROSCIENCE

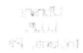

CIRCULATION, NEUROBIOLOGY AND BEHAVIOR

Proceedings of the Working Conference on Circulation, Neurobiology and Behavior held October 4-7, 1981, in Dallas, Texas, U.S.A.

Editors:

ORVILLE A. SMITH, Ph.D.
Professor of Physiology and Biophysics, Director, Regional Primate Research Center, University of Washington, Seattle, Washington, U.S.A.

RICHARD A. GALOSY, Ph.D.
Associate Professor of Cell Biology, University of Texas Health Science Center, Dallas, Texas, U.S.A.

STEPHEN M. WEISS, Ph.D.
Chief, Behavioral Medicine Branch, National Heart, Lung, and Blood Institute, National Institutes of Health, Bethesda, Maryland, U.S.A.

ELSEVIER BIOMEDICAL
New York · Amsterdam · Oxford

The cover illustration, representing the theme of the symposium, is a polygraph
record of heart rate, arterial blood pressure, normal renal blood flow, renal blood flow
in a denervated kidney and oxygen consumption, taken from an unanesthetized baboon
during a conditional emotional situation.

©1982 by Elsevier Science Publishing Co., Inc.

Published by:

Elsevier Science Publishing Co., Inc.
52 Vanderbilt Avenue, New York, New York 10017

Sole distributors outside the USA and Canada:

Elsevier Science Publishers B.V.
P.O. Box 211, 1000 AE, Amsterdam, The Netherlands

Library of Congress Cataloging in Publication Data

Working Conference on Circulation, Neurobiology, and Behavior (1981: Dallas, Tex.)
    Circulation, neurobiology, and behavior.
    (Developments in neuroscience; v. 15)

    Bibliography:
    Includes index.
    1. Nervous system, Vasomotor—Congresses. 2. Cardiovascular system—
    Diseases—Psychosomatic aspects—Congresses. I. Smith, Orville A.
    II. Galosy, Richard A. III. Weiss, Stephen M. IV. Title. V. Series.
QP109.W67   1981   612'.1   82-16261
ISBN 0-444-00759-8

Manufactured in the United States of America

Contents

BEHAVIOR AND SPECIFIC PATTERN OF CARDIOVASCULAR RESPONSES

CENTRAL NEURAL MECHANISMS LINKING
BEHAVIORAL AND CARDIOVASCULAR RESPONSES

TASK FORCE REPORTS ON HYPERTENSION, SUDDEN CARDIAC DEATH,
CORONARY ARTERY DISEASE, AND CARDIOMYOPATHY

Dedication

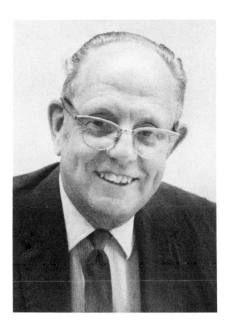

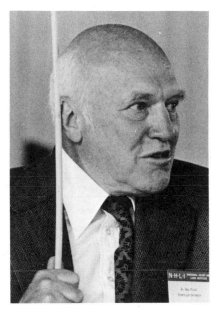

WALTER C. RANDALL   NEAL E. MILLER

To Walter C. Randall and Neal E. Miller, eminent Scientists and Educators who have contributed substantially to our understanding of Circulation, Neurobiology and Behavior.

Preface

As the biomedical community gains more insight into causes of the diseases that plague society, it becomes increasingly obvious that there is considerable overlap of information among disciplines that historically were treated as separate entities. Today rapid growth in knowledge and research techniques is revealing that behavioral factors play an important role in the etiologies of many diseases, several of which involve the cardiovascular system. A primary mediator of the relation between behavior and cardiovascular function is the nervous system. Out of this realization, multidisciplinary research efforts are attempting to explain a constellation of physiological phenomena in a broad context. These developments have made it necessary for many scientists to become more broadly based in their scientific expertise.

In this latter context, it was decided that it would be very important to collect the leaders in the fields of neurobiology, cardiovascular physiology and behavioral analysis in one location for a free and open exchange of research results and ideas. The result was a "working conference" held October 4-7, 1981 in Dallas, Texas, the proceedings of which are presented in this volume.

The volume is divided into four sections. In the first section, the central neural basis for regulation of circulatory control is specified in terms of current knowledge of neuroanatomical connections, electrophysiology, neurochemistry and neuropharmacology related to autonomic and especially cardiovascular control. In the second section, the focus is on the relation between behavior and the generation of specific patterns of cardiovascular responses accompanying those behaviors. The third section presents the central neural mechanisms that may be operative in linking behavior and cardiovascular adjustments. These include mechanisms such as modulation of the baroreflex, central command, and socially produced stress. The fourth section represents a unique attempt to relate this basic biologic information to the genesis of the major pathologic cardiovascular syndromes: hypertension, sudden cardiac death, coronary artery disease, and cardiomyopathy.

The volume represents an ambitious attempt to bring together in one place the most current material ranging across three broad disciplines. This information has been related to important clinical syndromes, and specific recommendations for further research with direct bearing on the clinical problem are presented.

Orville A. Smith, Richard A. Galosy and Stephen M. Weiss

Acknowledgments

We would like to thank Lewis Clarke, John Smith, and Carolyn Hamm of The University of Texas Health Science Center at Dallas, and Tim Engebretson, Joan Twiss, Margaret Mattson, and Katrina Johnson of the National Institutes of Health, for their considerable support and many hours they spent insuring the success of the conference. Special thanks are in order to the Behavioral Medicine Branch of the National Institutes of Health and Dr. Charles C. Sprague, President of The University of Texas Health Science Center at Dallas, for providing the funds and confidence that made the conference possible.

The task force reports represent a group effort, and we thank Sonja Haber of the National Institutes of Health for collecting and organizing these chapters. She was assisted by Gosha Ziajka and Elizabeth Sandler.

This volume was prepared at the Regional Primate Research Center at the University of Washington (supported by NIH grant RR00166), and we gratefully acknowledge the individuals who put it all together. We particularly thank Phyllis Wood for touching up numerous illustrations, Patricia Huling for meticulously preparing the camera-ready mats, and Kate Schmitt for editing the volume and coordinating the many phases of its production.

Participants and Contributors

DAVID ANDERSON
Department of Psychiatry, University of South Florida College of Medicine, Tampa, Florida

WILLIAM BAILEY
Rockefeller University, New York, New York

MICHAEL J. BRODY
Department of Pharmacology, University of Iowa College of Medicine, Iowa City, Iowa

C. ANDREW COMBS
Regional Primate Research Center, University of Washington, Seattle, Washington

KARL C. CORLEY, JR.
Department of Physiology, Medical College of Virginia, Richmond, Virginia

ISAAC L. CRAWFORD
Department of Neurology and Pharmacology, Southwestern Medical School, Dallas, Texas

KENNETH J. DORMER
Department of Physiology and Biophysics, University of Oklahoma, Oklahoma City, Oklahoma

ROBERT FOREMAN
Department of Physiology and Biophysics, University of Oklahoma, Oklahoma City, Oklahoma

RICHARD A. GALOSY
Department of Cell Biology, University of Texas Health Science Center, Dallas, Texas

GERARD L. GEBBER
Department of Pharmacology and Toxicology, Michigan State University, East Lansing, Michigan

RICHARD A. GILLIS

Department of Pharmacology, Georgetown University School of Medicine and Dentistry, Washington, D.C.

ALAN HARRIS

Department of Psychiatry and Behavioral Sciences, Johns Hopkins University School of Medicine, Baltimore, Maryland

JAMES P. HENRY

Department of Physiology, University of Southern California, Los Angeles, California

J. ALAN HERD

Sid W. Richardson Institute for Preventive Medicine, The Methodist Hospital, Houston, Texas

STUART HOBBS

Department of Physiology and Biophysics, University of Washington, Seattle, Washington

ALAN K. JOHNSON

Department of Psychology, University of Iowa, Iowa City, Iowa

JAMES A. JOSEPH

Gerontology Research Center, National Institute of Aging/NIH, Baltimore City Hospital, Baltimore, Maryland

MARC P. KAUFMAN

Department of Physiology, University of Texas Health Science Center, Dallas, Texas

JAMES LAWLER

Department of Psychology, University of Tennessee, Knoxville, Tennessee

ARTHUR D. LOEWY

Department of Anatomy and Neurobiology, Washington University School of Medicine, St. Louis, Missouri

JOHN W. MANNING

Department of Physiology, Emory University, Atlanta, Georgia

NEAL E. MILLER

Rockefeller University, New York, New York

JERE H. MITCHELL

Department of Medicine and Physiology, University of Texas, Southwestern Medical School, Dallas, Texas

BENJAMIN H. NATELSON

Department of Neuroscience, New Jersey Medical School, East Orange, New Jersey

MARC A. NATHAN

Department of Pharmacology, University of Texas Health Science Center, San Antonio, Texas

PAUL A. OBRIST

Department of Psychiatry, School of Medicine, University of North Carolina, Chapel Hill, North Carolina

DAVID C. RANDALL

Department of Physiology and Biophysics, University of Kentucky College of Medicine, Lexington, Kentucky

WALTER C. RANDALL

Department of Physiology, Loyola University, Stritch School of Medicine, Maywood, Illinois

DONALD J. REIS

Department of Neurology, Cornell University Medical School, New York, New York

LORING B. ROWELL

Department of Physiology and Biophysics, University of Washington, Seattle, Washington

EVELYN SATINOFF

Department of Psychology, University of Illinois, Champaign, Illinois

NEIL SCHNEIDERMAN

Department of Psychology, University of Miami, Coral Gables, Florida

LAWRENCE P. SCHRAMM
Department of Biomedical Engineering, Johns Hopkins University School of Medicine, Baltimore, Maryland

GARY E. SCHWARTZ
Department of Psychology, Yale University, New Haven, Connecticut

ALVIN SHAPIRO
University of Pittsburgh School of Medicine, Pittsburgh, Pennsylvania

JOHN B. SIMPSON
Department of Psychology, University of Washington, Seattle, Washington

JAMES E. SKINNER
Department of Neurology and Neuroscience Program, Baylor College of Medicine, Houston, Texas

ORVILLE A. SMITH
Regional Primate Research Center, University of Washington, Seattle, Washington

ROBERT B. STEPHENSON
Department of Physiology, Michigan State University, East Lansing, Michigan

H. LOWELL STONE
Department of Physiology and Biophysics, University of Oklahoma, Oklahoma City, Oklahoma

LARRY W. SWANSON
Salk Institute, La Jolla, California

JAYLAN TURKKAN
Department of Psychiatry and Behavioral Sciences, Johns Hopkins University School of Medicine, Baltimore, Maryland

ARTHUR J. VANDER
Department of Physiology, University of Michigan, Ann Arbor, Michigan

RICHARD L. VERRIER

Cardiovascular Research, Department of Nutrition, Harvard School of Public Health, Boston, Massachusetts

SUSAN WALGENBACH

Department of Physiology and Biophysics, Mayo Foundation, Rochester, Minnesota

LYNNE C. WEAVER

Department of Physiology, Michigan State University, East Lansing, Michigan

JAY WEISS

Rockefeller University, New York, New York

STEPHEN M. WEISS

Behavioral Medicine Branch, National Heart, Lung and Blood Institute, National Institutes of Health, Bethesda, Maryland

REDFORD B. WILLIAMS, JR.

Department of Psychiatry, Duke University Medical Center, Durham, North Carolina

CIRCULATION, NEUROBIOLOGY
AND BEHAVIOR

Central Neural Basis for
Control of the Circulation

Copyright 1982 by Elsevier Science Publishing Co.,Inc.
Smith, Galosy, and Weiss, editors
CIRCULATION, NEUROBIOLOGY, AND BEHAVIOR   3

Central Cardiovascular Pathways

ARTHUR D. LOEWY
Department of Anatomy and Neurobiology, Washington University School of Medicine, St. Louis, Missouri

INTRODUCTION

A growing field in neurobiology deals with the organization of central autonomic pathways. One area of particular interest has been to define those neural circuits that are involved in blood pressure control and to determine the neurotransmitters associated with them. In this chapter, a brief summary will be made of this area.

ORGANIZATION OF AUTONOMIC PREGANGLIONIC NEURONS

Sympathetic Preganglionic Neurons

Sympathetic preganglionic neurons arise from four sites within the spinal cord at the T1-L2 levels (Fig. 1): (1) intermediolateral cell column, (2) intercalated neurons in the intermediate gray matter (Rexed's (1954) lamina VII), (3) central autonomic neurons dorsal to the central canal, and (4) scattered cells in the lateral funiculus (Chung et al., 1975; Dalsgaard and Elfvin, 1979; Deuschl and Illert, 1978; Petras and Faden, 1978; Schramm et al., 1975). The greatest number of cells arise from the intermediolateral cell column (Deuschl and Illert, 1978) and are found concentrated in cell clusters that become continuous with the intercalated cells (Deuschl and Illert, 1978; Petras and Faden, 1978; Schramm et al., 1975).

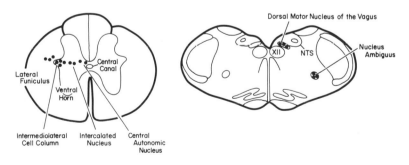

Fig. 1. Location of sympathetic preganglionic neurons (left) and parasympathetic cardiac neurons (right).

Petras and Faden (1978) observed that the sympathetic preganglionic neurons that innervate the paravertebral ganglia arise mainly from the intermediolateral cell column and lateral funiculus, while those that innervate the pre-aortic ganglia arise from the intercalated cells. Horseradish peroxidase (HRP) transport studies by Dalsgaard and Elfvin (1979) support this observation. The functional significance of this arrangement is not understood. Lebedev et al. (1976) found that the intercalated preganglionic cells conduct action potentials in the range of 0.98-1.7 m/sec (C fibers) and the neurons of the intermediolateral cell column conduct in the range of 3-10 m/sec (B-fibers).

Until recently, it was assumed that the transmitter released by the sympathetic preganglionic neurons was acetylcholine. Studies by Konishi et al. (1981) indicate that an enkephalin-like transmitter is also released in the inferior mesenteric ganglion; this release is blocked by naloxone. The enkephalin-like transmitter is released and causes presynaptic inhibition of the acetylcholine-containing fibers (Fig. 2).

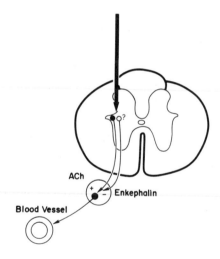

Fig. 2. Presynaptic inhibition of the acetylcholine preganglionic fibers, caused by enkephalin-like preganglionic sympathetic fibers (Konishi et al., 1981).

It is not yet known whether sympathetic preganglionic neurons contain both acetylcholine and an enkephalin-like substance as has been observed in sacral preganglionic neurons (Glazer and Basbaum, 1980). A peptide resembling luteinizing releasing hormone (LHRH) has been found in frog sympathetic ganglia (Jan and Jan, 1981), but not in mammals (Konishi et al., 1979). These results indicate the potential complexity of the sympathetic outflow.

Two other issues regarding the organization of the sympathetic preganglionic neurons have not yet been resolved: the first deals with the question of whether the axons of the sympathetic preganglionic neurons possess collaterals, and the second deals with whether there are local interneurons modulating the sympathetic outflow. Golgi studies by Rethelyi (1972) have failed to provide evidence that sympathetic preganglionic neurons have axonal collaterals. Since this question has not yet been addressed by making intracellular labeling with HRP, Lucifer yellow, or some other dye into electrophysiologically identified sympathetic preganglionic neurons, the significance of this negative result is still unclear. Lebedev et al. (1980) suggested that certain sympathetic preganglionic neurons have some type of recurrent inhibitory mechanism. Whether this is due to recurrent collaterals or some type of dendrodendritic mechanism (Gebber, 1980) is unknown. The second unresolved question deals with the existence of local interneurons. Studies by Gebber and McCall (1976) and McCall et al. (1977) indicate that there are neurons in the intermediomedial nucleus of the spinal cord whose firing pattern is related to the R wave of the electrocardiogram and that could not be antidromically activated by stimulation of the cervical or thoracic sympathetic nerves. These cells may be one set of local interneurons modulating the sympathetic outflow.

Parasympathetic Preganglionic Neurons

The site of origin of the cardiac vagal preganglionic neurons varies from one species of mammal to another (Nosaka et al., 1979). Kerr (1967, 1969) observed that following lesions of the dorsal motor nucleus in the cat, electrical stimulation of the cervical portion of the vagus nerve still caused cardioinhibition. Subsequently, McAllen and Spyer (1976) demonstrated in this species that the cardiac preganglionic neurons affecting heart rate arose solely from the nucleus ambiguus. They found that iontophoresis of the excitatory amino acid D,L-homocysteic acid onto a single cardiovagal cell caused bradycardia. Geis and Wurster (1980a) observed that after HRP injections in the heart of the cat, retrograde cell labeling was present in both the dorsal motor nucleus and the nucleus ambiguus. Later (1980b), they demonstrated that stimulation of the dorsal motor nucleus caused an increase in ventricular contractility while stimulation of the nucleus ambiguus caused a decrease in heart rate.

The central pathways that modulate the cardiovagal outflow have not been examined. It is known, however, that opioid receptors are localized in the nucleus ambiguus (Goodman et al., 1980) and enkephalin-like fibers have been described in this area (Finley et al., 1981b). Microinjections of morphine-like drugs (fentanyl and met-enkephalinamide) into the nucleus ambiguus of the dog cause bradycardia which was antagonized by naloxone (Laubie et al., 1979).

CARDIOVASCULAR AFFERENT INPUTS TO THE NUCLEUS TRACTUS SOLITARIUS

Baroreceptors and chemoreceptors of the carotid sinus and aortic arch provide direct inputs to the nucleus tractus solitarius (NTS). Using the transganglionic transport technique, the central projections of the carotid sinus nerve and the aortic depressor nerve have been studied in several species (Berger, 1979; Wallach and Loewy, 1980). Figure 3 shows the labeling pattern seen after incubating the aortic nerve of a rabbit in HRP. Since this nerve in the rabbit carries only barosensory information, this type of experiment indicates that the dorsomedial region of the NTS and to a lesser degree in the commissural nucleus receive baroreceptor information.

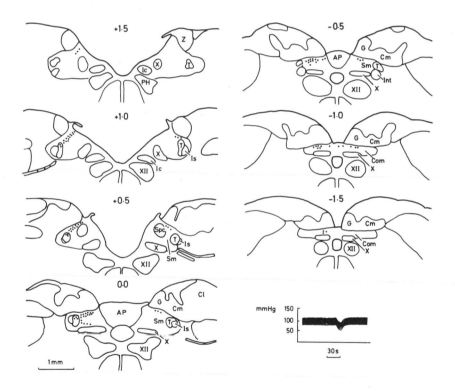

Fig. 3. After incubating the left aortic nerve of a rabbit in HRP transganglionic labeling is seen in the dorsomedial, medial and commissural regions of the nucleus tractus solitarius. (From Wallach and Loewy, 1980, with permission.)

Various neuropeptides have been localized in the nodose ganglion and NTS (Fig. 4), including substance P, vasoactive intestinal polypeptide, cholecystokinin, methionine-enkephalin, and somatostatin (Finley et al., 1981b; Ljungdahl et al., 1978; Lundberg et al.,

1978; Uhl et al., 1979). Haeusler and Osterwalder (1980) suggested that substance P may be the transmitter of the primary afferent fibers for the baroreceptor reflex. Their argument was based on the immunohistochemical findings of others who have localized substance P-like immunoreactivity in the carotid sinus and aortic arch, petrosal and nodose ganglia, and NTS, and on the observation by Gillis et al. (1980) that intracranial transection of IXth and Xth cranial nerves caused a decrease in substance P in the NTS. Haeusler and Osterwalder (1980) found that application of substance P or capsaicin (an agent that causes the release of substance P) to the NTS caused a decrease in blood pressure and heart rate. Talman and Reis (1981) could not confirm this result, and pointed out that the maximal amount of substance P they could get in solution and subsequently inject into the NTS without causing local distortion of the NTS was 0.7 n moles. This dose and volume was much less than that used by Haeusler and Osterwalder, and did not cause a decrease in blood pressure or heart rate.

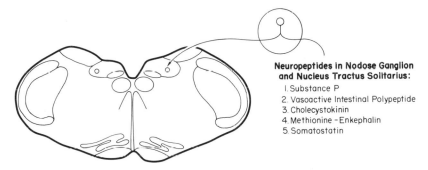

Neuropeptides in Nodose Ganglion and Nucleus Tractus Solitarius:
1. Substance P
2. Vasoactive Intestinal Polypeptide
3. Cholecystokinin
4. Methionine-Enkephalin
5. Somatostatin

Fig. 4. Various neuropeptides localized in the nodose ganglion and nucleus tractus solitarius.

Talman et al. (1980) provided evidence for a high affinity uptake system for glutamate in the NTS. They also found that microinjections of glutamate caused hypotension. On the basis of these findings and subsequent studies with the glutamate antagonist, glutamic diethyl ester (Talman et al., 1981), they suggested that L-glutamate may be a potential transmitter at the NTS.

Our group became interested in this problem. Dietrich et al. (in press) examined the levels of aspartate, glutamate, and GABA in various subnuclei of the NTS in the cat. L-glutamate was found to be particularly high in those regions of the NTS where the carotid sinus nerve and aortic depressor nerves appear to terminate, viz., the dorsal and commissural nuclei. Transection of the IXth and Xth cranial nerves caused a decrease in glutamate levels in these areas. These data support the idea that glutamate may be involved as a transmitter in this reflex.

8

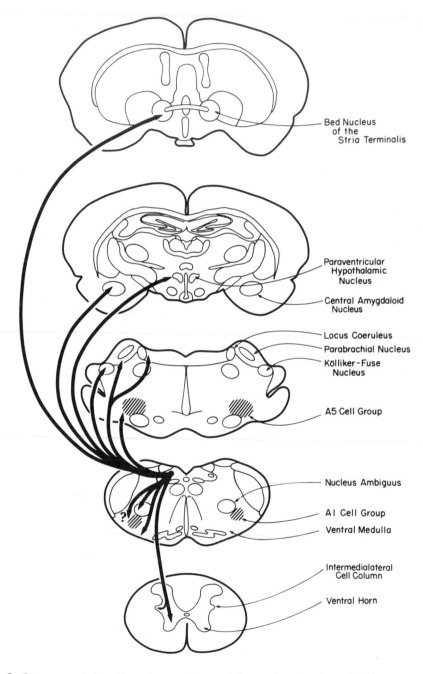

Bed Nucleus
of the
Stria Terminalis

Paraventricular
Hypothalamic
Nucleus

Central Amygdaloid
Nucleus

Locus Coeruleus

Parabrachial Nucleus

Kölliker-Fuse
Nucleus

A5 Cell Group

Nucleus Ambiguus

A1 Cell Group

Ventral Medulla

Intermedialateral
Cell Column

Ventral Horn

Fig. 5. Summary of the efferent connections of the nucleus tractus solitarius.

EFFERENT CONNECTIONS OF THE NUCLEUS TRACTUS SOLITARIUS

Afferent cardiovascular information is relayed from the NTS to a number of sites in the central nervous system (CNS). Figure 5 presents a schematic summary of the efferent connections of the NTS. Many of the projections are bilateral, but in this illustration only ipsilateral connections are shown for graphic clarity. The scheme is based on a series of autoradiographic studies which, for the most part, have been verified using the retrograde transport of HRP (Loewy and Burton, 1978; Ricardo and Koh, 1978). However, it should be stressed that these studies do not clarify the type of visceral information that is being relayed. For example, Loewy and Burton (1978) injected tritiated amino acids in regions of the NTS where cardiac activity could be recorded, but pointed out that some of the isotope may have spread to cells involved with other types of visceral information. Nevertheless, it is clear that the NTS may influence a number of sites in the CNS that project directly to the sympathetic preganglionic neurons (e.g., A5 catecholamine cell group, ventral medulla, Kolliker-Fuse nucleus, parvocellular division of the paraventricular hypothalamic nucleus) as well as nuclei that modulate the release of vasopressin because of their direct connections to hypothalamic magnocellular neurons (A1 catecholamine cell group and ventral medulla) (McKellar and Loewy, 1981). Some of these pathways seem to arise from norepinephrine- and epinephrine-containing cells. Others may arise from somatostatin, enkephalin, or neurotensin-like neurons (Finley et al., 1981b; Finley et al., 1981b; Ljungdahl et al., 1978; Uhl et al., 1979). The connections of these various neuropeptide- and catecholamine-containing NTS neurons are unknown.

REFERENCES

Berger, A.J. (1979) Distribution of carotid sinus nerve afferent fibers to solitary tract nuclei of the cat using transganglionic transport of horseradish peroxidase. Neurosci. Lett. 14, 53-58.

Chung, J.M., Chung, K. and Wurster, R.D. (1975) Sympathetic preganglionic neurons of the cat spinal cord: horseradish peroxidase study. Brain Res. 91, 126-131.

Dalsgaard, C.J. and Elfvin, L.G. (1979) Spinal origin of preganglionic fibers projecting onto the superior cervical ganglion and inferior mesenteric ganglion of the guinea pig, as demonstrated by the horseradish peroxidase technique. Brain Res. 172, 139-143.

Deuschl, G. and Illert, M. (1978) Location of lumbar preganglionic sympathetic neurones in the cat. Neurosci. Lett. 10, 49-54.

Dietrich, W.D., Lowry, O.H. and Loewy, A.D. (In press) The distribution of glutamate, GABA, and aspartate in the nucleus tractus solitarius of the cat. Brain Res.

Finley, J.C.W., Maderdrut, J.L. and Petrusz, P. (1981a) The immunocytochemical localization of enkephalin in the central nervous system of the rat. J. Comp. Neurol. 198, 541-565.

Finley, J.C.W., Maderdrut, J.L., Roger, L.J. and Petrusz, P. (1981b) The immunocytochemical localization of somatostatin-containing neurons in the rat central nervous system. Neuroscience 6, 2173-2192.

Gebber, G.L. (1980) Bulbospinal control of sympathetic nerve discharge; in Neural Control of Circulation, M.J. Hughes and C.D. Barnes, eds. Academic Press, New York, pp. 51-80.

Gebber, G.L. and McCall, R.B. (1976) Identification and discharge patterns of spinal sympathetic interneurons. Amer. J. Physiol. 231, 722-733.

Geis, G.S. and Wurster, R.D. (1980) Horseradish peroxidase location of cardiac vagal preganglionic somata. Brain Res. 182, 19-30.

Geis, G.S. and Wurster, R.D. (1980) Cardiac responses during stimulation of the dorsal motor nucleus and nucleus ambiguus in the cat. Circulat. Res. 46, 606-611.

Gillis, R.A., Helke, C.J., Hamilton, B.L., Norman, W.P. and Jacobowitz, D.M. (1980) Evidence that substance P is a neurotransmitter of baro- and chemoreceptor afferents in nucleus tractus solitarius. Brain Res. 181, 476-481.

Glazer, E.G. and Basbaum, A.I. (1980) Leucine enkephalin: localization in and axoplasmic transport by sacral parasympathetic preganglionic neurons. Science 208, 1479-1481.

Goodman, R.R., Snyder, S.H., Kuhar, M.J. and Young, W.S. III (1980) Differentiation of delta and mu opiate receptor localizations by light microscopic autoradiography. Proc. Nat. Acad. Sci. 77, 6239-6243.

Haeusler, G. and Osterwalder, R. (1980) Evidence suggesting a transmitter of neuromodulatory role for substance P at the first synapse of the baroreceptor reflex. Naunyn-Schmiedeberg's Arch. Pharmacol. 314, 111-121.

Jan, L.Y. and Jan, Y.N. (1981) Role of an LHRH-like peptide as a neurotransmitter in sympathetic ganglia of the frog. Fed. Proc. 40, 2560-2564.

Kerr, F.W.L. (1967) Function of the dorsal motor nucleus of the vagus. Science 157, 451-452.

Kerr, F.W.L. (1969) Preserved vagal visceromotor function following destruction of the dorsal motor nucleus. J. Physiol. (Lond.) 202, 755-769.

Konishi, S., Tsunoo, A. and Otsuka, M. (1979) Substance P and noncholinergic excitatory synaptic transmission in guinea pig sympathetic ganglia. Proc. Jap. Acad. B55, 525-530.

Konishi, S., Tsunoo, A. and Otsuka, M. (1981) Enkephalin as a transmitter for presynaptic inhibition in sympathetic ganglion. Nature 294, 80-82.

Laubie, M., Schmitt, H. and Vincent, M. (1979) Vagal bradycardia produced by microinjections of morphine-like drugs into the nucleus ambiguus in anaesthetized dogs. Eur. J. Pharmacol. 59, 287-291.

Lebedev, V.P., Petrov, V.I. and Skobelev, V.A. (1976) Antidromic discharges of sympathetic preganglionic neurons located outside of the spinal cord lateral horns. Neurosci. Lett. 2, 325-329.

Lebedev, V.P., Petrov, V.I. and Skobelev, V.A. (1980) Do sympathetic preganglionic neurones have a recurrent inhibitory mechanism? Pflügers Arch. 383, 91-97.

Ljungdahl, A., Hokfelt, T. and Nilsson, G. (1978) Distribution of substance P-like immunoreactivity in the central nervous system of the rat. I. Cell bodies and nerve terminals. Neuroscience 3, 861-943.

Loewy, A.D. and Burton, H. (1978) Nuclei of the solitary tract: efferent connections to the lower brain stem and spinal cord of the cat. J. Comp. Neurol. 181, 421-450.

Lundberg, J.M., Hokfelt, T., Nilsson, G., Terenius, L., Rehfeld, J., Elde, R., and Said, S. (1978) Peptide neurons in the vagus, splanchnic, and sciatic nerves. Acta Physiol. Scand. 104, 499-501.

McAllen, R.M. and Spyer, K.M. (1976) The location of cardiac vagal preganglionic motoneurones in the medulla of the cat. J. Physiol. (Lond.) 258, 187-204.

McCall, R.B., Gebber, G.L. and Barman, S.M. (1977) Spinal interneurons in the baroreceptor reflex arc. Amer. J. Physiol. 232, H657-H665.

McKellar, S. and Loewy, A.D. (1981) Organization of some brain stem afferents to the paraventricular nucleus of the hypothalamus in the rat. Brain Res. 217, 351-357.

Nosaka, S., Yamamoto, T. and Yasunaga, K. (1979) Localization of vagal cardioinhibitory preganglionic neurons within rat brain stem. J. Comp. Neurol. 186, 79-92.

Petras, J.M. and Faden, A.I. (1978) The origin of sympathetic preganglionic neurons in the dog. Brain Res. 144, 353-357.

Rethelyi, M. (1972) Cell and neuropil architecture of the interomediolateral (sympathetic) nucleus of the cat spinal cord. Brain Res. 46, 203-213.

Rexed, B. (1954) A cytoarchitectonic atlas of the spinal cord of the cat. J. Comp. Neurol. 100, 297-379.

Ricardo, J.A. and Koh, E.T. (1978) Anatomical evidence of direct projections from the nucleus of the solitary tract to the hypothalamus, amygdala and other forebrain structures in the rat. Brain Res. 153, 1-26.

Schramm, L.P., Adair, J.P., Stribling, J.M. and Gray, L.P. (1975) Preganglionic innervation of the adrenal gland of the rat: a study using horseradish peroxidase. Exp. Neurol. 49, 540-553.

Talman, W.T., Perrone, M.H. and Reis, D.J. (1980) Evidence for L-glutamate as the neurotransmitter of baroreceptor afferent nerve fibers. Science 209, 813-814.

Talman, W.T., Perrone, M.H., Scher, P., Kwo, S. and Reis, D.J. (1981) Antagonism of the baroreceptor reflex by glutamate diethyl ester, an antagonist to L-glutamate. Brain Res. 217, 186-191.

Talman, W.T. and Reis, D.J. (1981) Baroreflex actions of substance P microinjected into the nucleus tractus solitarii in rat: a consequence of local distortion. Brain Res. 220, 402-407.

Wallach, J.H. and Loewy, A.D. (1980) Projections of the aortic nerve to the nucleus tractus solitarius in the rabbit. Brain Res. 188, 247-251.

Uhl, G.R., Goodman, R.R. and Snyder, S.H. (1979) Neurotensin-containing cell bodies, fibers, and nerve terminals in the brain stem of the rat: immunohistochemical mapping. Brain Res. 167, 77-91.

Copyright 1982 by Elsevier Science Publishing Co.,Inc.
Smith, Galosy, and Weiss, editors
CIRCULATION, NEUROBIOLOGY, AND BEHAVIOR

Forebrain Neural Mechanisms Involved in Cardiovascular Regulation

L. W. SWANSON
The Salk Institute and The Clayton Foundation for Research--California Division, San Diego, California

INTRODUCTION

Two major divisions of the forebrain are thought to play important roles in the neural circuitry that regulates the cardiovascular (CV) system. The cerebral cortex is almost certainly involved in the mediation of changes in heart rate and blood pressure that accompany "psychogenic stress," because the responses are based on the perception and integration of sensory information and are often influenced by past experience. The hypothalamus, which is often considered to be the "head ganglion" of the visceral system, is of particular importance because cells in the paraventricular (PVH) and supraoptic (SO) nuclei release the hormone vasopressin into the blood stream of the posterior pituitary, and because it modulates autonomic reflexes in the lower brain stem and spinal cord.

We shall focus, in this brief review, on recent anatomical evidence that clarifies the organization of neural pathways involved in the integration of endocrine and autonomic responses from the hypothalamus, and in the relay of cognitive information from the cortical mantle to the hypothalamus and to lower autonomic centers. For many years the existence of such pathways was inferred from the results of physiological experiments, with little insight into their morphological substrate. Almost a century ago, Spencer (1894) showed that vasomotor responses could be elicited by electrical stimulation of prefrontal (orbital) cortical areas in a variety of species, including the monkey. This observation was essentially forgotten for almost 50 years, until a flood of similar experiments implicated a number of other parts of the telencephalon, including anterior regions of the cingulate gyrus (Smith, 1945), the amygdala (Kaada, 1951), where the elicited bradycardia was shown to be vagally mediated (Reis and Oliphant, 1964), and the septum (Ranson et al., 1935). On the other hand, the pioneering work of Karplus and Kreidl (1910) established that electrical stimulation of the hypothalamus produces a wide range of autonomic effects, including changes in the CV system, and this work was confirmed and greatly extended by Hess (1947) and by Ranson and colleagues (1939).

Recent anatomical evidence, based on the axonal transport of a variety of markers and on the immunohistochemical identification of transmitter-specific pathways, has begun to clarify the neural basis of these responses. For the sake of clarity, the following discussion will deal with three major topics: the origin of direct inputs from the forebrain to autonomic cell groups in the medulla and spinal cord, the afferent regulation of vasopressin secretion, and the integration of autonomic and neuroendocrine responses to baroreceptor information.

DIRECT PROJECTIONS TO AUTONOMIC CENTERS

As summarized in Figure 1, direct projections have been demonstrated from a surprising variety of cell groups in the forebrain to preganglionic cell groups and to the nucleus of the solitary tract (NTS), which relays inputs from the carotid sinus and aortic depressor nerves to other parts of the brain and spinal cord involved in the mediation of baroreceptor reflexes. Anterograde and retrograde axonal transport studies in the rat

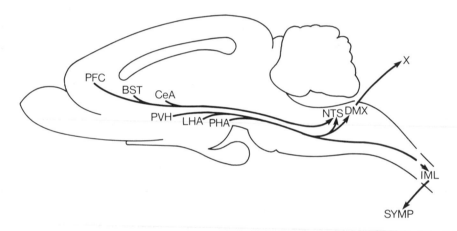

Fig. 1. Summary of the major cell groups in the forebrain that project directly to the dorsal vagal complex and to the intermediolateral column (IML) of the spinal cord, which gives rise to preganglionic fibers of the sympathetic (SYMP) system. The regions in the telencephalon send fibers to the nucleus of the solitary tract (NTS), while those in the hypothalamus also innervate the dorsal motor nucleus of the vagus (DMX) and the IML. The substantia innominata and zona incerta (not shown) may also contribute to these pathways. Other abbreviations: BST, bed nucleus of the stria terminalis; CeA, central nucleus of the amygdala; LHA, lateral hypothalamic area; PFC, prefrontal cortex; PHA, posterior hypothalamic area; PVH, paraventricular nucleus; X, vagus nerve.

indicate that pyramidal cells in the deeper layers of a rather broad expanse of the prefrontal cortex project bilaterally to the NTS, and perhaps in a limited way to the dorsal motor nucleus of the vagus as well (Van der Kooy et al., submitted). Similar methods have been used to show that cells in the central nucleus of the amygdala (Hopkins and Holstege, 1978; Post and Mai, 1980; Schwaber et al., 1980; Price and Amaral, 1981) project in much the same way to the dorsal vagal complex, as apparently do cells in adjacent parts of the substantia innominata and the bed nucleus of the stria terminalis (Schwaber et al., 1980). In summary, then, restricted parts of the prefrontal cortex, the amygdala, and the septal region (but not the cingulate gyrus) project directly to the NTS, and may thus influence the relay of afferent baroreceptor information to other parts of the CNS. It should be pointed out that these same telencephalic regions also project to the parabrachial nucleus in the dorsolateral pons (Hopkins and Holstege, 1978; Post and Mai, 1980; Price and Amaral, 1981; Krettek and Price, 1978; Swanson and Cowan, 1979), which is known to relay information from the NTS to a variety of structures in the forebrain, including the hypothalamus and the amygdala (Post and Mai, 1980; Saper and Loewy, 1980).

Several years ago it was shown with the HRP and autoradiographic methods (in the rat, cat and monkey) that fibers from the hypothalamus, unlike those from the telencephalic structures just considered, descend as far as the sympathetic cell groups in the spinal cord, as well as to the NTS and the dorsal motor nucleus of the vagus (Saper et al., 1976), and it was suggested that cells in the lateral and posterior hypothalamic areas, in the zona incerta, and, surprisingly, in the PVH itself contribute to these pathways. Since then attention has focused on the PVH because it is a compact cell group, and because it contains dense clusters of vasopressinergic and oxytocinergic cells that project to the posterior pituitary and may thus be involved in both the endocrine and autonomic modes of CV regulation. The results of these studies have been reviewed in detail elsewhere (Swanson and Sawchenko, 1980, in press), and will only be summarized here.

The PVH in the rat contains readily distinguishable magnocellular and parvocellular divisions, and is thus more complex on cytoarchitectonic grounds alone than the SO, which consists almost entirely of magnocellular neurosecretory neurons. It is now clear that most of the cells in the SO, and in the magnocellular division of the PVH, project to the posterior pituitary, and that both regions contain groups of cells that synthesize either oxytocin or vasopressin. In addition, however, cells concentrated in the parvocellular division of the PVH project to the portal system zone of the median eminence, where they are presumably in a position to influence the release of anterior pituitary hormones including ACTH (Makara et al., 1981), and to autonomic centers in the brain stem and spinal cord. Double-labeling studies with different retrogradely transported fluorescent markers (Swanson and Kuypers, 1980; Swanson et al., 1980) further indicate that essentially different, and topographically segregated, cell groups in the PVH project to the posterior pituitary, to the external lamina of the median eminence, and to the brain stem and spinal cord, although, interestingly, a substantial proportion of the cells that innervate the intermediolateral column in the spinal cord also appear to send a collateral to the dorsal vagal complex (Fig. 2). Single cells in the PVH may thus innervate both sympathetic and parasympathetic cell groups, while other cells release vasopressin in the posterior pituitary, or release vasopressin (and other as yet unidentified peptides) in the median eminence.

The descending pathway from the PVH appears to be rather substantial, as at least 1500 cells contribute to it (Swanson and Kuypers, 1980), and to be functionally hetero-geneous. Double-labeling studies based on the use of a retrogradely transported marker and the immunohistochemical localization of specific antigens indicate that essentially separate groups of cells that cross-react with antisera to oxytocin, vasopressin, somato-statin, leu-enkephalin, met-enkephalin, or tyrosine hydroxylase (and are presumably dopaminergic) all project to the dorsal vagal complex and to the spinal cord (Swanson et al., 1981; Sawchenko and Swanson, in press b). However, as these 6 cell types appear to account for only about a quarter of the cells in the PVH with descending projections, it seems likely that additional cell groups remain to be identified.

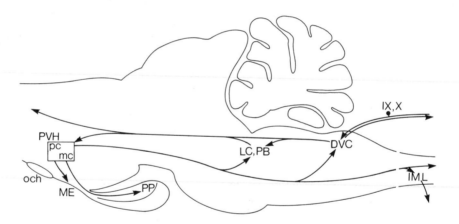

Fig. 2. Different cell groups in the magnocellular (mc) and parvocellular (pc) divisions of the paraventricular nucleus (PVH) project to the posterior pituitary (PP), to the median eminence (ME), and to several regions in the lower brain stem and spinal cord, including the dorsal vagal complex (DVC). The latter also receives visceral sensory information from the glossopharyngeal (IX) and vagus (X) nerves, and projects directly to parvocellular parts of the PVH. Other abbreviations: LC, locus ceruleus; PB, parabrachial nucleus. (From Swanson and Sawchenko, 1980, with permission.)

The course and distribution of oxytocin-stained fibers in the lower brain stem and spinal cord have been studied in some detail. These fibers, all of which appear to arise in the PVH (Swanchenko and Swanson, in press b), course initially through the medial forebrain bundle, and then descend through ventrolateral parts of the reticular formation to the dorsolateral funiculus of the spinal cord, where they can be followed as far caudally as the filum terminali (Swanson, 1977; Swanson and McKellar, 1979). Along the way, fibers leave this pathway to distribute within the Edinger-Westphal nucleus, the locus ceruleus and parabrachial nucleus (which also appear to receive an input that courses through the central gray), the dorsal vagal complex, and the intermediolateral column, central gray, and marginal zone of the spinal cord. Interestingly, oxytocin-stained fibers are selectively distributed within the dorsal vagal complex (including the dorsal motor nucleus; P.E. Sawchenko and L.W. Swanson, in preparation), and the intermediolateral column (Swanson and McKellar, 1979). For example, such fibers are particularly dense in spinal segments T_9-T_{11}, which contain many preganglionic neurons that are involved in the sympathetic innervation of the adrenal medulla and the kidney, and may thus play a role in the regulation of blood pressure and volume. Although the precise functional significance of these fibers remains to be determined, it is clear that descending fibers from a single hypothalamic nucleus can preferentially innervate a specific subset of preganglionic neurons.

NEURAL CONTROL OF VASOPRESSIN RELEASE

Quite recently the source of two neural inputs to the region of vasopressinergic cell bodies in the PVH and SO have been identified (Fig. 3). One arises in the A_1 region of the

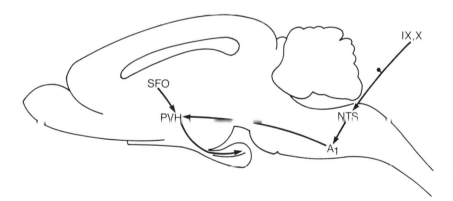

Fig. 3. Only two anatomically defined pathways are known to end among the magno-cellular neurosecretory neurons, in the paraventricular (PVH) and supraoptic (not shown) nuclei, that synthesize vasopressin (VAS) and release it into the blood stream of the posterior pituitary. One group of fibers, which is noradrenergic, arises in the A_1 region of the ventrolateral medulla. The A_1 region in turn receives an input from the nucleus of the solitary tract (NTS), and may thus relay baroreceptor information from the ninth and tenth cranial nerves to vasopressinergic cells in the PVH. The other group of fibers arises from cells in the subfornical organ (SFO), which appear to respond to circulating levels of angiotensin II.

ventrolateral medulla, just dorsal to the lateral reticular nucleus, and is predominantly noradrenergic (Sawchenko and Swanson, 1981a). This pathway may well be involved in the modulation of vasopressin (but not oxytocin) release by baroreceptor information (Share, 1974), since the A_1 region receives a dense input from the NTS (Sawchenko and Swanson, 1981a) (Fig. 3). The NTS itself projects directly to the PVH, but this pathway, which is also predominantly noradrenergic (Sawchenko and Swanson, 1981a), ends in parvocellular regions of the nucleus that project to the median eminence and back down to autonomic centers. It is thought that the ventrolateral medulla, including the A_1 region, contains a chemosensitive zone involved in CV regulation (see Winnergren and Oberg, 1980), and 6-OHDA lesions in this area produce hypertension (Blessing et al., 1981) and increased release of vasopressin (W.W. Blessing, personal communication). The other input arises in the subfornical organ (Miselis, in press), and innervates both oxytocinergic and vaso-pressinergic cell groups (Sawchenko and Swanson, 1981b). This pathway appears to be involved in the release of vasopressin due to increased levels of angiotensin II in the blood (Miselis, in press).

INTEGRATION OF AUTONOMIC AND ENDOCRINE RESPONSES

The autonomic component of baroreceptor reflexes appears to be mediated by circuits in the medulla and spinal cord, while the release of vasopressin depends on the modulation of neuroendocrine cells in the PVH and SO. How then are appropriate endocrine and autonomic responses coordinated in response to stimuli such as hemorrhage and dehydration? The answer to this question is still not entirely clear, but recent anatomical evidence has provided clues for further investigation. Perhaps the most interesting observations are related to the organization of the PVH, which receives baroreceptor (and undoubtedly other visceral sensory) information from the NTS (Ciriello and Calaresu, 1980). As alluded to above, this information appears to be relayed in large part by three predominantly noradrenergic cell groups, in the NTS (the A_2 group), the A_1 region, and the locus ceruleus (the A_6 group). These three pathways are closely interrelated since the NTS projects to the A_1 region, and noradrenergic fibers from the A_1 region innervate the NTS and the locus ceruleus (Sawchenko and Swanson, 1981a, in press a) (Fig. 4). These pathways appear to be organized such that the A_1 region influences vasopressin release as well as projections from the PVH to the median eminence and autonomic centers, the cells in the NTS (the A_2 group) influence projections from the PVH to the median eminence and autonomic centers, and cells in the locus ceruleus influence projections to the median eminence. Although these pathways are complex, the major point is that baroreceptor information from the NTS is relayed to preganglionic neurons of the sympathetic and parasympathetic systems through pathways of unknown biochemical specificity, and to the PVH (and SO) through a series of interrelated noradrenergic pathways. In addition, the PVH, which releases vasopressin in the posterior pituitary, projects back to the NTS and to preganglionic cell groups that may be involved in baroreceptor reflex modulation. In essence, a series of rather direct bidirectional pathways interrelate autonomic reflex circuitry in the brain stem and spinal cord, and neuroendocrine cell groups in the hypothalamus.

It should be pointed out that the circuitry outlined in Fig. 4 may also be involved in the coordination of peripheral and central responses to changes in arterial pressure. As reviewed elsewhere (Hartman et al., 1980), fibers from the locus ceruleus appear to change intracerebral capillary permeability to water, and thus play a role in the prevention of cerebral edema during periods of increased arterial pressure. The A_1 cell group may play a particularly important integrative role in the circuitry outlined in Fig. 4 because it projects to baroreceptor reflex circuitry (the NTS), to the locus ceruleus, and to vasopressinergic cell groups.

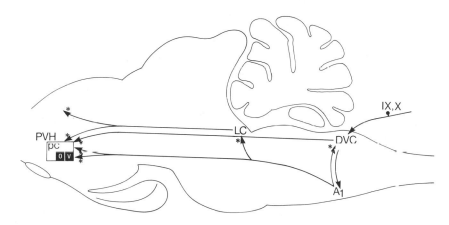

Fig. 4. Summary of the noradrenergic pathways (asterisks) that are known to link the dorsal vagal complex (DVC) with the paraventricular nucleus (PVH). Other abbreviations: LC, locus ceruleus; o, oxytocinergic cells; pc, parvocellular division of PVH; v, vasopressinergic cells.

CONCLUSION

Recent anatomical studies have begun to shed some light on the neural mechanisms in the brain stem and hypothalamus that serve to integrate autonomic and neuroendocrine responses to perturbations in blood pressure. They also indicate which neural pathways might be involved in the mediation of CV changes that accompany psychogenic stress. As noted above, several regions in the telencephalon, including parts of the prefrontal cortex, the amygdala, and the septum, are now known to project directly to the NTS, which of course plays a major role in the neural circuitry that modulates heart rate and blood pressure. All of these telencephalic regions can be regarded as integral components of the limbic system, and as such receive cognitive information from neocortical association fields. (For a review of the limbic system concept, and of specific connections between association cortex and limbic structures, see Swanson, in press.) It appears, therefore, that a series of relatively well-defined neural pathways involving the limbic system may relay cognitive information to the sensory nucleus of the vagus and to a variety of sites in the hypothalamus as well (Krettek and Price, 1978).

For the sake of completeness, it should be mentioned that motivated or goal-oriented behavioral responses are important for the maintenance of appropriate levels of body water, and thus of blood pressure. For example, thirst accompanies hemorrhage or dehydration, and leads to the ingestion of fluids. The neural circuitry that underlies the integration of behavioral and visceral responses to hypovolemia has been clarified in the last few years, and it appears that the subfornical organ, medial parts of the preoptic region, and the PVH are particularly important components of this circuitry, which is activated in part by circulating levels of angiotensin II (Swanson and Mogenson, 1981).

The anatomically defined circuitry outlined here has only recently been clarified, and detailed functional studies must be carried out to determine the precise role of each of its components in CV regulation. Important advances in our understanding of the central neural control of blood pressure can be expected in the next few years, along with insights into the pathophysiology of the various forms of hypertension, some of which may be due to abnormalities within this circuitry.

ACKNOWLEDGEMENTS

The original work described here was supported in part by grant NS16686 from the National Institutes of Health, and by grant DA11259 from ADAMHA. Dr. Swanson is a Clayton Foundation Investigator.

REFERENCES

Blessing, W.W., West, M.J. and Chalmers, J. (1981) Hypertension, bradycardia and pulmonary edema in the conscious rabbit after brainstem lesions coinciding with the A1 group of catecholamine neurons. Circulat. Res. 49, 949-958.

Ciriello, J. and Calaresu, F.R. (1980) Monosynaptic pathway from cardiovascular neurons in the nucleus tractus solitarii to the paraventricular nucleus in the cat. Brain Res. 193, 529-533.

Hartman, B.K., Swanson, L.W., Raichle, M.E., Preskorn, S.H. and Clark, H.B. (1980) Central adrenergic regulation of cerebral microvascular permeability and blood flow; anatomic physiologic evidence; in The Cerebral Microvasculature, H.M. Eisenberg and R.L. Suddith, eds., Plenum, New York, pp. 113-126.

Hess, W.R. (1947) Das Zwischenhirn. Schwalb, Basel.

Hopkins, D.A. and Holstege, G. (1978) Amygdaloid projections to the mesencephalon, pons and medulla oblongata in the cat. Exp. Brain Res. 32, 529-547.

Kaada, R.B. (1951) Somato-motor, autonomic and electrocorticographic responses to electrical stimulation of "rhinencephalic" and other structures in primates, cat and dog: a study of responses from the limbic, subcallosal, orbito-insular, piriform and temporal cortex, hippocampus-fornix and amygdala. Acta Physiol. Scand. 23 (Suppl. 83), 1-285.

Karplus, J.P. and Kreidl, A. (1910) Gehirn und Sympathicus. II. Ein Sympathicus-Zentrum in Zwischenhirn. Arch. Ges. Physiol. 135, 401-411.

Krettek, J.E. and Price, J.L. (1978) Amygdaloid projections to subcortical structures within the basal forebrain in the rat and cat. J. Comp. Neurol. 178, 225-254.

Makara, G.B., Stark, E., Karteszi, M., Palkovits, M. and Rappay, G.Y. (1981) Effects of paraventricular tensions on stimulated ACTH release and CRF in stalk-median eminence of the rat. Amer. J. Physiol. 240, E441-E446.

Miselis, R. (in press) The efferent projections of the subfornical organ of the rat: a circumventricular organ within a neural network subserving water balance. Brain Res.

Norgren, R. (1976) Taste pathways to hypothalamus and amygdala. J. Comp. Neurol. 166, 17-30.

Post, S. and Mai, J.K. (1980) Contribution to the amygdaloid projection field in the rat. A quantitative autoradiographic study. J. Hirnforsch. 21, 199-225.

Price, J.L. and Amaral, D.G. (1981) An autoradiographic study of the projections of the central nucleus of the monkey amygdala. J. Neurosci. 1, 1242-1259.

Ranson, S.W., Kabat, H., and Magoun, H.W. (1935) Autonomic responses to electrical stimulation of hypothalamus, preoptic region and septum. Arch. Neurol. Psychiat. 33, 467-477.

Ranson, S.W. and Magoun, H.W. (1939) The hypothalamus. Ergebn. Physiol. 41, 56-163.

Reis, D.J. and Oliphant, M.C. (1964) Bradycardia and tachycardia following electrical stimulation of the amygdaloid region in monkey. J. Neurophysiol. 27, 893-912.

Saper, C.B. and Loewy, A.D. (1980) Efferent connections of the parabrachial nucleus in the rat. Brain Res. 197, 291-317.

Saper, C.B., Loewy, A.D., Swanson, L.W. and Cowan, W.M. (1976) Direct hypothalamo-autonomic connections. Brain Res. 117, 305-312.

Sawchenko, P.E. and Swanson, L.W. (1981a) Central noradrenergic pathways for the integration of hypothalamic neuroendocrine and autonomic responses. Science 214, 685-687.

Sawchenko, P.E. and Swanson, L.W. (1981b) The distribution and cells of origin of some afferent projections to the paraventricular and supraoptic nuclei in the rat. Soc. Neurosci. Abst. 7, 325.

Sawchenko, P.E. and Swanson, L.W. (in press a) The organization of noradrenergic pathways from the brainstem to the paraventricular and supraoptic nuclei in the rat. Brain Res. Rev.

Sawchenko, P.E. and Swanson, L.W. (in press b) Immunohistochemical identification of neurons in the paraventricular nucleus of the hypothalamus that project to the medulla or to the spinal cord in the rat. J. Comp. Neurol.

Schwaber, J.S., Kapp, B.S. and Higgins, G. (1980) The origin and extent of direct amygdala projections to the region of the dorsal motor nucleus of the vagus and the nucleus of the solitary tract. Neurosci. Lett. 20, 15.

Share, L. (1974) Blood pressure, blood volume, and the release of vasopressin; in Handbook of Physiology, sect. 7, ViV, part 1, E. Knobil and W.H. Sawyer, eds. American Physiological Society, Washington, pp. 243-255.

Smith, W.K. (1945) The functional significance of the rostral cingular cortex as revealed by its responses to electrical excitation. J. Neurophysiol. 8, 241-255.

Spencer, W.G. (1894) The effect produced upon respiration by feradic excitation of the cerebrum in the monkey. Phil. Trans. Ser. B 185, 609-657.

Swanson, L.W. (1977) Immunohistochemical evidence for a neurophysin-containing autonomic pathway arising in the paraventricular nucleus of the hypothalamus. Brain Res. 128, 356-363.

22

Swanson, L.W. (in press) The hippocampus and the concept of the limbic system; in Molecular, Cellular and Behavioral Biology of the Hippocampus, W. Seifert, ed. Academic Press, New York.

Swanson, L.W. and Cowan, W.M. (1979) The connections of the septal region in the rat. J. Comp. Neurol. 186, 621-656.

Swanson, L.W. and Kuypers, H.G.J.M. (1980) The paraventricular nucleus of the hypothalamus: cytoarchitectonic subdivisions and the organization of projections to the pituitary, dorsal vagal complex and spinal cord as demonstrated by retrograde fluorescence double-labeling methods. J. Comp. Neurol. 194, 555-570.

Swanson, L.W. and McKellar, S. (1979) The distribution of oxytocin- and neurophysin-stained fibers in the spinal cord of the rat and monkey. J. Comp. Neurol. 188, 87-106.

Swanson, L.W. and Mogenson, G.J. (1981) Neural mechanisms for the functional coupling of autonomic, endocrine and somatomotor responses in adaptive behavior. Brain Res. Rev. 3, 1-34.

Swanson, L.W. and Sawchenko, P.E. (1980) Paraventricular nucleus: a site for integration of neuroendocrine and autonomic mechanisms. Neuroendocrinology 31, 410-417.

Swanson, L.W. and Sawchenko, P.E. (in press) Hypothalamic integration: organization of the paraventricular and supraoptic nuclei. Ann. Rev. Neurosci.

Swanson, L.W., Sawchenko, P.E., Berod, A., Hartman, B.K., Helle, K.B. and Van Orden, D.E. (1981) An immunohistochemical study of the organization of catecholaminergic cells and terminal fields in the paraventricular and supraoptic nuclei of the hypothalamus. J. Comp. Neurol. 196, 271-285.

Swanson, L.W., Sawchenko, P.E., Wiegand, S.J. and Price, J.L. (1980) Separate neurons in the paraventricular nucleus project to the median eminence and to the medulla or spinal cord. Brain Res. 197, 207-212.

Van der Kooy, D., McGinty, J.F., Koda, L.Y., Gerfen, C.R. and Bloom, F.E. (submitted) Visual cortex: direct projections from prefrontal cortex to the solitary nucleus.

Winnergren, G. and Oberg, B. (1980) Cardiovascular effects elicited from the ventral surface of medulla oblongata in the cat. Pflügers Arch. 387, 189.

Ganglionic, Spinal and Medullary Substrates for Functional Specificity in Circulatory Regulation

LAWRENCE P. SCHRAMM
The Johns Hopkins University School of Medicine, Baltimore, Maryland

INTRODUCTION

Several excellent and comprehensive reviews on the neural regulation of the circulation have been published in the last decade (Koizumi and Brooks, 1972; Calaresu et al., 1975; Wurster, 1977; Randall, 1977; Abboud et al., 1981). Therefore, this chapter will focus on a single issue, the progress achieved and problems encountered in attaching specific neural structures to specific cardiovascular (CV) regulatory functions.

A CV physiologist well may wonder why some neurobiologists who profess an interest in the regulation of blood pressure, blood volume and cardiac output spend so much of their time investigating sympathetic silent periods, somato-sympathetic reflexes and brain stem catecholaminergic nuclei. Those of us who choose to work on the neural regulation of the circulation must contend with several problems. The first is a universal problem in neurobiology, the difficulty of ascribing functions to structures. The basic physiological roles of the heart and blood vessels are clear to the CV physiologist. But what can the neurobiologist say, for certain, about the circulatory functions of the A2 cell group, the dorsolateral funicular sympathoinhibitory pathway, and sympathetic ganglionic reflex pathways? In other words, we have a catalog of neural structures and phenomena that we are quite certain play roles in circulatory regulation. However, we are still in the process of matching neural structures and neural phenomena to CV functions.

A second problem that is especially acute for, if not unique to, the autonomic neurobiologist is the **naming** of functions. Neurobiologists working with somatic control can, at least, describe the output of their system in three-dimensional space. CV control, as a subset of metabolic control, operates in a metabolic space whose dimensions are only conjectural. We often wonder whether a particular neural system is regulating a pressure, a volume, a flow, a delivery of material to a tissue, the removal of material from a tissue, or, more likely, some combination of these.

Should we be attempting to relate central nervous system (CNS) structures of poorly understood **neural** function to poorly defined **circulatory** functions? I believe we should. When we make progress with neural mechanisms, our search for the significance of peripheral mechanisms is better focused. The improved view of peripheral regulatory function, in turn, leads to more perceptive investigations of neural systems. This recursive process has led to slow but significant progress in our understanding of neural factors in circulatory regulation. At the same time, CV physiologists have succeeded in describing circulatory adjustments that are increasingly specific to their associated metabolic and somatic behaviors. Understanding the neural mechanisms by which this specificity is generated is probably our most challenging task.

FUNCTIONAL ORGANIZATION IN THE SYMPATHETIC PERIPHERY

I begin with a discussion of the sympathetic periphery for two reasons. First, no matter what degree of functional specificity is generated by central systems, it can only be expressed through peripheral autonomic nerves. Second, the history of concepts of peripheral sympathetic organization and functions is extremely instructive. Until the early nineteenth century, many believed the sympathetic nervous system to be isolated from the CNS. Its role was to maintain "sympathy" between the body's organs and tissues. Information passing via sympathetic nerves to a given organ controlled that organ's function with respect to the state of the other organs and tissues, and information passing from a given organ informed other organs and tissues of its state. This concept implied a high degree of specificity of function if the needs of all of the innervated tissues were to be served.

As the connections between the central and sympathetic nervous systems became increasingly clear, an important change took place in concepts of sympathetic function. At first, scientists still attributed a high degree of functional specificity to sympathetic innervation. For instance, Charles Bell (1830) said this system controlled "those thousand secret operations of a living body we call constitutional." At the same time, he made it clear that this control was mediated by the peripheral connections of the sympathetics. Involvement of "higher" functions with sympathetic control was unusually pathological, and he said, "when, by circuitous influence, the mind does operate on the vital functions, we know what disturbance is produced."

By the early twentieth century there was anatomical evidence for an enormous divergence of information in the sympathetic ganglia. It was reasonable for physiologists to conclude that few centrally organized patterns of sympathetic behavior could share a network in which one preganglionic neuron synapsed on hundreds of postganglionic neurons. However, the observable patterns of sympathetic output had become too numerous and too well differentiated to be accounted for by a purely divergent sympathetic nervous system. Physiologists came to the rescue by demonstrating that activation of sympathetic postganglionic neurons required convergent excitatory input from multiple preganglionic neurons (Blackman and Purves, 1969). Thus ganglionic output possesses the necessary degree of divergence to provide innervation to virtually every organ and tissue in the body, and ganglionic input may possess the necessary degree of convergence to generate the large variety of observed patterns of output.

About the time that autonomic neurobiologists were becoming comfortable with the idea that ganglionic mechanisms could account for the transduction of highly specific central patterns of sympathetic control, evidence began to accumulate that implied that, in some cases, functional specificity may actually be generated at ganglionic levels. Szurszewski and Weems (1976) and Kreulen and Szurszewski (1979) have shown that sensory neurons, presumably lying in the intestinal wall and sensitive to stretch, project centrally and make very powerful excitatory synapses on prevertebral postganglionic neurons. These connections probably form the substrate for ganglionic mechanisms controlling intestinal tone or motility. If similar sensory neurons also excited postganglionic neurons regulating the vasculature, then similar controls might help integrate intestinal motility and local intestinal circulation, or intestinal secretion and circulation. Ganglionically organized relations between circulation and function can be envisioned in many other tissues. Indeed, peripheral interactions involving more than one organ or tissue may also be imagined. For instance, changes in hepatic function might, via ganglionic mechanisms, initiate adjustments in mesenteric or renal circulation.

Should such peripheral controls turn out to be of significance in circulatory regulation, we would have to return to the sympathetic nervous system some of the autonomy attributed to it in the last century. Indeed, ganglia would become an important element in a regulatory hierarchy that would progress from tissue level autoregulation to ganglionic-level coordination of certain organs and tissues to the generation of overall adaptive patterns by the CNS.

If ganglionic mechanisms may be seen as a way of interposing specific local patterns of circulatory regulation on more general, centrally commanded patterns, they may also be seen in a somewhat more sinister light. A centrally mediated circulatory adjustment to one organ or tissue, in itself benign, might lead to undesirable secondary adjustments in other organs or tissues. We may pay for increased flexibility of function with increased modes of potential malfunction.

FUNCTIONAL SYMPATHETIC ORGANIZATION AT SPINAL LEVELS

Attaching functional significance to spinal sympathetic systems presents special difficulties. Spinal systems are distant enough from the medullary site of primary baroreceptor and chemoreceptor input that the information they receive from supraspinal levels has already been heavily processed. To complicate matters further, because of the interposed sympathetic ganglia, preganglionic neurons lose the organ and tissue specificity possessed by postganglionic neurons. Ironically, only the adrenal preganglionic neurons are anatomically organ-specific. And their function is global!

Despite these difficulties, some significant steps have been taken toward delineating functional categories of preganglionic neurons. For instance, Jänig and colleagues (see Jänig and Szulczyk, 1981, for review) have used the clever strategy of identifying preganglionic neurons whose responses to a variety of stimuli match those of anatomically or functionally identified postganglionic vasoconstrictor fibers to muscle and to skin. Each behaved differently with respect to baroreceptor, chemoreceptor, and nociceptor activation. Fibers to muscle decreased their activity during baroreceptor activation and increased their activity during chemoreceptor and nociceptor activation. Fibers to skin exhibited little change in activity in response to baroreceptor activation, and decreased their activity in response to chemoreceptor and nociceptor activation. Preganglionic fibers with similarly differentiated responses to these three inputs could be identified and were assumed to play specific muscle and cutaneous vasoconstrictor roles. In addition, preganglionic fibers that, upon electrical stimulation, activated postganglionic cutaneous vasoconstrictor, muscle vasoconstrictor, sudomotor and piloerector fibers, had somewhat different conduction velocities. These results led Jänig to conclude that a considerable degree of functional specificity is coded straight through the sympathetic ganglia. To the extent that this is the case, the identification of those tissues affected by given preganglionic neurons and the description of their roles in particular regulatory activities may be facilitated.

The sympathetic preganglionic neuron receives inputs from spinal afferents, from intrinsic spinal systems, and from supraspinal systems. The relations between these inputs are poorly understood. For instance, it is not clear to what extent commands originating at supraspinal levels are mediated via direct connections to preganglionic neurons or via activation or inhibition of intrinsic spinal systems. Although the difficulty of maintaining animals with chronically transected spinal cords has limited research on this question, the results that have been obtained lead us to believe that intrinsic spinal systems may be more important than commonly believed. For instance, Kirchner et al. (1975) electrically stimulated portions of the spinal cord thought to contain sympathoexcitatory and sympathoinhibitory pathways descending from supraspinal levels. They were still able to elicit responses from these areas weeks after spinal transection, indicating the presence of functional intrinsic systems. Hopefully, the role(s) of these intrinsic systems will be clarified during the current explosion of interest in spinal sympathetic systems.

Despite the outstanding contributions made by the laboratories of John Coote, Robert Wurster, Michael Illert, Horst Seller, and many others, confusion and controversy still abound over the functions of those pathways that seem to descend, from supraspinal levels, upon the interneurons and sympathetic preganglionic neurons of the intermediate zone of the thoracic spinal cord. Most studies of descending pathways have begun operationally. A circulatory variable is measured, a spinal locus is stimulated and/or damaged, and the circulatory effects of these manipulations are observed. For instance, Barman and Wurster (1975) electrically stimulated dorsolateral funicular (DLF) sympatho-excitatory regions and measured heart rate and vascular resistance in cerebral, renal and hindlimb vascular beds. The DLF appeared to be somatotopically and viscerotopically organized with respect to the evoked vasoconstrictions and tachycardia.

There are at least three interpretations of this study, all of which have important implications for functional specificity of sympathetic control. First, if we accept the authors' contention that the observed responses resulted from stimulation of pathways descending from supraspinal levels, the data suggest that organs and tissue may be spatially represented in these pathways. One implication of this interpretation is that patterns of circulatory control that require selective vasoconstriction and vasodilation of tissue must be generated largely at supraspinal levels and conducted, relatively unaltered, to the appropriate vascular beds.

Second, and still assuming that descending pathways were stimulated, we might conclude that the pathways were organized functionally rather than somatotopically or viscerotopically. For instance, hindlimb vasoconstriction may have been a component of an arterial pressure regulatory mechanism and renal vasoconstriction may have been a component of a blood volume regulatory mechanism. This interpretation implies that spinal and/or ganglionic systems are capable of organizing complex patterns of circulatory control, and that these patterns need only be triggered or excited by supraspinal systems.

Third, the possibility exists that Barman and Wurster stimulated the axons of ascending primary or secondary afferent fibers, which made excitatory collateral connections on preganglionic neurons or on excitatory spinal interneurons. These afferent pathways, like the putative descending pathways, could be either viscerotopically or functionally organized. They could also be components of the intrinsic spinal systems discussed above.

Continuing studies in Wurster's laboratory (see for instance Geis et al., 1978) have sought to determine the physiological role of these dorsolateral funicular systems. Evidence to date indicates that these systems are not involved in the maintenance of normal blood pressure, but they are important in the circulatory responses to exercise and other stresses. However, it has not yet been possible to determine whether these effects are mediated by the transmission of supraspinally generated patterns or by the activation of spinally generated patterns of sympathetic output.

The functional roles of spinal sympathoinhibitory systems have also been explored. Perhaps of greatest interest to the CV physiologist are studies on pathways involved in baroreceptor-mediated sympathoinhibition. It is now generally agreed that at least a portion of this sympathoinhibition is generated by the excitation of medullospinal pathways which have their inhibitory effects in the intermediate zone of the spinal cord

(Taylor and Gebber, 1975; McLachlan and Hirst, 1980; Coote et al., 1981). There is much less agreement on the spinal locus of the descending sympathoinhibitory pathways. Coote et al. (1981) have found that chemical or surgical lesions of the DLF reduce baroreceptor-induced sympathoinhibition. On the other hand, Dembrowsky et al. (1981) using cold blockade could not find evidence for a baroreceptor role of the dorsolateral funiculus.

Certainly, the delineation of the pathway(s) that convey baroreceptor-mediated sympathoinhibition would be an important step, not only in understanding circulatory control, but in understanding central autonomic organization. However, it may not be an easy task, for the spinal level of inhibition may be mediated by several pathways. The surgical and pharmacological interventions used to date obviate fine quantitative estimates of the relative importance of different candidate pathways. This is especially true since the locations of spinal sympathoinhibitory pathways are ill-defined, and their destruction often alters both spontaneous sympathetic activity and baroreceptor-induced changes in sympathetic activity. Thus, we have both technical and conceptual problems. We must find more discrete, hopefully reversible, methods for blocking spinal pathways. We must learn to take into account changes in baseline sympathetic activity when we implement blockade. And we must squarely face the possibility that baroreceptor-mediated sympathoinhibition may be a "function" shared by multiple pathways.

FUNCTIONAL SPECIFICITY AT BRAIN STEM LEVELS

The brain stem is truly a crossroads for CV control. Not only does this region receive ascending input from spinal levels and descending information from suprabulbar systems, it receives direct barosensory and chemosensory information from the vasculature. It even contains its own chemosensory regions (Ferrario et al., 1979; Feldberg, 1980). Much of this information is integrated by neurons, each of which may receive diverse inputs. This multimodality of brain stem neurons leads to two questions. First, can the firing rate of autonomic neurons which appear to receive such diverse inputs be precisely regulated? Second, is it possible that neurons with such heterogeneous inputs may have relatively specific functions, and is there any hope that we will be able to identify these functions?

That brain stem neurons are capable of generating extremely precise outputs is demonstrated by the control of the cardiac vagal preganglionic neurons. These cholinergic neurons lie in the medulla, and their axons project to intracardiac, cholinergic, postganglionic neurons. Cardiac vagal preganglionic neurons receive indirect excitatory input from baroreceptors (McAllen and Spyer, 1978b). They receive a GABAergic inhibitory input that is so powerful that it can largely override baroreceptor excitation (Quest and Gebber, 1972; Barman and Gebber, 1979; Williford et al., 1980). It is probably this latter input that permits a pronounced tachycardia in the face of elevated arterial pressure during certain emotional states. Firing of the cardiac vagal preganglionic neurons is also modulated by input from so-called "respiratory neurons," leading to respiration-related, cardiac arrhythmias (McAllan and Spyer, 1978b). Do these multiple inputs to cardiac vagal preganglionic neurons predispose them to frequent and capricious changes in firing rate? Apparently not. McAllen and Spyer (1978a) demonstrated that iontophoretic excitation of a **single** cardiac vagal preganglionic neuron within the physiological range of firing rate decreased heart rate in cats by 10 to 30 beats per minute. Since the heart receives input from hundreds of these neurons, we must conclude that, under ordinary conditions, the complex spectrum of inputs to cardiac vagal preganglionic neurons results in a very smoothly and precisely regulated output. On the other hand, the surprising potency of vagal output, demonstrated by the work of McAllen and Spyer, warns us of the potential danger of severe disruptions in cardiac rhythm should brain stem integrative mechanisms fail.

Finally, what can be said about the functional specificity of brain stem reticular neurons? It is clear that in the reticular formation one can record from neurons whose firing rates correlate with a variety of afferent signals from baroreceptor, chemoreceptor, pulmonary and nonpulmonary somatic receptors. In addition, the firing rates of a very large proportion of neurons in some reticular regions are either positively or negatively correlated with sympathetic activity (Gebber, 1980; Barman and Gebber, 1981). The dilemma in "naming" these neurons may be dramatized by polarizing the thinking of a number of laboratories into two schools.

The view of the first school is represented in Figure 1, showing three reticular neurons. Each neuron has a readily named output to a nonrespiratory somatic moto-neuron, a respiratory motoneuron, or a sympathetic preganglionic neuron. Each receives input from baroreceptor, chemoreceptor, somatic and respiratory afferents. However, the inputs are distributed unequally to each reticular neuron according to its "function." Small changes in this afferent distribution and weak interactions between reticular neurons of specific function (not shown) may occur.

The second school (Koepchen et al., 1975) envisages a much more plastic system in which individual reticular neurons play different roles depending on the metabolic or behavioral state of the animal. This view is represented in Figures 2 and 3. The same neuron is illustrated regulating activity of a sympathetic preganglionic neuron based on baroreceptor and chemoreceptor input (Fig. 2) and regulating respiratory activity based on chemoreceptor and respiratory afferents (Fig. 3).

The issue represented by these two schools represents less a raging controversy than an example of how neurobiologists go about their business. For instance, it is reminiscent of the long-standing issue in somatic neurophysiology of whether individual cortical neurons are organized by muscle or by movement. The issue will be clarified by the

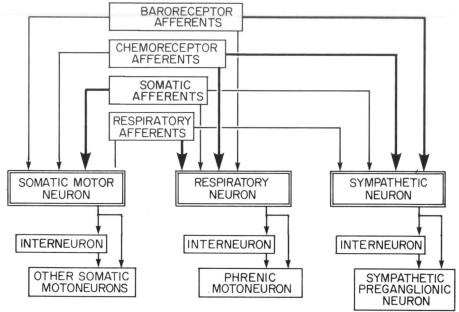

Fig. 1. Three neurons of the reticular formation (somatic, respiratory, and sympathetic). Each neuron has well-defined afferent and efferent projections which are stable over time and over a variety of metabolic states.

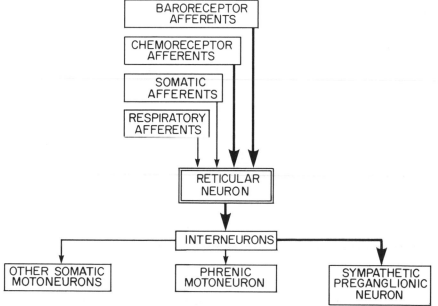

Fig. 2. A neuron of the reticular formation serving to control the activity of a sympathetic preganglionic neuron based on baroreceptor and chemoreceptor afferents.

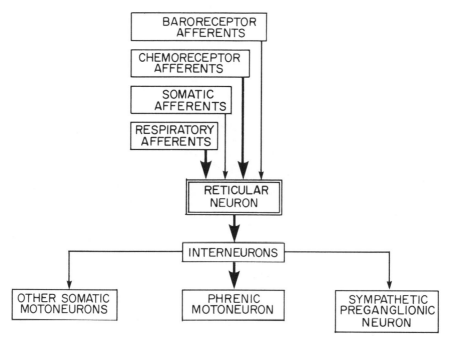

Fig. 3. Same neuron illustrated in Figure 2 controlling respiration based on chemo-receptor and respiratory afferents.

simultaneous correlation of an increased number of inputs and outputs with firing rates of reticular neurons. The issue will also be clarified by recording neuronal activity during more carefully observed and controlled patterns of circulatory regulation. However, we must also be prepared for the issue itself to evolve. For, as noted throughout this chapter, our idea of "function" is extremely vague. Fortunately, most laboratories are prepared to substitute "temperature regulatory," "muscle vasoconstrictor," or perhaps "cardiomotor" for "sympathetic," or vice versa, as the evidence better defines the role of a neuron.

CONCLUSION

There now seems to be an abundance of neural pathways and mechanisms to account for the observed precision and functional specificity of CV regulation. However, progress has been slow in relating specific neural processes and pathways to specific CV regulatory functions, both because of the state of our knowledge of central autonomic regulation and because of the difficulty in naming the regulatory functions. Future progress will depend not only on technical accomplishments, but on our willingness to explore alternative definitions of regulated variables.

ACKNOWLEDGMENTS

This chapter was prepared with support from NIH Grant HL16315. I thank Ms. Evelyn McCann for processing the manuscript.

REFERENCES

Abboud, F.M., Fozzard, H.A., Gilmore, J.P. and Reis, D.J. (1981) Disturbances in Neurogenic Control of the Circulation. American Physiological Society, Bethesda.

Barman, S.M. and Gebber, G.L. (1979) Picrotoxin and bicuculline-sensitive inhibition of cardiac vagal reflexes. J. Pharm. Exp. Ther. 209, 67-72.

Barman, S.M. and Gebber, G.L. (1981) Problems associated with the identification of brain stem neurons responsible for sympathetic nerve discharge. J. Autonom. Nerv. Syst. 3, 369-378.

Barman, S.M. and Wurster, R.D. (1975) Visceromotor organization within descending spinal sympathetic pathways in the dog. Circulat. Res. 37, 209-214.

Bell, C. (1830) The Nervous System of the Human Body. Longman, Rees, Orme, Brown and Green, London.

Blackman, J.G. and Purves, R.D. (1969) Intracellular recordings from ganglia of the thoracic sympathetic chain of the guinea-pig. J. Physiol. (Lond.) 203, 173-198.

Calaresu, F.R., Faiers, A.A. and Mogenson, G.J. (1975) Central neural regulation of heart and blood vessels in mammals. Progr. Neurobiol. 5, 1-35.

Coote, J.H., Macleod, V.H., Fleetwood-Walter, S.M., and Gilbey, M.P. (1981) Baroreceptor inhibition of sympathetic activity at the spinal site. Brain Res. 220, 81-93.

Dembrowsky, K., Lackner, K., Czachurski, J. and Seller, H. (1981) Tonic catecholaminergic inhibition of the spinal somato-sympathetic reflexes originating in the ventrolateral medulla oblongata. J. Autonom. Nerv. Syst. 3, 277-290.

Feldberg, W. (1980) Cardiovascular effects of drugs acting on the ventral surface of the brain stem; in Central Interaction Between Respiratory and Cardiovascular Control Systems, H.P. Koepchen, S.M. Hilton, and A. Trzebski, eds. Springer-Verlag, Berlin, pp. 47-55.

Ferrario, C.M., Barnes, K.L., Szilagyi, J.E. and Brosnihan, K.B. (1979) Physiological and pharmacological characterization of the area postrema pressor pathways in the normal dog. Hypertension 1, 235-245.

Gebber, G.L. (1980) Central oscillators responsible for sympathetic nerve discharge. Amer. J. Physiol. 234, H143-H155.

Geis, G.S., Barratt, G. and Wurster, R.D. (1978) Role of the descending pressor pathway in the conscious and pentobarbital-anesthetized dog. Amer. J. Physiol. 234, H152-H156.

Jänig, W. and Szulczyk, P. (1981) The organization of lumbar preganglionic neurons. J. Autonom. Nerv. Syst. 3, 177-191.

Kirchner, F., Wyszogrodski, I. and Polosa, P. (1975) Some properties of sympathetic neuron inhibition by depressor area and intraspinal stimulation. Pflüger's Arch. 357, 349-360.

Koepchen, H.P., Langhorst, P. and Seller, H. (1975) The problem of identification of autonomic neurons in the lower brainstem. Brain Res. 87, 375-393.

Koizumi, K. and Brooks, C. McC. (1972) The integration of autonomic system reactions: a discussion of autonomic reflexes, their control and their associations with somatic reactions. Ergebn. Physiol. 67, 1-68.

Kreulen, D.L. and Szurszewski, J.H. (1979) Reflex pathways in the abdominal prevertebral ganglia: evidence for a colo-colonic inhibitory reflex. J. Physiol. (Lond.) 295, 21-32.

McAllen, R.M. and Spyer, K.M. (1978a) Two types of vagal preganglionic motoneurons projecting to the heart and lungs. J. Physiol. (Lond.) 282, 353-364.

McAllen, R.M. and Spyer, K.M. (1978b) The baroreceptor input to cardiac vagal motoneurons. J. Physiol. (Lond.) 282, 365-374.

McLachlan, E.M. and Hirst, G.D.S. (1980) Some properties of preganglionic neurons in upper thoracic spinal cord of the cat. J. Neurophysiol. 43, 1251-1265.

Quest, J.A. and Gebber, G.L. (1972) Modulation of baroreceptor reflexes by somatic afferent nerve stimulation. Amer. J. Physiol. 222, 1251-1259.

Randall, D.C. (1977) Neural control of the heart in the intact nonhuman primate; in Neural Regulation of the Heart, W.C. Randall, ed. Oxford University Press, New York, pp. 381-408.

Szurszewski, J.H. and Weems, W.A. (1976) A study of peripheral input to and its control by post-ganglionic neurones of the inferior mesenteric ganglion. J. Physiol. (Lond.) 256, 541-556.

Taylor, D.G. and Gebber, G.L. (1975) Baroreceptor mechanisms controlling sympathetic nervous rhythms of central origin. Amer. J. Physiol. 228, 1002-1013.

Williford, D.J., Hamilton, B.L. and Gillis, R.A. (1980) Evidence that a GABAergic mechanism at nucleus ambiguus influences reflex-induced vagal activity. Brain Res. 193, 584-588.

Wurster, R.D. (1977) Spinal sympathetic control of the heart; in Neural Regulation of the Heart, W.C. Randall, ed. Oxford University Press, New York, pp. 213-246.

Electrophysiology of Cardiovascular Response Patterns

JOHN W. MANNING
Emory University School of Medicine, Department of Physiology, Atlanta, Georgia

INTRODUCTION

Knowledge of regulation and control of cardiac and vascular functions is basic to understanding the pathophysiology in, and the treatment of, heart and blood vessel diseases. Recent fundamental research has illuminated both local tissue control mechanisms and brain functions in cardiovascular (CV) control. This new information has helped explain (1) the contribution of behavioral and emotional responses to the hypertensive state and coronary occlusive conditions in predisposed personalities (Henery and Meehan, 1981); (2) the role of autonomic innervation in concert, when present, with centrally acting drugs in control of heart rate and in the genesis of ventricular arrhythmias (Schwartz et al., 1978; Malliani et al., 1980); (3) the adaptation of cardiac afferent receptors in hypervolemic stages of heart failure, which yields an abnormal circulatory state because of the suppressed reflex-engaged neurohormonal response (Zucker and Gilmore, 1981); (4) the beneficial action of agents such as cardiac glycosides, which enhance the sensitivity of atrial receptors under these conditions (Abboud et al., 1981); and (5) regardless of the etiology of hypertension, the progressive hypertrophy of blood vessel walls that resets upward the blood pressure control system (Folkow, 1981).

I will focus here on brain function and CV control. The homeostatic control of the CV system was thought to be in the domain of the medullary vasomotor centers, which were appropriately named vasoconstrictor, vasodilator, cardiac accelerator and depressor (Peiss, 1965). These brain stem areas maintained normal vascular tone and heart rate, thereby producing an appropriate blood pressure. Central nervous structures related to emotional state, limbic and diencephalic systems, as well as peripheral inputs detecting environmental changes were ostensibly integrated in and relayed through these centers. In spite of the known independence of vascular adjustment, such as in thermoregulatory responses, the medullary center so dominated thinking that it still appears in medical textbooks as a primary control site (Guyton, 1981).

I shall attempt to give a general overview of CV control that focuses on cephalad structures engaged during a circulatory state change. In the past decade there has been an expansion and a redefinition of neural elements that participate in the control and regulation of CV state (Loewy and McKellar, 1980). The long-established concepts of functionally named centers of the reticular formation can no longer be considered the sole sites of integration of circulatory reflexes (Spyer, 1981). Cortical, cerebellar, diencephalic-brain stem and spinal mechanisms play a role to yield integrated responses (Fig. 1). A variety of afferent inputs interact at different sites such that information emanating from command loci associated with emotion or voluntary activity modifies the blood pressure control system to produce a varied but precise pattern of autonomic responses (Manning, 1980). The information that allows for the description of a control system with multi-access to many dispersed integrating sites comes from (1) neuroanatomical studies (Loewy, this volume); (2) evidence of visceral afferent engagement of hypothalamic structures, some with neuroendocrine function (Adair and Manning, 1975; Brody et al., 1980), that activate limbic subsystems to yield stereotyped autonomic and behavior pattern responses (Folkow, 1981); and (3) the pervasive occurrence of neuropeptide-neuromodulators in the CNS and their action on areas important in blood pressure control (Ganten et al., 1981b).

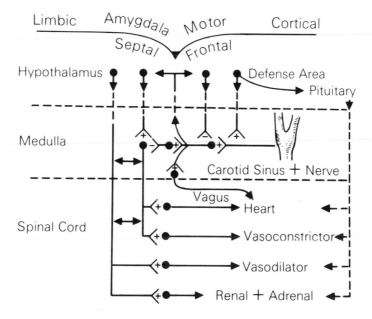

Fig. 1. Scheme depicting a distributed system for CV control focusing on the carotid baroreceptor as a prototype of visceral afferent input. Information from the ninth nerve arrives at multiloci throughout the brain stem and hypothalamus. Diencephalic systems under the influence of cortical and limbic projections affect medullary and spinal autonomic outflow, activate hypothalamic-hypophyseal release mechanisms, and engage the pituitary-adrenal axis. (Modified from Manning, 1980.)

HYPOTHALAMIC AND NEUROENDOCRINE INFLUENCE

It has long been known that stimulation of hypothalamic sites results in changes in vascular and cardiac parameters depending on the area activated (see Korner, 1979). Spyer (1972) recorded unit responses in the anterior hypothalamus to arterial baroreceptor stimulation. Stimulation of this same area evoked a fall in blood pressure with bradycardia. Indeed, Hilton and Spyer (1971) proposed this anterior extent of the brain stem to be part of the neural network used in baroreflex adjustment. Others (Adair and Manning, 1975; Thomas and Calaresu, 1972) have likewise recorded unitary responses to sinus nerve stimulation in the medial and posterior hypothalamus. Activation of the posterior area markedly attenuates incoming afferent activity in the sinus nerve as well as postsynaptic events in the nucleus tractus solitarius (Weiss and Crill, 1969). Thus such a brain stem system, in addition to receiving information and generating an appropriate autonomic response, also includes intrinsic feedback in that the area of the hypothalamus impinged upon by baroreceptor afferents can generate a response in the medullary area limiting the amount of information to be accepted (Fig. 1). It is important to note that the inhibition is not 100% and that the noninhibited medullary responses to sinus nerve stimulation continue to relay afferent information, however modified. The activation of such an intrinsic brain stem circuit becomes important for the full expression of autonomic-behavior responses.

Similarly, Menninger and Frazier (1972) recorded unitary activity in the supraoptic periventricular and lateral hypothalamic nuclei to atrial stretch. The importance of this vagal afferent projecting system is in relating detectors of the capacitance component of the circulation to the hypothalamic structures known to participate in salt and water metabolism. The significance of the atrial mechanoreceptors in the reflex inhibition of the ADH is well established. The actions on renal sympathetics are considered by Weaver elsewhere in this volume. A change in the reflex sensitivity, decreased afferent activity, is seen with chronic atrial distention as in congestive heart failure, and leads to an inappropriate elevation of catecholamines, renin, aldosterone and antidiuretic hormone (Zucker and Gilmore, 1981; Ammons et al., in press).

BRAIN PEPTIDES AND BLOOD PRESSURE REGULATION

I will just mention a few thoughts on the rapidly expanding field of neuropeptides that modulate central mechanisms regulating blood pressure. First, peptides such as enkephalins, substance P, angiotensin and somatostatin are localized in brain areas involved in CV control. Second, neuropeptides are known to modify an animal's thermoregulation. Third, a few are capable of altering catecholamine metabolism, release and uptake. Fourth, some brain peptides act as releasing factors for hypothalamic hormones (Ganten et al., 1981a).

Although there is controversy on the matter, one can use angiotensin as an example. Stimulating the biosynthesis of angiotensin II in the brain stimulates hypothalamic receptors to increase drinking behavior, and to enhance the release of ADH, adreno-corticotropic hormone, and the adrenergic transmitter. The cascade of factors, including the release of aldosterone which results in salt retention, leads to a slow but long-lasting increase in blood pressure (Ganten et al., 1981b).

AUTONOMIC RESPONSES ASSOCIATED WITH PATTERNS OF BEHAVIOR

Two contrasting autonomic response patterns are elicited by stimuli applied to selected hypothalamic sites. One, defense reaction, gives rise to increases in blood pressure, cardiac output, and heart rate accompanied by vasoconstriction in renal, intestinal and skin vascular beds. The hallmark of the pressor response is a cholinergic vasodilation in muscle beds (Hilton, 1974). In the unanesthetized animal the stimulus evokes a behavioral posture of attack. Zanchetti and colleagues (1976) found that the conscious animal, when faced with the challenge of an aggressive attack, responded with three types of behavior: (1) supportive fighting, which entailed hindlimb movements and yielded CV changes typical of the defense response; (2) nonsupportive fighting, in which vasoconstriction and tachycardia were noted with the absence of active muscle dilation and hindquarter movements; and (3) immobile confrontation, consisting of no-fight response, with widespread vasoconstriction and a fall in heart rate. The first two fighting postures must use brain stem systems already mentioned to modify the incoming baroreceptor information in order to effectively alter cardiac parameters in face of rising systemic pressures. In a series of reflex interaction experiments, Lisander (1970) has demonstrated the ability of hypothalamic and cerebellar mechanisms to reset the baroreflex response curve.

The other pattern mimics baroreflex depressor response in many aspects and is accompanied by a general somatic state of inhibition. Similar activity is obtained by stimulation of the lateral septal area. The response has been labeled the "playing possum" or "playing dead" reaction (Folkow and Neil, 1971).

The vascular and somatic responses elicited by nasopharyngeal stimulation, including the early components of the "diving response" and those of the "smoke response," have been shown to involve suprapontine pathways to activate the full integrated response (Korner, 1979).

From limbic structures, an array of cardiac and vascular changes are admitted. Thus from the basolateral amygdala decreases in blood pressure and heart rate, both parameters are reversed by stimulation in the central amygdaloid. All such stimulations are accompanied by altered respiratory patterns. We will be hearing more on this subject, for these visceral responses are best understood when viewed from the amygdaloid attack behavior on one hand and anxiety posture on the other (Henery and Meehan, 1981).

Differences in the mode of limbic-hypothalamic participation in vascular control are discerned from studies on the major rat strains inbred for primary hypertension. Thus the Okamoto-Aoki spontaneous hypertensive rat (SHR) seems to express the genetic predisposition in early life by a neurohormonal activity pattern nearly identical to a state of increased alertness. The young SHR consistently responds with a more intense and prolonged tachycardia and pressor response to acute alerting stimuli than similarly treated paired controls (Folkow, 1981).

Contrast the findings of Bianchi et al. (1975) in the Milan hypertensive strain (MHS), which spontaneously develops a fairly benign "volume variant" of primary hypertension in early life. No central hyperactivity is noted in the young MHS, which exhibits accentuated vagal tone in a reduced heart rate accompanied by a modest stroke volume increase. The comparison focuses on two different elements: (1) an accentuated pressor influence by the psychosocial stimuli that evoke an aroused or emotional response, and (2) a volume-dependent pressor state induced by habitual salt intake that exceeds renal capacity.

REFERENCES

Abboud, F.M., Thames, M.D. and Mark, A.L. (1981) Role of cardiac afferent nerves in regulation of circulation; in Disturbance in Neurogenic Control of the Circulation, F.M. Abboud et al., eds. Waverly Press, Baltimore, pp. 65-86.

Adair, J.R. and Manning, J.W. (1975) Hypothalamic modulation of baroreceptor afferent unit activity. Amer. J. Physiol. 229, 1357-1364.

Ammons, W.S., Koyama, S. and Manning, J.W. (in press) Neural and vascular interaction in renin response to graded renal nerve stimulation. Amer. J. Physiol. (Regulat. Integrat. Comp. Physiol.)

Bianchi, G., Baer, P.G., Fox, U., Puzzi, L., Pagetti, D. and Giovonetti, A.M. (1975) Changes in renin, water balance and sodium balance during development of high blood pressure in genetically hypertensive rats. Circulat. Res. (Suppl. 1), 36-37.

Brody, M.J., Haywood, J.R. and Touw, K.B. (1980) Neural mechanism in hypertension. Ann. Rev. Physiol. 42, 441-453.

Folkow, B. (1981) Central and peripheral mechanism in spontaneous hypertension in rats. Res. Publ. Ass. Res. Nerv. Ment. Dis. 59, 257-272.

Folkow, B. and Neil, E. (1971) Circulation. Oxford Press, New York, pp. 307-363.

Ganten, D., Speck, G., Schelling, P. and Unger, Th. (1981a) The brain renin-angiotensin system. Adv. Biochem. Psychopharmacol. 28, 359-372.

Ganten, D., Unger, Th., Scholkens, B., Rascher, W., Speck, G. and Stock, G. (1981b) Role of neuropeptides in regulation of blood pressure; in Disturbances in Neurogenic Control of the Circulation, F.M. Abboud, H. Fozzard, J. Gilmore and D. Reis, eds. Waverly Press, Baltimore, pp. 139-152.

Guyton, A.C. (1981) Textbook of Medical Physiology (6th Edition). W.B. Saunders Co., Philadelphia, pp. 239-241.

Henery, J. and Meehan, J. (1981) Psychosocial stimuli, physiological specificity and cardiovascular disease. Res. Publ. Ass. Res. Nerv. Ment. Dis. 59, 305-334.

Hilton, S.M. (1974) The role of the hypothalamus in the organization of patterns of cardiovascular responses; in Recent Studies of Hypothalamic Function, K. Lederis and K.E. Cooper, eds. S. Karger, Basel, pp. 306-314.

Hilton, S.M. and Spyer, K.M. (1971) Participation of the anterior hypothalamus in the baroreceptor reflex. J. Physiol. (Lond.) 218, 271-293.

Korner, P.I. (1979) Central nervous control of cardiovascular function; in Handbook of Physiology, Sec. 1. The Cardiovascular System, Vol. 1., pp. 691-739.

Lisander, B. (1970) Factors influencing the autonomic components of the defense reaction. Acta Physiol. Scand. 78, 1-42.

Loewy, A.D. and McKellar, S. (1980) The neuroanatomical basis of central cardiovascular control. Fed. Proc. 39, 2490-2503.

Malliani, A., Schwartz, P.J. and Zanchetti, A. (1980) Neural mechanisms in life-threatening arrhythmias. Amer. Heart. J. 100, 705-715.

Manning, J.W. (1980) Central cardiovascular control: a distributed neural network. Fed. Proc. 39, 2485-2486.

Menninger, R.P. and Frazier, D.T. (1972) Effects of blood volume and atrial stretch on hypothalamic single-unit activity. Amer. J. Physiol. 223, 288-293.

Peiss, C.N. (1965) Concepts of cardiovascular regulation; past, present, future; in Nervous Control of the Heart. W.C. Randall, ed. Williams and Wilkins, Baltimore, pp. 153-197.

Schwartz, P.J., Brown, A.M., Malliani, A. and Zanchetti, A. (1978) Neural mechanisms in cardiac arrhythmias; in Perspectives in Cardiovascular Research, Vol. 2, P.J. Schwartz, A.M. Brown, A. Malliani and A. Zanchetti, eds. Raven Press, New York.

Spyer, K.M. (1972) Baroreceptor sensitive neurons in the anterior hypothalamus of the cat. J. Physiol. (Lond.) 224, 245-257.

Spyer, K.M. (1981) Neural organisation and control of the baroreceptor reflex. Rev. Physiol. Biochem. Pharmacol. 38, 23-124.

Thomas, M.R. and Calaresu, F.R. (1972) Responses of single units in the medial hypothalamus to electrical stimulation of the carotid sinus nerve in the cat. Brain Res. 44, 49-62.

Weiss, G.K. and Crill, W.E. (1969) Carotid sinus nerve: primary afferent depolarization evoked by hypothalamic stimulation. Brain Res. 16, 269-272.

Zanchetti, A., Baccelli, G. and Mancia, G. (1976) Fighting, emotions and exercise: cardiovascular effects in the cat; in Regulation of Blood Pressure by the Central Nervous System, Part 2, G. Onesti, M. Fernandes and K.E. Kim, eds. Grune, New York, pp. 87-103.

Zucker, I.H. and Gilmore, J.P. (1981) Atrial receptor modulation of renal function in heart failure; in Disturbances in Neurogenic Control of the Circulation. F.M. Abboud, ed. American Physiological Society, Bethesda, pp. 1-16.

Neurotransmitters Involved in the Central Nervous System Control of Cardiovascular Function

RICHARD A. GILLIS
Department of Pharmacology, Georgetown University Schools of Medicine and Dentistry, Washington, DC

INTRODUCTION

There are a large number of neurotransmitters that are known to act in the central nervous system (CNS) to produce changes in cardiovascular (CV) function. These include catecholamines, notably norepinephrine; acetylcholine; serotonin; gamma-aminobutyric acid (GABA); glycine; glutamic acid; and several of the peptides. Evidence documenting their importance in the CNS control of CV function has been obtained from several types of studies: injecting each of the above substances into the CNS (i.e., into the ventricular system, or into brain tissue) while monitoring several indices of CV function; injecting specific antagonists of the neurotransmitters into the CNS while monitoring several indices of CV function; injecting either the agonist or antagonist into the CNS while monitoring reflex-induced changes in several indices of CV function; and injecting either agonist or antagonist into the CNS while monitoring changes in CV function induced by electrical stimulation of specific brain nuclei (e.g., locus ceruleus) or tracts (e.g., medial forebrain bundle). The neurally mediated changes in CV function produced by these types of studies are, in some cases, of great interest *per se*, such as the coronary constriction evoked by injecting the GABA antagonist drug picrotoxin into the brain ventricles (Segal et al., in press **a**). The real excitement about these studies, however, is the information they afford on endogenous CNS neurotransmitters playing a role in CV control, and the CNS sites where drugs exert their CV effects. Results of these studies provide strong evidence that norepinephrine, acetylcholine, serotonin, GABA, glutamic acid, and substance P are neurotransmitters or neuromodulators acting in the CNS to influence CV function. They also strongly suggest that the ventral surface of the medulla, area postrema, anteroventral third ventricle, and nucleus ambiguus comprise important pathways for CV control, and are important sites to consider in the determination of drug action.

EVIDENCE FOR CATECHOLAMINES

To determine whether central catecholaminergic nerves comprise part of the central connections of the autonomic nervous system, investigators have injected drugs such as 6-hydroxydopamine (an agent that produces selective chemical lesions of noradrenergic neuron terminals) directly into the brain and monitored arterial blood pressure and heart rate of normotensive and hypertensive animals. One conclusion from these studies is that central catecholaminergic nerves seem to have little importance in the maintenance of resting arterial blood pressure (Chalmers, 1975). A second conclusion is that catecholaminergic nerves are implicated in the development of some animal models of DOCA-salt, genetic, and neurogenic hypertension (Chalmers and Wurtman, 1971; Finch et al., 1972; Haeusler et al., 1972; Chalmers et al., 1974; Doba and Reis, 1974; Erinoff et al., 1975). Destruction of noradrenergic neurons prevents these forms of hypertension. A third conclusion is that catecholaminergic neurons are involved in the hypertensive response produced by electrical stimulation of the posterior hypothalamus (Haeusler, 1975) and the A5 catecholamine cell group (Loewy et al., 1979). Destruction of noradrenergic neurons counteracts these pressor responses. A fourth conclusion is that catecholaminergic nerves in the nucleus tractus solitarius (NTS) affect the lability of arterial pressure (Snyder et al., 1978). Destruction of noradrenergic neurons causes the arterial pressure to become extremely labile.

Experiments performed with local application of catecholamine-receptor stimulating agents indicate that activation of catecholaminergic receptors in the NTS and in the anterior hypothalamic-preoptic region causes hypotension and bradycardia (Struyker-Boudier et al., 1974; Zandberg et al., 1979). Activation of catecholaminergic receptors in the posterior hypothalamic nucleus results in hypertension (Kobinger, 1978). The blood pressure response resulting from activation of catecholaminergic receptors at the spinal cord level is controversial. Data from some studies indicate excitation of sympathetic preganglionic neurons (Neumayer et al., 1974; Taylor and Brody, 1976), while data from other studies indicate inhibition of sympathetic preganglionic neurons (Coote and MacLeod, 1974, 1977; Guyenet and Cabot, 1981). The catecholaminergic receptor responsible for the hypotensive effect of these agents appears to be a postsynaptic $alpha_2$-adrenoceptor (Guyenet and Cabot, 1981; Timmermans et al., 1981).

The studies above deal with the role of central catecholaminergic nerves and receptors on sympathetic outflow to the periphery. In terms of parasympathetic outflow, it can be concluded that these nerves in the NTS do not mediate baroreceptor-induced activation of the cardiac vagus (Snyder et al., 1978). However, they may modulate baroreceptor-induced activation of the cardiac vagus. Evidence for this was the finding that destruction of the catecholamine innervation of the NTS with 6-hydroxydopamine does not alter the magnitude of reflex-induced vagal bradycardia but does reduce the gain of this response (Snyder et al., 1978). Central catecholaminergic nerves may play a role in resting cardiac vagal tone, as destruction of these neurons has been reported to increase parasympathetic outflow to the heart (Doba and Reis, 1974; Chalmers, 1975).

EVIDENCE FOR ACETYLCHOLINE

In terms of the importance of CNS cholinergic neurons in the control of CV function, it appears that activity in this neurotransmitter system exerts no tonic effect over arterial pressure of normotensive animals (Lang and Rush, 1973; Buccafusco and Brezenoff, 1978; Brezenoff and Caputi, 1980). This conclusion is based on the findings that atropine and mecamylamine, which block muscarinic and nicotinic receptors, respectively, and hemicholinium-3, which inhibits the synthesis of acetylcholine, have no effect on resting arterial pressure when injected into the lateral cerebral ventricle. Furthermore, a cholinergic mechanism does not seem to be involved in the elevated blood pressure of spontaneously hypertensive rats, as neither atropine nor mecamylamine injected into the lateral cerebral ventricle had any effect on the basal level of arterial pressure and heart rate in these animals (Brezenoff and Caputi, 1980). This conclusion is not firm, however, as intracerebroventricular injection of hemicholinium-3 has been shown to lower arterial pressure in this animal model of hypertension (Brezenoff and Caputi, 1980). In addition, data obtained with physostigmine- and oxotremorine-induced pressor responses suggest that the spontaneous release of acetylcholine at certain central sites is increased in spontaneously hypertensive rats but not in renal hypertensive and DOCA-salt hypertensive rats (Kubo and Tatsumi, 1979).

Evidence from studies with localized administration of drugs that affect the cholinergic synapse suggests that endogenous acetylcholine in the posterior hypothalamic nucleus can act via muscarinic receptors to elevate blood pressure (Buccafusco and Brezenoff, 1979). A similar cholinergic mechanism seems also to exist in some region of the brain stem (Brezenoff and Jenden, 1970). Interestingly, endogenous acetylcholine on the ventral surface of the medulla has been shown to have the opposite effect on arterial pressure. Acetylcholine at this site (i.e., Schlaefke's area) has been shown to act via muscarinic receptors to lower arterial blood pressure (Guertzenstein, 1973; Wennergren and Oberg, 1980; Feldberg, 1980).

In terms of parasympathetic outflow, there are data indicating that a CNS cholinergic synapse comprises part of the reflex vagal pathway, and that muscarinic receptors mediate transmission at this synapse (Rozear et al., 1968; Lee et al., 1972; Petti et al., 1979; Canputi et al., 1980). This was shown by noting blockade of reflex-induced vagal bradycardia by intracerebroventricular injections of ℓ-hyoscyamine, ethybenztropine, propantheline, and hemicholinium-3.

EVIDENCE FOR SEROTONIN

The importance of CNS serotonergic neurons in the control of CV function is controversial. At present, no conclusion can be drawn on whether this neurotransmitter system exerts a tonic effect over arterial pressure of normotensive animals. This is because investigators testing this point using p-chlorophenylalanine, which inhibits the synthesis of serotonin, or 5,6- and 5,7-dihydroxytryptamine, which produce selective lesions of terminals of serotonergic neurons, report an increase in arterial pressure (Ito and Schanberg, 1972), a decrease in arterial pressure (Wing and Chalmers, 1974), and no change in arterial pressure (Helke, 1978). Possible reasons for these conflicting data have been suggested by Chalmers (1975) and Kuhn et al. (1980). Serotonergic nerves may be involved in development of neurogenic hypertension, as central administration of 5,6-dihydroxytryptamine has been shown to prevent the increases in arterial pressure and heart rate produced by sinoaortic denervation and to reverse them when they are already established (Wing and Chalmers, 1974). Serotonergic nerves may also be involved in the development of DOCA-salt hypertension (Finch, 1975; Buckingham et al., 1976), as treatment with 5,6-dihydroxytryptamine and p-chlorophenylalanine reduced arterial pressure in these animals. In the spontaneously hypertensive rat, inhibition of brain serotonin synthesis has produced two effects: hypotension in one case (Jarrott et al., 1975), and further increased arterial pressure in the other (DeJong et al., 1975). Destruction of serotonergic neurons with 5,6-dihydroxytryptamine seemed to have little effect on renal hypertension (Wing and Chalmers, 1974).

Experiments performed with local application of serotonin and electrical stimulation of the dorsal and median raphe nuclei indicate that activation of serotonin receptors in the anterior hypothalamus-preoptic region and NTS causes hypertension. Smits and Struyker-Boudier (1976) reported that injection of serotonin into the anterior hypothalamic-preoptic area caused an increase in arterial pressure. This effect was counteracted by pretreatment with the serotonin receptor blocking agent, methysergide. Kuhn and colleagues (1980) reported that electrical stimulation of the dorsal and median raphe nuclei produces an increase in arterial pressure. This pressor response was attenuated by injections of the serotonin antagonist, 2-bromolysergic acid diethylamide (BOL) into the anterior hypothalamic-preoptic area. These results suggest that activation of the raphe nuclei leads to a pressor effect as a result of a stimulation-evoked release of serotonin in the anterior hypothalamic-preoptic area. Wolf and colleagues (1981) reported that injection of serotonin into the NTS also caused an increase in arterial pressure, an effect that was counteracted by the serotonin antagonists, BOL and metergoline. They pointed out that enhanced serotonergic activity causes an increase in blood pressure in regions where enhanced catecholaminergic activity causes a decrease in blood pressure. This may also be true of sympathetic preganglionic neurons; serotonin has been shown to produce an excitatory effect (deGroat and Ryall, 1967), whereas norepinephrine has been shown to produce an inhibitory effect (Timmermans et al., 1981). It should be noted, however, that electrical stimulation of the medullary raphe causes inhibition of sympathetic preganglionic neurons (Cabot et al., 1979).

In terms of parasympathetic outflow, there is evidence that serotonin may inhibit reflex-induced increases in cardiac vagal tone. Lin and Chern (1979) reported that elevating brain serotonin with 5-hydroxytryptophan produced a significant reduction in reflex bradycardia in response to an elevation in arterial pressure. In contrast, depleting serotonin with either p-chlorophenylamine or 5,7-dihydroxytryptamine led to an enhancement in reflex-induced bradycardia.

EVIDENCE FOR GABA

In contrast to the lack of a definitive role for CNS noradrenergic, cholinergic and serotonergic neurons in the maintenance of resting arterial blood pressure, data obtained with drugs that interfere with CNS GABAergic transmission indicate that CNS GABAergic neurons are important in the maintenance of resting blood pressure. Blockade of CNS GABAergic transmission with bicuculline and picrotoxin causes increases in arterial pressure and sympathetic outflow (DiMicco, 1978; Gillis et al., 1980). Increases in sympathetic outflow also occur after GABA synthesis is inhibited with thiosemicarbozide (Taylor et al., 1977). Local application of bicuculline and picrotoxin to the ventral surface of the medulla (Schlaefke's area) also results in an increase in arterial pressure (Feldberg, 1976; Yamada et al., in press). Recently we have found that intravenously and centrally administrered picrotoxin to chloralose-anesthetized cats will produce sympathetically-mediated coronary artery constriction (Segal et al., in press).

Results obtained with drugs that directly activate GABA receptors (GABA, muscimol, imidazole-4-acetic acid) indicate that CNS administration of these agents decreases sympathetic outflow and arterial pressure (Antonaccio and Taylor, 1977; Williford et al., 1980; Antonaccio and Snyder, 1981). This is true for resting arterial pressure and sympathetic nervous discharge as well as for pressor and sympathetic discharge evoked by electrical stimulation of the posterior hypothalamus (Antonaccio et al., 1978). In addition, activation of CNS GABA receptors will counteract vasoconstrictor responses induced by bilateral carotid occlusion (Wennergren and Oberg, 1980; Sweet et al., 1979). The CNS site of action for these effects of GABA seems to be the ventral surface of the medulla (Schlaefke's area) (Wennergren and Oberg, 1980; Feldberg, 1980; Yamada et al., in press b; Bousquet et al., 1978; Williford et al., 1981). Finally, the effect of GABA on arterial pressure and heart rate is accompanied by pronounced respiratory depression (Yamada et al., in press b). This is not surprising, as the ventral surface of the medulla contains chemosensitive sites that influence respiratory drive (Schlaefke, 1981).

Central GABAergic mechanisms also have an important effect on cardiac vagal tone. For example, bicuculline and picrotoxin block inhibition of reflex-induced vagal bradycardia elicited by stimulation of the lateral hypothalamus (Barman and Gebber, 1979), suggesting that GABA may be the transmitter responsible for inhibition of reflex-induced vagal bradycardia. Blockade of GABA receptors results in an increase in resting vagal tone (DiMicco et al., 1979). In addition, stimulation of GABA receptors completely prevents reflex-induced vagal bradycardia evoked by raising the arterial pressure with phenylephrine (Williford et al., 1980a). The brain site where GABA is thought to be important for inhibiting vagal activity is the nucleus ambiguus (DiMicco et al., 1979; Williford et al., 1980b).

EVIDENCE FOR GLYCINE

Most of the data obtained with glycine center on effects produced at the ventral surface of the medulla (Schlaefke's area). Glycine applied to this site produces a decrease in arterial pressure (Wennergren and Oberg, 1980; Guertzenstein and Silver, 1974). This is reflected by decreases in arteriole resistance in both skeletal muscle and kidney (Wennergren and Oberg, 1980). In addition, there is a pronounced vasodilatation in the mesenteric bed (Hilton, 1979). Interestingly, the circulatory response elicited by stimulation of the defense area of the amygdala or hypothalamus is reduced, particularly the rise in arterial pressure and mesenteric vasoconstriction. From these findings, Hilton (1979) proposes that "the glycine-sensitive neurons on, or near, the ventral surface of the medulla may be the origin of the final common path for the visceral components of the defense reaction."

EVIDENCE FOR GLUTAMIC ACID

Interest in glutamic acid centers around the possibility that this substance may be the neurotransmitter released by baroreceptor afferent nerves at their site of termination in the intermediate third of the NTS. Evidence for this can be found in the recent studies by Reiss and colleagues: (1) microinjection of glutamic acid into the NTS of the rat resulted in hypotension and bradycardia (Talman et al., 1980, 1981); (2) microinjection of an antagonist of L-glutamic acid, glutamic acid diethylester into the NTS produced hypertension and tachycardia (Talman et al., 1981), and also prevented the hypotension and bradycardia produced by L-glutamic acid; (3) removal of vagal afferent fibers synapsing in the NTS by extirpating the nodose ganglion partially inhibited high affinity uptake of ^{3}H-L-glutamate in the NTS (Reis et al., 1981); and (4) electrical stimulation of vagal afferent fibers caused release of ^{3}H-glutamic acid in the NTS (Reis et al., 1981).

EVIDENCE FOR PEPTIDES

A number of peptides have been studied (e.g., angiotensin II, bradykinin, vasopressin, thyrotropin-releasing hormone), and others remain to be studied (e.g., cholecystokinin, oxytocin). Most thoroughly studied is angiotensin II (reviewed by Fitzsimons, 1980). Briefly, angiotensin II-like immunoreactivity has been demonstrated in axons and nerve terminals in the brain and spinal cord of the rat, and distribution of this peptide was widespread (Fuxe et al., 1976). Furthermore, angiotension II has been shown to act on several structures in the CNS , resulting in increases in arterial pressure. The sensitive sites for the pressor response include the area postrema in the dog, cat and rabbit (Gildenberg et al., 1963; Dickinson and Yu, 1967; Fitzsimons, 1980), the anteroventral third ventricle in the rat (Hoffman and Phillips, 1976; Buggy et al., 1977), and the subnucleus medialis of the midbrain in dog and cat (Deuben and Buckley, 1970). Pressor responses elicited from the area postrema may depend, in part, on the presence of endogenous opioid peptides (Szilagyi and Ferrario, 1981), while pressor responses elicited from the anteroventral third ventricle may depend, in part, on the presence of vasopressin (Fitzsimons, 1980). The studies dealing with the anteroventral third ventricle and angiotensin II have evolved into studies focused on examining the role of this brain region in the development and maintenance of hypertension in a number of rat models. This brain area seems to play a role in renal hypertension and DOCA-salt hypertension (Brady et al., 1978).

Interest in substance P also centers around the possibility that this agent is released by baroreceptor (and chemoreceptor) afferent nerves at their site of termination in the NTS. Evidence that substance P may be a neurotransmitter is based on the findings that: (1) substance P-like immunoreactivity (SP-I) is present in the parts of the NTS where baro- and chemoreceptor fibers terminate, and in the petrosal and nodose ganglia (Gillis et al., 1980; Helke et al., 1980); (2) denervation of the IXth and Xth cranial nerves results in significant reduction in SP-I in the parts of the NTS where baro- and chemoreceptor fibers terminate (Gillis et al., 1980; Helke et al., 1980); (3) substance P immunoreactive fibers are present in the carotid body (Jacobowitz and Helke, 1980); and (4) local application of substance P and capsaicin to the NTS produces hypotension and bradycardia (Haeusler and Osterwalder, 1980).

The presence of both enkephalins and opiate receptors in the NTS, nucleus ambiguus and dorsal motor nucleus of the vagus (Elde et al., 1976; Atweh and Kuhar, 1977) raises the question of whether enkephalins play a role in central CV regulation. This has been tested in normotensive animals by administering the opioid receptor antagonist drug, naloxone. Administration of this agent has no effect on arterial blood pressure unless either opioid peptides have been injected, afferent sensory pathways from viscera have been interrupted, excessive stress from the surgical procedures has been incurred, or shock has been induced by transection of the spinal cord or injection of endotoxin (Dashwood and Feldberg, 1980; Faden and Holaday, 1980; Faden et al., 1980). Under these circumstances, naloxone does produce a pressor response presumably because of antagonism of the CNS effects of injected opioids or endogenously released opioid peptides. Injection of opioid peptides into the CNS of dogs has been shown to produce hypotension, bradycardia and a reduction in sympathetic nerve activity (Laubie et al., 1977). Interestingly, injection of opioid peptides into the CNS of rats increases arterial pressure and heart rate, indicating a species difference in the response to these agents (Bellet et al., 1980).

In dogs, stimulation of opioid receptors causes enhancement of parasympathetic outflow to the heart, and this seems to occur at nucleus ambiguus (Laubie et al., 1979). Activation of these receptors by endogenous opioids has been postulated by Faden and colleagues (1980) to be responsible for some of the hypotension following spinal cord transection. These investigators suggest that activation of opioid receptors at nucleus ambiguus results in a depression of myocardial contractility which is mediated through cholinergic vagal efferent pathways.

SUMMARY

The intent of this review was not to be exhaustive, but to highlight some of the evidence suggesting that a particular neurotransmitter might be important in the CNS control of CV function. In undertaking this task, I have become keenly aware of the importance of neurotransmitter action at the ventral surface of the medulla, particularly Schlaefke's area, in influencing CV function. Indeed, as pointed out by Feldberg (1976), this region may be an important site of action for drugs known to influence arterial pressure through a CNS mechanism. Our own preliminary data indicate that cardio-respiratory depression induced by pentobarbital is due to this agent acting through a GABAergic system at the ventral surface of the medulla (Yamada et al., in press b). Additional studies of this region combining techniques described above with anatomical and biochemical approaches should enhance our understanding of cardio-respiratory control.

ACKNOWLEDGMENTS

The author's own studies were supported by NIH grants NS12566 and HL28406 and by a Grant-in-Aid from the American Heart Association with funds contributed in part by the American Heart Association, Nation's Capitol Affiliate, and a grant from McNeil Pharmaceutical.

REFERENCES

Antonaccio, M.J., Kerwin, L. and Taylor, D.G. (1978) Effects of central GABA receptor agonism and antagonism on evoked diencephalic cardiovascular responses. Neuropharmacology 17, 597-603.

Antonaccio, M.J. and Snyder, D.W. (1981) Redutions in blood pressure, heart rate and renal sympathetic nervous discharge after imidazole-4-acetic acid: mediation through central γ-aminobutyric acid (GABA) receptor stimulation. J. Pharmacol. Exp. Ther. 218, 200-205.

Antonaccio, M.J. and Taylor, D.G. (1977) Involvement of central GABA receptors in the regulation of blood pressure and heart rate of anesthetized cats. Eur. J. Pharmacol. 46, 283-287.

Atweh, F. and Kuhar, M.J. (1977) Autoradiographic localization of opiate receptors in rat brain. I. Spinal cord and lower medulla. Brain Res. 124, 53-67.

Barman, S.M. and Gebber, G.L. (1979) Picrotoxin and bicuculline-sensitive inhibition of cardiac vagal reflexes. J. Pharmacol. Exp. Ther. 209, 67-72.

Bellet, M., Elghozi, J.L., Meyer, P., Pernollet, M.G. and Schmitt, H. (1980) Central cardiovascular effects of narcotic analgesics and enkephalins in rats. Brit. J. Pharmacol. 71, 365-369.

Bousquet, P., Feldman, J., Bloch, R. and Schwartz, J. (1978) Action hypotensive ventrobulbaire du muscimol. C.R. Soc. Biol. 172, 770-773.

Brady, M.J., Fink, G.D., Buggy, J., Haywood, J.R., Gordon, F.J. and Johnson, A.K. (1978) The role of the anteroventral third ventricle (AV3V) region in experimental hypertension. Circulat. Res. 43 (Suppl 1), I2-I13.

Brezenoff, H.E. and Caputi, A.P. (1980) Intracerebroventricular injection of hemicholiniums lowers blood pressure in conscious spontaneously hypertensive rats, but not in normotensive rats. Life Sci. 26, 1037-1045.

Brezenoff, H.E. and Jenden, D.J. (1970) Changes in arterial blood pressure after microinjecions of carbachol into the medulla and IVth ventricle of the rat brain. Neuropharmacology 9, 341-348.

Buccafusco, J.J. and Brezenoff, H.E. (1978) The hypertensive response to injection of physostigmine into the hypothalamus of the unanesthetized rat. Clin. Exp. Hypertension 1, 219-227.

Buccafusco, J.J. and Brezenoff, H.E. (1979) Pharmacological study of a cholinergic mechanism within the rat posterior hypothalamic nucleus which mediates a hypertensive response. Brain Res. 165, 295-310.

Buckingham, R.E., Hamilton, T.C. and Moore, R.A. (1976) Prolonged effects of p-chlorophenylamine on the blood pressure of conscious normotensive and doca/saline hypertensive rats. Brit. J. Pharmacol. 56, 69-75.

Buggy, J., Fink, G.D., Johnson, A.K. and Brady, M.J. (1977) Prevention of the development of renal hypertension by anteroventral third ventricular tissue lesions. Circulat. Res. 40 (Suppl. 1), 110-117.

Cabot, J.B., Wild, J.M. and Cohen, D.H. (1979) Raphe inhibition of sympathetic preganglionic neurons. Science 203, 184-186.

Caputi, A.P., Rossi, F., Carney, K. and Brezenoff, H.E. (1980) Modulatory effect of brain acetylcholine on reflex-induced bradycardia and tachycardia in conscious rats. J. Pharmacol. Exp. Ther. 215, 309-316.

Chalmers, J.P. (1975) Brain amines and models of experimental hypertension. Circulat. Res. 36, 469-480.

Chalmers, J.P., Dollery, C.T., Lewis, P.J. and Reid, J.L. (1974) The importance of central adrenergic neurones in renal hypertension in rabbits. J. Physiol. (Lond.) 238, 403-411.

Chalmers, J.P. and Wurtman, R.J. (1971) Participation of central noradrenergic neurons in arterial baroreceptor reflexes in the rabbit. Circulat. Res. 28, 480-491.

Coote, J.H. and MacLeod, V.H. (1974) The influence of bulbospinal monoaminergic pathways on sympathetic nerve activity. J. Physiol. (Lond.) 241, 453-475.

Coote, J.H. and MacLeod, V.H. (1977) The effect of intraspinal microinjections of hydroxydopamine on the inhibitory influence exerted on spinal sympathetic activity by the baroreceptors. Pflügers Arch. 371, 277.

Dashwood, M.R. and Feldberg, W. (1980) Release of opioid peptides in anaesthetized cats. Brit. J. Pharmacol. 68, 796-703.

de Groat, W.C. and Ryall, R.W. (1967) An excitatory action of 5-hydroxytryptamine on sympathetic preganglionic neurones. Exp. Brain Res. 3, 299-305.

De Jong, W., Nijkamp, F.P. and Bohus, B. (1975) Role of noradrenaline and serotonin in the central control of blood pressure in normotensive and spontaneously hypertensive rats. Arch Int. Pharmacodyn. 213, 272-284.

Deuben, R.R. and Buckley, J.P. (1970) Identification of a central site of action of angiotensin II. J. Pharmacol. Exp. Ther. 175, 139-145.

Dickinson, C.J. and Yu, R. (1967) Mechanisms involved in the progressive pressor response to very small amounts of angiotensin in conscious rabbits. Circulat. Res. 20-21 (Suppl. 2), 157-163.

DiMicco, J.A. (1978) Neurocardiovascular Effects of the GABA Antagonists Picrotoxin and Bicuculline in the Cat: Evidence for the Involvement of GABA in Central Cardiovascular Control, Ph.D. Thesis.

DiMicco, J.A., Gale, K., Hamilton, B.L. and Gillis, R.G. (1979) Evidence that a GABAergic mechanism at nucleus ambiguus influences reflex-induced vagal activity. Brain Res. 193, 584-588.

Doba, N. and Reis, D.J. (1974) Role of central and peripheral adrenergic mechanisms in neurogenic hypertension produced by brainstem lesions in rat. Circulat. Res. 34, 293-301.

Elde, R., Hokfelt, T., Johansson, O. and Terenius, L. (1976) Immunohistochemical studies using antibodies to leucine-enkephaline: initial observations on the nervous system of the rat. Neuroscience 1, 349-351.

Erinoff, L., Heller, A. and Oparil, S. (1975) Prevention of hypertension in the SH rat: effects of differential central catecholamine depletion. Proc. Soc. Exp. Biol. 150, 748-754.

Faden, A.I. and Holaday, J.W. (1980) Naloxone treatment of endotoxin shock: stereo-specificity of physiologic and pharmacologic effects in the rat. J. Pharmacol. Exp. Ther. 212, 441-447.

Faden, A.I., Jacobs, T.P. and Holaday, J.W. (1980) Endorphin-parasympathetic interaction in spinal shock. J. Autonom. Nerv. Syst. 2, 295-304.

Feldberg, W. (1976) The ventral surface of the brain stem: a scarcely explored region of pharmacological sensitivity. Neuroscience 1, 427-441.

Feldberg, W. (1980) Cardiovascular effects of drugs acting on the ventral surface of the brain stem; in Central Interaction Between Respiratory and Cardiovascular Control Systems, H.P. Koepchen, S.M. Hilton and A. Trzebski, eds. Springer-Verlag, Berlin, 47-55.

Finch, L. (1975) The cardiovascular effects of intraventricular 5,6-dihydroxytryptamine in conscious hypertensive rats. Clin. Exp. Pharmacol. Physiol. 2, 503-508.

Finch, L., Haeusler, G. and Thoenen, H. (1972) Failure to induce experimental hypertension in rats after intraventricular injection of 6-hydroxydopamine. Brit. J. Pharmacol. 44, 356-357.

Fitzsimons, J.T. (1980) Angiotensin stimulation of the central nervous system. Rev. Physiol. Biochem. Pharmacol. 87, 117-167.

Fuxe, K., Ganten, D. Hokfelt, T. and Bolme, P. (1976) Immunohistochemical evidence for the existence of angiotensin II-containing nerve terminals in the brain and spinal cord in the rat. Neurosci. Lett. 2, 229-234.

Gildenberg, P.L., Ferrario, C.M. and McCubbin, J.W. (1963) Two sites of cardiovascular action of angiotensin II in the brain of the dog. Clin. Sci. 44, 417-420.

Gillis, R.A., DiMicco, J.A., Williford, D.J., Hamilton, B.L. and Gale, K.N. (1980) Importance of CNS GABAergic mechanisms in the regulation of cardiovascular function. Brain Res. Bull. 5 (Suppl. 2), 303-315.

Gillis, R.A., Helke, C.J., Hamilton, B.L., Norman, W.P. and Jacobowitz, D.M. (1980) Evidence that substance P is a neurotransmitter of baro- and chemoreceptor afferent in nucleus tractus solitarius. Brain Res. 181, 476-481.

Guertzenstein, P.G. (1973) Blood pressure effects obtained by drugs applied to the ventral surface of the brain stem. J. Physiol. (Lond.) 229, 395-408.

Guertzenstein, P.G. and Silver, A. (1974) Fall in blood pressure produced from discrete regions of the ventral surface of the medulla by glycine and lesions. J. Physiol. (Lond.) 242, 489-503.

Guyenet, P.G. and Cabot, J.B. (1981) Inhibition of sympathetic preganglionic neurons by catecholamines and clonidine: mediation by an α-adrenergic receptor. J. Neurosci. 1, 908-917.

Haeusler, G. (1975) Cardiovascular regulation by central adrenergic mechanisms and its alteration by hypotensive drugs. Circulat. Res. 36-37, 1223-1232.

Haeusler, G., Finch, L. and Thoenen, H. (1972) Central adrenergic neurones and the initiation and development of experimental hypertension. Experientia 28, 1200-1203.

Haeusler, G. and Osterwalder, R. (1980) Evidence suggesting a transmitter or neuromodulatory role for substance P at the first synapse of the baroreceptor reflex. Naunyn-Schmiedeberg's Arch. Exp. Path. Pharmak. 314, 111-121.

Helke, C.J. (1978) The Role of Monoaminergic Neurotransmitter Systems in the Arrhythmogenic Effects of Digitalis, Ph.D. Thesis.

Helke, C.J., O'Donohue, T.L. and Jacobowitz, D.M. (1980) Substance P as a baro- and chemoreceptor afferent neurotransmitter: immunocytochemical and neurochemical evidence in the rat. Peptides 1, 1-9.

Hilton, S.M. (1979) The defense reaction as a paradigm for cardiovascular control; in Integrative Function of the Autonomic Nervous System, K. Koizumi and A. Sato, eds. Elsevier/North-Holland, pp. 443-449.

Hoffman, W.E. and Phillips, M.I. (1976) Regional study of cerebral ventricle sensitive sites to angiotensin II. Brain Res. 110, 313-330.

Ito, A. and Schanberg, S.M. (1972) Central nervous system mechanisms responsible for blood pressure elevation induced by p-chlorophenylalamine. J. Pharmacol. Exp. Ther. 181, 65-74.

Jacobowitz, D.M. and Helke, C.J. (1980) Localization of substance P immunoreactive nerves in the carotid body. Brain Res. Bull. 5, 195-197.

Jarrott, B., McQueen, A., Gradf, L. and Louis, W.J. (1975) Serotonin levels in vascular tissue and the effects of a serotonin synthesis inhibitor on blood pressure in hypertensive rats. Clin. Exp. Pharmacol. Physiol. (Suppl. 2), 201-205.

Kobinger, W. (1978) Central α-adrenergic systems as targets for hypotensive drugs. Rev. Physiol. Biochem. Pharmacol. 81, 40-100.

Kubo, T. and Tatsumi, M. (1979) Increased pressure responses to physostigmine in spontaneously hypertensive rats. Naunyn-Schmiedeberg's Arch. Exp. Path. Pharmak. 306, 81-83.

Kuhn, D.M., Wolf, W.A. and Lovenberg, W. (1980a) Pressor effects of electrical stimulation of the dorsal and median raphe nuclei in anesthetized rats. J. Pharmacol. Exp. Ther. 214, 403-409.

Kuhn, D.M., Wolf, W.A. and Lovenberg, W. (1980b) Review of the role of the central serotonergic neuronal system in blood pressure regulation. Hypertension 2, 243-255.

Lang, W.J. and Rush, M.L. (1973) Cardiovascular responses to injections of cholinomimetic drugs into the cerebral ventricles of unanaesthetized dogs. Brit. J. Pharmacol. 47, 196-205.

Laubie, M., Schmitt, H. and Vincent, M. (1979) Vagal bradycardia produced by microinjections of morphine-like drugs into the nucleus ambiguus in anesthetized dogs. Eur. J. Pharmacol. 59, 287-291.

Laubie, M., Schmitt, H., Vincent, M. and Remond, G. (1977) Central cardiovascular effects of morphinomimetic peptides in dogs. Eur. J. Pharmacol. 46, 67-71.

Lee, T.M., Kuo, J.S. and Chai, C.Y. (1972) Central integrating mechanism of the Bezold-Jarisch and baroreceptor reflex. Amer. J. Physiol. 222, 713-720.

Lin, M.T. and Chern, S.I. (1979) Effect of brain 5-hydroxytryptamine alterations on reflex bradycardia in rats. Amer. J. Physiol. 236, R302-R306.

Loewy, A.D., Gregorie, E.M., McKellar, S. and Baker, R.P. (1979) Electrophysiological evidence that the A5 catecholamine cell group is a vasomotor center. Brain Res. 178, 196-200.

Neumayr, R.J., Hare, B.D. and Franz, D.N. (1974) Evidence for bulbospinal control of sympathetic preganglionic neurons by monoaminergic pathways. Life Sci. 14, 793-806.

Petti, C.A., Williams, T.P., Helke, C.J. and Gillis, R.A. (1979) Evidence for involvement of a CNS cholinergic mechanism in reflex-induced vagal bradycardia in the cat. Neurosci. Abstr. 5, 48.

Reis, D.J., Perrone, M.H. and Talman, W.T. (1981) Glutamic acid as the neurotransmitter of baroreceptor afferents in the nucleus tractus solitarii: possible relationship to neurogenic hypertension; in Central Nervous System Mechanisms in Hypertension, J.P. Buckley and C.M. Ferrario, eds. Raven Press, N.Y., pp. 37-48.

Rozear, M., Bircher, R.P., Chai, C.Y. and Wang, S.C. (1968) Effects of intracerebroventricular ℓ-hyoscyamine, ethylbenztropine and procaine on cardiac arrhythmias induced in dogs by pentylenetetrazol, picrotoxin or deslanoside. Int. J. Neuropharmacol. 71, 1-6.

Schlaefke, M.E. (1981) Central chemosensitivity: a respiratory drive. Rev. Physiol. Biochem. Pharmacol. 90, 172-244.

Segal, S.A., Pearle, D.L. and Gillis, R.A. (in press a) Coronary spasm in the cat produced by increasing central sympathetic outflow to the heart. Amer. J. Cardiol.

Segal, S.A., Pearle, D.L. and Gillis, R.A. (in press b) Coronary spasm produced by picrotoxin in cats. Eur. J. Pharmacol.

Smits, J.F. and Struyker-Boudier, H.A. (1976) Intra-hypothalamic serotonin and cardiovascular control in rats. Brain Res. 111, 422-427.

Snyder, D.W., Nathan, M.A. and Reis, D.J. (1978) Chronic lability of arterial pressure produced by selective destruction of the catecholamine innervation of nucleus tractus solitarii in the rat. Circulat. Res. 43, 662-671.

Struyker-Boudier, H.A.J., Smeets, G.W., Brouwer, G.M. and van Rossum, J.M. (1974) Hypothalamic adrenergic receptors in cardiovascular regulation. Neuropharmacology 13, 837-846.

Sweet, C.S., Wenger, H.C. and Gross, D.M. (1979) Central antihypertensive properties of muscimol and related γ-aminobutyric acid agonist and the interactions of muscimol with baroreceptor reflexes. Canad. J. Physiol. Pharmacol. 57, 600.

Szilagyi, J.E. and Ferrario, C.M. (1981) Central opiate system modulation of the area postrema pressor pathway. Hypertension 3, 313-317.

Talman, W.T., Perrone, M.H. and Reis, D.J. (1980) Evidence for L-glutamate as a neurotransmitter of primary baroreceptor afferent nerve fibers. Science 209, 813-815.

Talman, W.T., Perrone, M.H., Scher, P., Kwo, S. and Reis, D.J. (1981) Antagonism of the baroreceptor reflex by glutamate diethyl ester, an antagonist to L-glutamate. Brain Res. 217, 186-191.

Taylor, D.G., Arbour, K.A. and Antonaccio, M.J. (1977) Effects of bicuculline and thiosemicarbazide on inhibition of reflex and spontaneous sympathetic nerve potentials in the cat. Neurosci. Abstr. 3, 25.

Taylor, D.G. and Brody, M.J. (1976) Spinal adrenergic mechanisms regulating sympathetic outflow to blood vessels. Circulat. Res. 38 (Suppl. II), 10.

Timmermans, P.B.M.W.M., Schoop, A.M.C., Kwa, H.Y. and van Zwieten, P.A. (1981) Characterization of α-adrenoceptors participating in the central hypotensive and sedative effects of clonidine using yohimbine, rauwolscine and corynanthine. Eur. J. Pharmacol. 70, 7-15.

Wennergren, G. and Oberg, B. (1980) Cardiovascular effects elicited from the ventral surface of medulla oblongata in the cat. Pflügers Arch. 387, 189-195.

Williford, D.J., Hamilton, B.L., Dias Souza, J., Williams, T.P., DiMicco, J.A. and Gillis, R.A. (1980a) CNS GABAergic mechanism influencing arterial pressure and heart rate in the cat. Circulat. Res. 47, 80-88.

Williford, D.J., Hamilton, B.L., DiMicco, J.A., Norman, W.P., Yamada, K.A., Quest, J.A., Zavadil, A. and Gillis, R.A. (1981) Central GABAergic mechanisms involved in the control of arterial blood pressure; in Central Nervous System Mechanisms in Hypertension, J.P. Buckley and C.M. Ferrario, eds. Raven Press, N.Y., pp. 49-60.

Williford, D.J., Hamilton, B.L. and Gillis, R.A. (1980b) Evidence that a GABAergic mechanism at nucleus ambiguus influences reflex-induced vagal activity. Brain Res. 193, 584-588.

Wing, L.M.H. and Chalmers, J.P. (1974) Participation of central serotonergic neurones in the control of the circulation of the unanaesthetized rabbit. Circulat. Res. 35, 504-513.

Wolf, W.A., Kuhn, D.M. and Lovenberg, W. (1981) Blood pressure responses to local application of serotonergic agents in the nucleus tractus solitarii. Eur. J. Pharmacol. 69, 291-299.

Yamada, K.A., Hamosh, P. and Gillis, R.A. (1981) Respiratory depression produced by activation of GABA receptors in hindbrain of cat. J. Appl. Physiol. 51, 1278-1286.

Yamada, K.A. Hamosh, P., and Gillis, R.A. (in press a) Cardio-respiratory depression induced by pentobarbital acting through a GABAergic system at the ventral surface of the medulla. Fed. Proc.

Yamada, K.A., Norman, W.P., Hamosh, P. and Gillis, R.A. (in press b) Medullary ventral surface GABA receptors affect respiratory and cardiovascular function. Brain Res.

Zandberg, P., De Jong, W. and De Wied, D. (1979) Effect of catecholamine-receptor stimulating agents on blood pressure after local application in the nucleus tractus solitarii of the medulla oblongata. Eur. J. Pharmacol. 55, 43-56.

Behavior and Specific Patterns
of Cardiovascular Responses

Behavioral-Cardiovascular Interaction

PAUL A. OBRIST, KATHLEEN C. LIGHT, ALAN W. LANGER,
ALBERTO GRIGNOLO, AND JOHN P. KOEPKE
University of North Carolina, Chapel Hill, North Carolina

INTRODUCTION

In this chapter we will review our research on what we refer to as the behavioral-cardiovascular interaction. Our initial focus was on myocardial events, but more recently it has been extended to the mechanisms of blood pressure (BP) control. In turn, these efforts have raised questions concerning fundamental homeostatic regulatory processes and how these might be modified by the organism-environment interaction. As a result, we have pursued not only cardiovascular (CV) phenomena, but also renal functioning. Our overall objective is to elucidate the ways by which the behavioral-cardiac interaction may be relevant to the hypertensive process. However, we have not worked with a hypertensive population but rather with normotensive young human males (18-20 years old) and, to a lesser extent, with the conscious dog preparation. This choice of subjects was necessitated by our interest in deciphering the basic mechanisms of CV control in the behaving organism that might be distorted by an existing disease process. Also, we believe insight into the hypertensive process requires, among other things, a prospective research strategy whereby the disease process is studied nearer to its inception than to its end point.

This chapter will review our work as it has progressed over the past 18 years. One unique characteristic of our research is the use of pharmacological antagonists to tease out neurogenic influences in this young adult healthy human population. While such interventions have their limitations, they nonetheless have provided some important insights into the manner in which behavioral events are translated into CV activity. We believe these insights are critical to deciphering the hypertensive process.

BEHAVIORAL-MYOCARDIAL INTERACTIONS

While we have used heart rate (HR) consistently in all of our efforts, we have also attempted to assess myocardial contractility with such indirect measures as carotid dP/dt and, more recently, systolic time intervals such as the pre-ejection period. The latter is probably the better of these contractility measures since it can be calibrated and may provide a more sensitive picture of adrenergic influences. The cardiac output has been evaluated in a limited number of dogs, and we are currently in the process of developing the technology for its measurement in humans using a noninvasive rebreathing technique.

The data foster several generalities. For one thing, there can be a complex interplay among the two cardiac innervations that seems to be influenced by qualitative differences among conditions (behavioral events), with vagal influences being dominant under some conditions and sympathetic influences more pronounced under other conditions. Furthermore, there are vast individual differences in the extent to which the innervations, particularly the sympathetic innervation, translate life's events into myocardial responsivity.

The first observation to note originated from the classical aversive conditioning paradigm in which the focus was on phasic or short-term HR changes associated with discrete events such as a conditioned stimulus (Obrist et al., 1965). The anticipatory response was biphasic, an increase followed by a decrease in HR, with the latter maximizing at the point where the aversive unconditioned stimulus was expected. However, when the vagal innervation of the heart was pharmacologically blocked, the initial acceleratory component was no longer observed; rather, the HR was accelerated at the point where the aversive stimulus was expected or where, with an intact innervation, the rate was most decelerated (Fig. 1). Thus, in anticipation of an intensely aversive event, changes in HR (both increases and decreases) were under vagal control, with the increased vagal excitation following the initial momentary loss of vagal restraint, literally masking sympathetic acceleratory effects. Vagal control of HR in other obviously stressful situations has been indicated in certain circumstances with both rodents (e.g., Hofer, 1970) and humans (e.g., Engel, 1971). Thus, the effects of behavioral challenges are not just a matter of mediation by the adrenergic innervations.

One other series of observations should be noted with regard to vagal influences on phasic HR changes. Whether vagal influences lessen or increase, they covary directly with somatomotor (striate muscle) activity. The somatic acts are usually subtle and not extensive, involving mouth and eye movements, and small changes in posture and respiratory activity. Thus, during periods of vagally mediated HR acceleration such somatic acts increase momentarily, while during periods of vagally mediated deceleration they cease. The degree of covariance is pronounced, suggesting that such vagally mediated HR effects involve central nervous system (CNS) control mechanisms that are involved in the control of striate muscle activity, as during exercise (Obrist, 1981). If so, these vagally mediated HR changes may not be subject to our behavioral manipulations independently of what is done with the striate musculature. In this respect, they do not provide unclouded windows into internal behavioral states of the organism involved with emotion or motivation. The covariation of vagal influences on HR and somatomotor

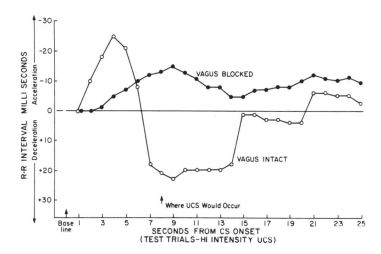

Fig. 1. Second-by-second HR changes on test trials during classical conditioning with an intact and blocked vagal innervation using a high-intensity unconditioned stimulus. (From Obrist et al., 1965, with permission.)

activity also point to one mechanism that might be involved in some aspects of myocardial control of the behaving organism.

The results of a succeeding study (Obrist et. al., 1974) illustrate a more complex interaction of the innervations, but perhaps more importantly suggest that sympathetic influences become manifest when the individual can exert some control over environmental events. The behavioral paradigm was modified from one in which the individual had no control over the receipt of aversive stimuli, i.e., classical aversive conditioning, to one in which some aspect of the subject's behavior could exert control over whether an aversive stimulus was received or not, i.e., shock avoidance. In this case, avoidance of aversive stimuli was made contingent on the adequacy of the subject's performance on a simple reaction-time task. On each trial, the subject was given an 8-sec "preparatory period," i.e., the time from a "get-ready" signal to the "respond" signal. If an aversive stimulus was to be given, it would occur 8 sec after the sensory-motor response. The pharmacological manipulation in this study involved giving one group of subjects the beta-adrenergic blocking agent propranolol.[1]

Figure 2 presents the average HR change over a 30-sec period commencing at the ready signal for the two groups of subjects (i.e., intact and blocked), using all trials on which shocks were avoided (which is most of them). During the 8-sec preparatory period and for several seconds after response execution, HR showed comparable changes in both groups characterized by first an increase, then a decrease, and then another increase in

60

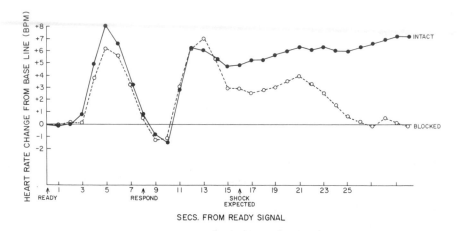

Fig. 2. Second-by-second HR changes with intact and blocked sympathetic innervations during a signaled shock-avoidance reaction-time task. Based on trials in which shock was not delivered. (From Obrist et al., 1974, with permission.)

rate, suggesting that this triphasic HR response was exclusively under vagal control. Shortly before shock expectation and for the remainder of the 30-sec measurement period, sympathetic influences on HR became evident, since it remained elevated with an intact innervation but returned to baseline values with the adrenergic innervations blocked. Thus, we did not see a masking of sympathetic effects as with classical conditioning, but rather an initial vagal influence followed by a sympathetic influence.

In this study, carotid dP/dt was also evaluated and evidenced a parallel effect with HR, at which point sympathetic influences were seen. Finally, these sympathetic influences did not systematically covary with somatomotor activity, as did vagal influences, suggesting the involvement of still other CNS mechanisms. This independence of adrenergic and somatomotor activity has since been seen repeatedly, and most directly when O_2 consumption was measured (see later discussion).

More recent data also suggest the significance of the "control" dimension.[2] In these studies, we shifted from an analysis of phasic to one of tonic myocardial effects. This involved averaging events during any one experimental task over blocks of time in relation to some resting baseline where average values are obtained in a like manner.

The first study (Obrist et al., 1978) evaluated the control dimension in two ways. One was to manipulate task difficulty during a shock avoidance task using an unsignaled reaction time procedure. One condition made the avoidance criterion almost impossible to meet, thus fostering the feeling of having no control. A second condition provided partial success in avoidance, thus permitting some control. Both increases in HR and carotid dP/dt were more sustained when subjects maintained some control than when the avoidance criterion was impossible to meet. This same study also used two other potent stressors over which the subject had no control, the cold pressor and viewing a pornographic film. With both tasks, HR and carotid dP/dt changes were significantly less than with shock avoidance (Figs. 3 and 4). Finally, neurogenic mechanisms were evaluated under these conditions with beta-adrenergic blockade. The results confirmed that the larger HR and carotid dP/dt changes observed with shock avoidance involved a more appreciable adrenergic component (Figs. 3 and 4).

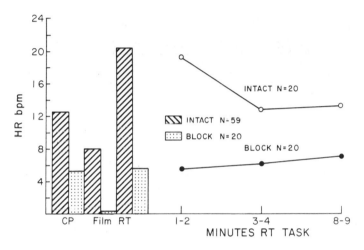

Fig. 3. Change from baseline in tonic levels of HR with intact and blocked sympathetic innervations. Left: changes averaged over 90 sec of cold pressor and the first 2 min of film and shock avoidance tasks. Right: changes in first 9 min of shock avoidance task. (From Obrist et al., 1978, with permission.)

A second study (Light and Obrist, 1980a) evaluated the control dimension by using a yoked control procedure with a shock avoidance task. In addition to HR and carotid dP/dt, we evaluated a measure that includes most of the pre-ejection period (PEP), R wave to carotid pulse wave interval or transit time.[3] Avoiders, in contrast to yoked or non-avoiders, evidenced greater increases in HR and carotid dP/dt, and changes in the transit time measure suggestive of a decrease in PEP. A third study (Light and Obrist, 1982) again manipulated task difficulty with a sensorimotor task, but used monetary (appetitive) reinforcers rather than aversive stimuli, and measured the PEP directly. Again, the condition that provided some control in contrast to consistent failure, or no control, evoked a more sustained increase in HR and the PEP, with the latter being the more sensitive to this manipulation. Finally, in a recently completed study by K.C. Light, decreases in PEP during a sensorimotor task, again using appetitive reinforcers, were found to be attenuated by beta-adrenergic blockade.

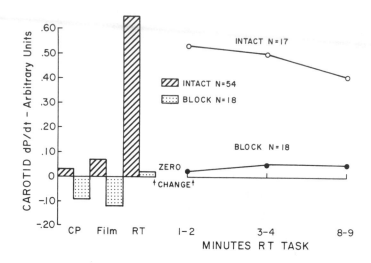

Fig. 4. Change from baseline in tonic levels of carotid dP/dt with intact and blocked sympathetic innervations. Left: changes averaged over 90 sec of cold pressor and the first 2 min of film and shock avoidance tasks. Right: changes in first 9 min of shock avoidance task. (From Obrist et al., 1978, with permission.)

    In summary, this line of inquiry indicated that tasks in which individuals have some control of challenging or threatening events, in contrast to those in which no control is possible (unavoidable pain or unobtainable financial incentives) or tasks in which they are only passively engaged (viewing an erotic movie), evoke more appreciable beta-adrenergic influences on the myocardium.[4] However, this generalization requires some qualifications based on the following observations. First, there is a wide range of individual differences in myocardial reactivity. Second, the effects of the control-no control dimension are most pronounced in the more reactive subjects, and hardly evident in the less reactive subjects. Third, even though the more reactive subjects show greater differences among conditions, they are more reactive to almost any novel or challenging event, even if they have little control over it. Fourth, the individual differences in myocardial reactivity primarily reflect differences in beta-adrenergic activation.

    These observations are based on several studies, and the following overview synthesizes some aspects of the data (Obrist, 1981). For this purpose, the discussion will be restricted to HR effects since data are available on more subjects with this measure of myocardial performance. Also, we shall reference all effects to a resting baseline condition, which follows participation in the study usually by 1-2 weeks, when the subject knowingly comes to the laboratory just to rest. This is referred to as follow-up baseline or as "baseline acclimated" (Fig. 5). We also obtain a baseline from a resting period occurring on the first occasion the subject comes to the laboratory and just before exposure to the experimental procedures. This is referred to as a pre-task baseline or "baseline-non-acclimated" (Fig. 5). The differences between these two resting baselines are important because the first, or non-acclimated, baseline is appreciably elevated in some individuals relative to the second, or acclimated, baseline. In other individuals, these two baselines are comparable and low.

Figure 5 summarizes the principal effects we wish to note. It presents the average HR during the two baselines, the cold pressor and a shock avoidance task, in three groups of subjects. Two of the groups have an intact sympathetic innervation and represent the upper and lower quartile in HR reactivity, defined as the difference between the acclimated baseline and shock avoidance. The third group consists of subjects whose beta-adrenergic innervations were pharmacologically blocked. No acclimation baseline was obtained on these subjects since their HR was already depressed during the non-acclimated baseline.

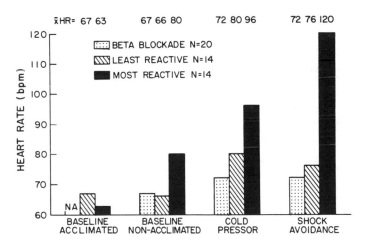

Fig. 5. Mean HR under four conditions as a function of reactivity to shock avoidance: innervations intact with two groups and beta-adrenergic innervations blocked with one group--see text for details.

The important details to note are as follows. The least and most reactive subjects with an intact innervation evidenced similar levels of HR during the acclimated baseline and had HR values comparable to baseline with pharmacological blockade. However, the reactive subjects showed higher HR levels under all other conditions including the initial or non-acclimated baseline and cold pressor. On the other hand, the non-reactive subjects were similar to subjects with beta blockade. They showed no difference between baseline conditions and equally small elevations of HR during the cold pressor and shock avoidance.

The differences between reactive and non-reactive subjects during shock avoidance were appreciable, i.e., 57 vs. 9 bpm. Finally, had we used the initial or non-acclimated baseline as our reference point, we would have appreciably underestimated HR reactivity during both tasks in the reactive subjects, but not in the least reactive subjects.

The importance of beta-adrenergic influences to these individual differences in myocardial reactivity was reinforced by the results of still another study (Light, 1981). Subjects were divided into those evidencing the higher and lower HR during two challenging procedures, a competitive reaction-time task using financial incentives and a difficult mental arithmetic task. These procedures were then repeated several months later with a beta-adrenergic blocking agent given to half the subjects in each group. Blockade reduced the HR more in those subjects with the initial higher values and, in the process, minimized the individual differences in reactivity. In those subjects whose innervations remained intact, HR was not altered in either group on this repeat exposure to the tasks.

Therefore, the data suggest that behavioral influences on myocardial performance involve two interacting influences. First, the task requirements have some influence on whether adrenergic influences are evoked; second, this in turn is influenced by some as yet undefinable predisposition on the part of some individuals to react beta-adrenergically.

BLOOD PRESSURE AND BEHAVIORAL-MYOCARDIAL INTERACTIONS

We have assessed BP changes in our paradigms for two different reasons. In one context, it was of secondary concern to the problem at hand. For example, where we observed vagally mediated decreases in HR during anticipation of aversive stimuli, we wondered if the myocardial effect was secondary to baroreceptor influences triggered by anticipatory increases in BP. In another case, we were concerned whether phasic increases in carotid dP/dt might reflect a decrease in afterload as would be suggested by a lowered diastolic blood pressure (DBP). In both instances, BP was measured invasively from the radial artery in small samples of subjects, and the evidence indicated that it had little influence on either event. Thus, with respect to neurogenic mechanisms, these chronotopic and ionotopic effects would seem to reflect a direct CNS influence on the myocardium.

In three more recent experiments, we also measured BP invasively to assess the reliability of noninvasive automated BP monitoring devices and, in one instance, to assess the relation between BP and R wave to pulse wave transit time, and pulse wave to pulse wave transit time (e.g., see Pollak and Obrist, 1982). The results of these studies are not particularly relevant to the present purposes other than to verify that our noninvasive BP measurement technology is reasonably reliable. However, after examining these direct pressure readings, we were struck by the lability of the BP in this normotensive population. For example, in one study using nine medical students, the average range of resting values was 31 mm Hg for SBP ($\bar{x}$ SD = 7.5) and 22 mm Hg for DBP ($\bar{x}$ SD = 4.7). Such variability is important since the resting BP is commonly assumed to be a more or less static event.

Our other interests in BP reflect the primary thrust of our current work on the hypertensive process. We have been measuring BP in all studies since we began evaluating the influence of the "control" dimension on tonic levels of myocardial activity. Since the experimental procedures proved to influence the SBP and DBP in different ways, each aspect of BP will be discussed separately.

SBP was found to be influenced in a manner similar to myocardial events. It increased most during the control task, differed appreciably among individuals, and covaried with HR, such that the HR "reactors" were almost always the SBP "reactors." Figure 6 illustrates the SBP changes during the same tasks in the same subjects whose data are depicted in Figures 3 and 4. Recall that this study involved a shock avoidance task, the cold pressor, and viewing a pornographic movie, with the beta-adrenergic innervations intact in one group and blocked in another. As with HR and carotid dP/dt, SBP increased more during shock avoidance than the other two tasks, and remained more elevated when some control of the aversive stimuli was possible than when it was not (not shown in Figure 6). Beta-adrenergic blockade reduced the SBP increase more during shock avoidance than either of the other two tasks, as it did with HR and carotid dP/dt.

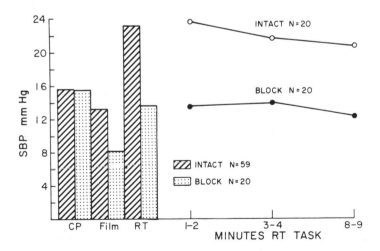

Fig. 6. Change from baseline in tonic levels of SBP with intact and blocked sympathetic innervations. Left: changes averaged over 90 sec of the cold pressor and the first 2 min of the film and the shock avoidance task. Right: changes in the first 9 min of the shock avoidance task. (From Obrist et al., 1978, with permission.)

This parallel between myocardial and SBP effects was seen in still other ways. First, when we manipulated control of aversive stimuli with a yoked procedure (Light and Obrist, 1980a), in subjects who had some control, the SBP increased most as did HR and decreases in R wave to pulse transit time. Second, increases in SBP covaried directly with increases in HR and carotid dP/dt and inversely with decreases in R wave to pulse wave interval. These relations are most evident when evaluated within subjects using data points from baseline and task conditions. For example, the average correlation (r) between SBP and R wave to pulse wave transit time was -.78 in one sample of 53 subjects. Beta-adrenergic blockade reduced the average correlation to -.28 (Obrist et al., 1979). Third, the extent to which individual differences in SBP and myocardial reactivity covary is seen in different ways. For example, the subjects showing the greatest changes in HR during shock avoidance (Fig. 5) had an average increase in SBP of 46 mm Hg, while the least reactive subjects had an increase of only 16 mm Hg. Beta-adrenergic influences on these individual differences in SBP reactivity were most directly revealed when we evaluated the effects of blockade in subjects showing the highest and lowest HR levels during appetitive reaction-time and mental arithmetic tasks (Light, 1981). The blocking agent resulted in an appreciable decrease in SBP only in those subjects with an elevated HR, having no effect on SBP in those with a less elevated HR.

In summary, our evidence consistently points to a marked degree of covariation between task-induced myocardial and SBP effects. Both events are influenced in a like manner by the individual's degree of control over challenging environmental events, but individual differences are pronounced and subjects who show greater myocardial reactivity also show greater SBP reactivity.

In contrast, the DBP was influenced in a manner somewhat opposite that of the SBP: in conditions and individuals where beta-adrenergic influences were maximum, the DBP changed least, whereas under conditions and with individuals in which beta-adrenergic influences were less, the DBP increased more and was more comparable to changes seen in SBP. This is illustrated in Figure 7, which shows data on the same tasks and individuals as in Figures 3, 4 and 6. With an intact innervation, DBP increased less during shock avoidance than during the cold pressor and film, quite the opposite of HR, carotid dP/dt and SBP. However, beta blockade changed this picture: while HR, carotid dP/dt and SBP changes were attenuated during shock avoidance, DBP was increased. Under the other conditions, blockade had a lesser effect on either aspect of the BP and on myocardial events. The DBP changed least in subjects who showed the greatest myocardial and SBP changes under conditions such as shock avoidance which maximize beta-adrenergic effects. These results suggest that increased beta-adrenergic excitation results not only in increased myocardial performance but also in vascular vasodilation, as Forsyth (1976) observed while measuring regional blood flows in rhesus macaques engaged in a shock-avoidance task. The result is that vascular resistance is minimally changed, resulting in little change in DBP. However, we have preliminary data (Light, 1981) indicating that individuals who showed maximal beta-adrenergic effects, and hence minimal DBP changes, also had appreciably increased alpha-adrenergic drive, the effects of which were masked by the beta-adrenergic vasodilatory influences. This was seen when we compared HR, SBP and DBP during competitive reaction-time tasks and difficult mental arithmetic problems using financial incentives, first with the innervations intact and then with the beta receptors blocked. Subjects showing higher levels of HR and SBP with an intact innervation evidenced larger increases in DBP following blockade, even though their HR and SBP were most reduced. It is as if there is a trade-off in such reactive individuals between adrenergic vasodilatory and constrictive effects, resulting in little change in vascular resistance. Thus, the control of the BP in these behavioral paradigms seems to involve an array of interacting events among the myocardium and vasculature, with both individual difference dimensions and situational components having an influence on BP control. More conclusive evidence awaits the measurement of cardiac output and regional vascular resistance.

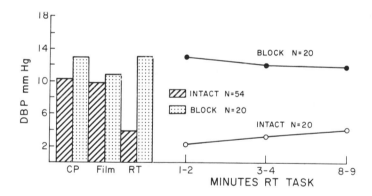

Fig. 7. Changes from baseline in tonic levels of DBP with intact and blocked sympathetic innervations. Left: changes averaged over 90 sec of cold pressor and the first 2 min of film and shock avoidance tasks. Right: changes in first 9 min of shock avoidance task. (From Obrist et al., 1978, with permission.)

BEHAVIORAL-CARDIAC INTERACTIONS AND THE HYPERTENSIVE PROCESS

Borderline hypertension has been found to have a certain predictive value for an eventual established hypertension (Julius, 1977). Furthermore, a number of borderline hypertensives show increased beta-adrenergic drive on the myocardium (Julius and Esler, 1975). In regard to our own work, these observations raised the question of whether behaviorally evoked increased beta-adrenergic excitation might be involved as an etiological route in the hypertensive process and, specifically, whether those individuals showing beta-adrenergic hyperresponsivity may be at greater risk for developing an established hypertension. A definitive answer awaits a more extensive evaluation of several issues involving long-term follow-up studies. To justify such efforts, we decided to use a "temporary end-point"--namely, the incidence of hypertension in the parents of our subject population. We chose this strategy because offspring of hypertensive parents have been demonstrated to be more apt to become hypertensive than offspring of normo-tensives parents (e.g., Schweitzer et al., 1967). Therefore, we reasoned that the incidence of parental hypertension should be greater in our more reactive subjects, if behavioral evoked beta-adrenergic hyperresponsivity was relevant to the etiological process.

We have examined this relation in several studies and in each have found a greater incidence of hypertension in the parents of those subjects showing greater HR and SBP reactivity, particularly when the individual has some control in the task, such as shock avoidance. The most extensive of these studies (Hastrup et al., 1982) involved 104 subjects for which we had interpretable data on both parents. During a shock avoidance task, both level of HR and change score from baseline were directly related to the incidence of parental hypertension. For example, of the 34 parents identified as hypertensive, 30 had sons whose average HR during shock avoidance was above the median value. Similar but less pronounced trends have been found for HR reactivity as well as for levels and change of SBP. Current studies are yielding similar results.

Several other aspects of these data warrant comment. One, we did not find a significant relation when using tasks that did not give the subject some control of laboratory events, such as the cold pressor (Hastrup et al., 1982). This seems to reinforce the significance of beta-adrenergic mechanisms in the etiological process, since such tasks evoke lesser beta-adrenergic effects. This latter conclusion was reinforced in one other manner using subjects from the original study. For approximately 60 of these subjects, we were able to obtain BP values under conditions more common to clinical evaluation (casual values). The values were found to relate to parental hypertension, provided that the subject also evidenced greater HR and SBP reactivity under laboratory conditions. In other words, a casual marginal elevation of the BP, which was found on at least one occasion in about half of the subjects, did not consistently relate to parental hypertension unless the subject was reactive to our laboratory procedures (Light and Obrist, 1980b). Such results suggest that a casual elevation of the pressure takes on greater significance once we have insight into BP control mechanisms. However, a note of caution is necessary. These latter observations involving the cold pressor and the evaluation of the casual SBP were made on a relatively small sample of subjects, and the work needs replication as well as a more systematic evaluation.

A second important aspect of these data is that in this subject population, the BP and HR values obtained once these subjects are acclimated to the laboratory relate only minimally to the incidence of parental hypertension. It is necessary to expose these subjects to a behavioral challenge before the relation becomes evident. Such an observation bears on the significance of behavioral factors in the etiological process and is analogous in ways to Lawler's observations (Lawler et al., 1981) that, in genetically prone hypertensive rats, the hypertension does not become evident until the rats are exposed to a challenging behavioral task.

The potential significance of behavioral factors to the hypertensive process is seen in our subject population in one other manner. When these subjects first came to the laboratory and were not acclimated to our procedures, approximately 20% evidenced resting SBP of 140 mm Hg or greater, which by some standards qualifies them as borderline hypertensive. Several other characteristics of these subjects are worth noting. First, they also evidenced a more elevated resting HR. Second, they were more apt to have a hypertensive parent. Third, on follow-up and once acclimated to the laboratory, their resting SBP and HR were usually markedly reduced, and comparable to the SBP and HR of remaining subjects, who evidenced similar low baselines under both conditions. This all suggests that just the novelty of the situation, i.e., their first exposure to the laboratory, triggers increased beta-adrenergic excitation, even in the "resting" state.

Finally, we might note that at this stage of our work we have not found any significant relation between DBP and the family history. It could be argued that this is contrary to what one might expect in light of the role an elevated vascular resistance plays in established hypertension. Also, some recent work has demonstrated that adolescent offspring of hypertensive parents evidence an elevated DBP both at rest and when challenged with a behavioral task (Falkner et al., 1979). There is as yet no ready solution to this apparent dilemma. One possibility is as follows: The etiological routes in the hypertensive process differ. If one route involves an initial beta-adrenergic influence, then it is not surprising that in our subject population beta-adrenergic excitation minimizes alpha-adrenergic influences on the vasculature, and hence the DBP is minimally elevated. In time, these beta-adrenergic influences on the vasculature lessen due to any number of events (such as autoregulation of blood flow, vascular structural changes, beta-adrenergic blunting, vascular water logging) to permit the manifestation of an increased vascular resistance. Consistent with this possibility is the clinical observation that young adults considered to be borderline hypertensive can show an elevated SBP but a normotensive DBP (e.g., Safar et al., 1973). On the other hand, where an elevated vascular resistance appears early in the progression of the disease process, as suggested by the Falkner et al. (1979) study, it may be a reflection of a different etiological route than when an appreciable beta-adrenergic component is present. Falkner's method of selecting subjects on the basis of DBP level does not rule out this possibility.

In summary, our studies evaluating the relation between parental hypertension and behaviorally induced myocardial and SBP reactivity encourage us to elucidate further the nature and significance of beta-adrenergic mechanisms. One fundamental question concerns why beta-adrenergic mechanisms may have a significant role in the etiological process. We have directed some attention to the question and would like to close this chapter by describing a working hypothesis and some relevant data. The data in this case are derived from both the conscious dog preparation and our young adult population. The dog is used since the initial efforts required a technology that could not be used with humans. We are now modifying that technology. This work also returns to us the theme of this workshop and book--the neurobiology of the circulation.

THE CONCEPT OF METABOLIC APPROPRIATENESS--
A WORKING HYPOTHESIS AND SOME DATA

Hypertension has been considered a disorder of regulation (e.g., Weiner, 1977). In this context, we have begun to evaluate two ways in which normal BP control may be disrupted by our experimental challenges, disturbances which have been viewed as contributing to the pathological elevation of the BP. These hypothesized disruptions involve the cardiac output (CO) and the renal handling of sodium (Lund-Johansen, 1979; Guyton, 1980). Specifically, we conceptualize the issue in the following manner. With both myocardial and renal functioning, the disorder of regulation reflects an inefficiency in the maintenance of critical metabolic processes. While metabolic homeostasis is being maintained, the inefficiency is expressed as (1) a cardiac output that is excessive relative to O_2 and other cellular requirements, and (2) renal "sluggishness" in maintaining sodium (Na) balance, favoring a positive balance. The latter could also act to facilitate further an increase in the CO (Guyton, 1980).

Our concern is to demonstrate that behavioral events can at least acutely modify myocardial and renal events in this manner. For this purpose, we need a means to establish what an efficient adjustment should be. We cannot assume that any particular myocardial or renal adjustment to an experimentally imposed behavioral task is not simply a reflection of some "necessary" change in metabolic requirements. For example, when dogs are exposed to a shock avoidance task, they become somatically active as illustrated by struggling or less extensive somatic acts such as shifting posture or even panel pressing (Obrist and Webb, 1967). Such acts would be expected to increase O_2 consumption and hence to evoke an elevation of the CO. Since our concern is whether an elevation of the CO associated with a behavioral challenge might be excessive relative to any increase in O_2 consumption, a most direct way to assess this would be to compare the relation between myocardial events and O_2 consumption during exercise with that found during a behavioral challenge such as shock avoidance. Thus, in both humans and dogs, we have used the exercise relation as a yard stick in evaluating the metabolic appropriateness of the myocardial adjustment.

In regard to renal functioning, there did not seem to be an obvious yard stick. In the first study with dogs, we used exercise as a companion task, expecting that either Na balance would be unaltered or, at most, there would be some Na retention as a means of protecting against the nonrenal loss of Na, as through salivation associated with panting. Since this proved not to be the case (i.e., Na excretion increased), in succeeding studies with dogs we used the resting baseline excretion rate as our reference point. In addition, we are evaluating in humans whether individual differences in Na excretion relate to myocardial reactivity as well as the incidence of hypertension in the parents. Any relation among these events would also suggest that we are dealing, albeit indirectly, with an inefficient metabolic adjustment.

Up to this point, our most definitive evidence has come from dogs. In the first study (Langer et al., 1979) we evaluated the relation between CO (measured with an electro-magnetic blood flow probe) and the arterio-venous blood oxygen content difference (A-V O_2d) during both treadmill exercise and shock avoidance. Relative to exercise, the avoidance task resulted in elevations of CO which were disproportionately greater than might be expected on the basis of any increase in the A-V O_2d or oxygen consumption. For example, one dog showed similar levels of CO while exercising on the treadmill at 3 mph and during avoidance. Yet his A-V O_2d was 24% less, and similar to the A-V O_2d observed while resting, when the CO was appreciably less. Comparable effects were found with HR. Such data are indicative of tissue overperfusion, which has been viewed as contributing to an elevated vascular resistance via autoregulatory mechanisms (Guyton, 1980). We have not yet evaluated beta-adrenergic influences while measuring both the CO and A-V O_2d. But we have evaluated these influences in another study with dogs, and found appreciable beta-adrenergic influences on left ventricular dP/dt, HR and CO during shock avoidance (Grignolo et al., 1981).

In humans, we have just completed our first study measuring O_2 consumption (A.W. Langer, unpublished results). Heart rate was the only myocardial event obtained since the technology for measuring CO is undeveloped. Subjects were studied during both exercise and shock avoidance, either with an intact sympathetic innervation or with beta-adrenergic blockade. The data have not been completely evaluated but the results thus far are consistent with what we see in dogs. Average HR and O_2 consumption during baseline and both exercise and avoidance are illustrated in Figure 8 for one subject with an intact innervation, and in Figure 9 for a subject with a blocked innervation. With an intact innervation, shock avoidance evoked a higher level of HR than exercise, while O_2

consumption was appreciably greater during exercise. With a blocked innervation, neither HR nor O_2 consumption were altered by the avoidance task, but both increased appreciably during exercise. While the subject whose data are shown in Figure 8 demonstrated a somewhat extreme effect, average values for the intact group as a whole showed little or no change in O_2 consumption and a modestly accelerated HR during avoidance. Average values for the blocked group, as with the subject depicted in Figure 9, showed essentially no change.

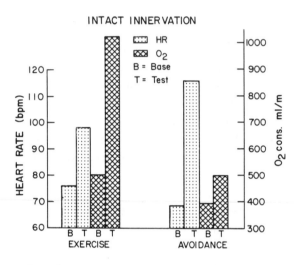

Fig. 8. Mean heart rate (stippled bars) and oxygen consumption (hatched bars) in one subject with myocardial innervations intact during baseline (B) and exercise and avoidance (T).

Renal functioning has been evaluated by obtaining excretion rates of water and Na. With dogs, this involved first expanding their plasma volume with saline, and then evaluating the effects of shock avoidance once excretion rates had become stabilized. In the first study (Grignolo et al., 1982), shock avoidance resulted in a decreased excretion rate of both water and Na, compared with control baseline conditions, while exercise resulted in increased excretion rates. The decrease in excretion rates was most pronounced when the avoidance procedure evoked the greater HR increase. Since neither the glomerular filtration rate (GFR) nor free water clearance were noticeably affected by avoidance, the Na retention seems to reflect a tubular reabsorptive process.

In a follow-up to these studies with dogs, we have evaluated both beta- and alpha-adrenergic mechanisms. Beta-adrenergic blockade completely attenuated the decrease in both water and Na retention, while alpha-adrenergic blockade, if anything, extended the decreased excretion rates into a follow-up baseline-recovery period (Koepke, 1981 and

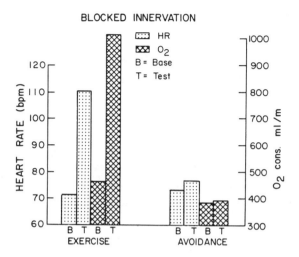

Fig. 9. Mean heart rate (stippled bars) and oxygen consumption (hatched bars) in one subject with the myocardial innervations blocked during baseline (B) and exercise and avoidance (T).

unpublished observations). In both studies, the influence of beta-adrenergic mechanisms is also suggested by the observation that excretion rates covary directly with HR reactivity.

Our study of renal functioning has not progressed as far in humans as it has in dogs. The first relevant observation is that plasma renin was significantly higher in subjects showing higher HR during a reaction-time task using competition for financial incentives (Light, 1981 and unpublished observations). We have also begun work evaluating water and Na excretion during our behavioral challenges. We have encountered some methodological problems, namely obtaining stable baseline excretion rates, but now have settled on a means for stabilizing rates through the controlled ingestion of water and some simple dietary restraints. Nineteen subjects have so far participated in the 5-hr procedure. Eight were controls who were not exposed to our experimental challenges but served to test the effectiveness of our procedures in stabilizing excretion rates and as a reference point for the experimental subjects. The latter were exposed during the fourth hour of the procedure to a variety of challenging tasks using nonaversive reinforcers. Some show evidence of decreased Na excretion following the experimental tasks which extended into the follow-up recovery hour. This decrease in excretion is most consistently seen in subjects who have a hypertensive parent.

In summary, our work evaluating the relations among myocardial and metabolic processes presents a consistent picture. In dogs, we have reasonably definitive evidence that a behavioral challenge such as shock avoidance disrupts both myocardial and renal functioning, so that the CO is elevated in excess to any increase in O_2 consumption, while at the same time Na is being retained. Both events seem to involve beta-adrenergic mechanisms. Results in humans are less definitive, but are consistent with our working hypothesis and, as with dogs, they suggest that similar neurogenic mechanisms are involved.

CONCLUSIONS

The research reviewed would seem to justify certain conclusions with regard to behavioral-cardiovascular interactions. (1) Both sympathetic and parasympathetic innervations of the heart are involved in mediating the means by which life's events are translated into myocardial adjustments. (2) Sympathetic effects are more readily evoked by environmental events over which the organism has some control. (3) There are appreciable individual differences in beta-adrenergic-mediated myocardial events, which are directly related to the SBP and the incidence of hypertension in the parents of our young adult normotensive subjects. (4) The efficiency with which the myocardium and kidney adjust to metabolic requirements can be compromised by behavioral challenges, and this seems to involve beta-adrenergic mechanisms.

ACKNOWLEDGMENTS

This research was supported by grant MH07995 from the National Institute of Mental Health, and grants HL18976, HL23718, and HL24643 from the National Institutes of Health.

NOTES

1. In human studies involving pharmacologic blockade of the myocardial sympathetic innervations, we used intravenously administered propranolol. Our initial reason was that it was the only beta-blocker permitted with humans. We have continued its use, in contrast to more cardio-selective agents, such as metoprolol, which are now cleared for use with humans, because we want to evaluate beta-adrenergic influences on the vasculature as well as the myocardium. We have found little evidence that the CV effects seen with propranolol are secondary to alterations in behavioral states caused by its influence on the CNS. For example, performance in reaction time tasks is no different with or without blockade (Obrist et al., 1978). Also see section on "Blood pressure and behavioral-myocardial interactions" for a discussion of effects of propranolol on diastolic blood pressure, an effect that is hard to attribute to a direct central action.

2. The control dimension can also be viewed with respect to active versus passive coping, whereby control of challenging events evokes active coping while lack of control evokes passive coping behavioral strategies.

3. The sensitivity of this measure to adrenergic influences on the myocardium has been evaluated with pharmacological intervention. With an intact innervation, R wave to carotid pulse wave interval decreased during a shock avoidance task by -17.8 msec, but by only -3.4 msec with the beta-adrenergic innervation blocked (Obrist et al., 1979).

4. A fundamental question is, why should the control of events influence the relative dominance of the myocardial sympathetic innervations? One teleological proposal is that adrenergic effects dominate under conditions where control is possible because they prepare or mobilize the organism for a dissipation of energy, i.e., action, as with flight or fight. Vagal influences dominate or sympathetic effects are less prominent under conditions in which action is not possible (no control) since there is nothing gained by a mobilization of those visceral processes that would expedite action.

REFERENCES

Engel, G.L. (1971) Sudden and rapid death during psychological stress. Ann. Intern. Med. 74, 771-782.

Falkner, B., Onesti, G., Angelakos, E.T., Fernandes, M. and Langman, C. (1979) Cardiovascular response to mental stress in normal adolescents with hypertensive parents. Hemodynamics and mental stress in adolescents. Hypertension 1, 23-30.

Forsyth, R.P. (1976) Effects of propranolol on stress-induced hemodynamic changes in monkeys; in Beta-adrenoceptor Blocking Agents, P.R. Saxena and R.P. Forsyth, eds. North-Holland, Amsterdam, pp. 317-322.

Grignolo, A., Light, K.C. and Obrist, P.A. (1981) Beta-adrenergic influence on cardiac dynamics during shock-avoidance in dogs. Pharmacol. Biochem. Behav. 14, 313-339.

Grignolo, A., Koepke, J.P. and Obrist, P.A. (in press) Renal function and cardiovascular dynamics during treadmill exercise and shock avoidance in dogs. Amer. J. Physiol.

Guyton, A.C. (1980) Arterial Blood Pressure and Hypertension. W.B. Saunders, Philadelphia.

Hastrup, J.L., Light, K.C. and Obrist, P.A. (in press) Parental hypertension and cardiovascular response to stress in healthy young adults. Psychophysiology.

Hofer, M.A. (1970) Cardiac and respiratory function during sudden prolonged immobility in wild rodents. Psychosom. Med. 32, 633-647.

Julius, S. (1977) Borderline hypertension: epidemiologic and clinical implications; in Hypertension: Physiopathology and Treatment, J. Genest, E. Koiw and O. Kuchel, eds. McGraw-Hill, New York, pp. 630-640.

Julius, S. and Esler, M.D. (1975) Autonomic nervous cardiovascular regulation in borderline hypertension. Amer. J. Cardiol. 36, 685-696.

Koepke, J.P., Grignolo, A. and Obrist, P.A. (1981) Decreased urine and sodium excretion rates during unsignaled shock avoidance in dogs: role of beta-adrenergic receptors. Fed. Proc. 40, 553.

Langer, A.W., Obrist, P.A. and McCubbin, J.A. (1979) Hemodynamic and metabolic adjustments during exercise and shock avoidance in dogs. Amer. J. Physiol.: Heart Circulat. Physiol. 5, H225-H230.

Langer, A.W., Hutcheson, J.S., Charlton, J.D., McCubbin, J.A. and Obrist, P.A. (1981) On-line minicomputerized measurement of respiratory gas exchange during exercise. Fed. Proc. 40 (Abstract).

Lawler, J.E., Barker, G.F., Hubbard, B.S. and Schaub, R.G. (1981) Effects of stress on blood pressure and cardiac pathology in rats with borderline hypertension. Hypertension 3, 496-505.

Light, K.C. (1981) Cardiovascular responses to effortful active coping: implications for the role of stress in hypertension development. Psychophysiology 18, 216-225.

Light, K.C. and Obrist, P.A. (1980a) Cardiovascular response to stress: effects of opportunity to avoid, shock experience and performance feedback. Psychophysiology 17, 243-252.

Light, K.C. and Obrist, P.A. (1980b) Cardiovascular reactivity to behavioral stress in young males with and without marginally elevated casual systolic pressures: a comparison of clinic, home and laboratory measures. Hypertension 2, 802-808.

Light, K.C. and Obrist, P.A. (1982) Cardiovascular response: relationships to task difficulty, exercise and behavioral traits. Submitted for publication, 1982.

Lund-Johansen, P. Spontaneous changes in central hemodynamics in essential hypertension--a 10 year study; in Hypertension--Determinants, Complications and Intervention, G. Onesti and C.R. Klimt, eds. Grune and Stratton, New York, pp. 201-209.

Obrist, P.A. (1981) Cardiovascular Psychophysiology: A Prespective. Plenum, New York.

Obrist, P.A., Gaebelein, C.J., Shanks-Teller, E., Langer, A.W., Grignolo, A., Light, K.C. and McCubbin, J.A. (1978) The relationship between heart rate, carotid dP/dt, and blood pressure in humans as a function of the type of stress. Psychophysiology 15, 102-115.

Obrist, P.A., Lawler, J.E., Howard, J.L., Smithson, K.W., Martin, P.L. and Manning, J. (1974) Sympathetic influences on the heart in humans: effects on contractility and heart rate of acute stress. Psychophysiology 11, 405-427.

Obrist, P.A., Light, K.C., McCubbin, J.A. and Hoffer, J.L. (1979) Pulse transit time: relationship to blood pressure and myocardial performance. Psychophysiology 16, 292-301.

Obrist, P.A. and Webb, R.A. (1967) Heart rate during conditioning in dogs: relationship to somatic-motor activity. Psychophysiology 4, 7-34.

Obrist, P.A., Wood, D.M. and Perez-Reyes, M. (1965) Heart rate during conditioning in humans: effects of UCS intensity, vagal blockade, and adrenergic block of vasomotor activity. J. Exp. Psychol. 70, 32-42.

Pollak, M.H. and Obrist, P.A. (in press) Pulse transit time and ECG Q-wave to pulse wave interval as indices of beat-by-beat blood pressure changes. Psychophysiology.

Safar, M.E., Weiss, Y.A., Levenson, J.A., London, G.M. and Milliez, P.L. (1973) Hemodynamic study of 85 patients with borderline hypertension. Amer. J. Cardiol. 31, 315-319.

Schweitzer, M.D., Gearing, F.R. and Perera, G.A. (1967) Family studies of primary hypertension: their contributions to the understanding of genetic factors; in The Epidemiology of Hypertension, J. Stamler, R. Stamler and T.N Pullman, eds. Grune and Stratton, New York, pp. 28-38.

Weiner, H. (1977) Psychobiology and Human Disease. Elsevier, New York.

Neural Basis for Differential Cardiovascular Control

LYNNE C. WEAVER
Department of Physiology, Michigan State University, East Lansing, Michigan

INTRODUCTION

Fifty years ago, Cannon (1932) stated that the autonomic nervous system was instrumental for warm-blooded vertebrates to maintain physiological homeostasis within a widely and rapidly changing environment. Earlier, he suggested that animals and man were capable of adjusting to variations in their surrounding temperature and oxygen tensions, and to emotional stress or demands for physical exertion particularly because of influences of the sympathetic nervous system (1915). Such adaptations were proposed to be accomplished by a unitary "en masse" activation of all sympathetic nerves. The extensive anatomical divergence of preganglionic neurons within the sympathetic chains previously reported by Langley (1899) supported such a concept. However, cardiac function and resistance of different vascular beds are not identical during sleep, ingestion or various emotional states. How does the sympathetic nervous system contribute to such adjustments? Do sympathetic nerves always discharge "en masse"? Does divergence within the sympathetic chains lead to undiscriminated neural influences on all organs? Evidence from recent and older literature suggests that it does not. Some of Langley's experiments illustrated discrete sympathetic organization (1892). For example, changes in diameter of the pupil are not necessarily accompanied by altered blood flow to the head; Langley demonstrated that preganglionic neurons causing dilation of the pupil emerged mostly from the first thoracic segment, whereas those causing vasoconstriction of the ear emerged more from the fourth segment. Apparently this discreteness of central organization is maintained throughout the sympathetic chains and ganglia and leads to specific rather than generalized organ responses.

Evidence suggesting patterned or fractionated control of different neuroeffector organs can be found throughout the cardiovascular literature. In 1961, Folkow et al. demonstrated that muscle blood flow was decreased more than renal blood flow during occlusion of the carotid arteries. This differential effect of the arterial baroreceptors was exaggerated in the presence of hypocapnia and was less distinct during hypercapnia. Folkow et al. suggested that

> . . . a differentiation in the discharge of the sympathetic vasoconstrictor fibers is made possible by the fact that the different medullary pools, controlling the functionally different vascular beds, exhibit different thresholds to excitatory stimuli. Such a mechanism makes it possible that the vascular regions can be quantitatively differently engaged even by primarily undifferentiated excitatory and inhibitory influences, but it also allows for mass activations.

In another report of patterned blood flow responses to various stimuli, Mancia et al. (1975) documented greater carotid baroreceptor influences on hind limb than renal blood flow and, conversely, greater cardiopulmonary vagal afferent influences on renal than hind limb blood flow. Important advances were made when patterned blood flow responses were observed in unanesthetized, behaving animals. Smith et al. (1979) found that conscious baboons, in anticipation of an electric shock, exhibit a "conditioned emotional response" consisting, in part, of an initial neurogenic renal vasoconstriction, which is not demonstrable in terminal aortic blood flow. These data suggest that the sympathetic outflow to the kidney is affected by an excitatory reflex that is not distributed to neurons controlling lower abdominal or hind limb vasculature. That such specificity exists in the conscious state allays the concern that patterns of reflexes are the consequence of unequal neuronal excitability due to anesthesia or other perturbations of normal physiology in the acutely prepared experimental animal.

In many circumstances, however, differential blood flow patterns may be caused by differences in local control of vascular beds rather than differential sympathetic activation. Further elucidation of neuronal mechanisms underlying fractionated cardiovascular responses to any stimulus requires documentation of differential involvement of the sympathetic nervous system. The presence of differential control can be established only by observing patterned neuronal responses to the stimuli that produce patterned cardiovascular responses. Few electrophysiological investigations have been specifically designed to determine differential sympathetic responses. Ninomiya and coworkers (1971, 1975) investigated sympathetic responses to arterial baroreceptor activation in anesthetized cats, and found that arterial baroreceptors cause greater inhibition of splenic than cardiac, renal or intestinal sympathetic nerve activity. These results illustrate that preferential reflex influences on different components of sympathetic outflow can exist. Sympathetic patterning in response to visceral afferent stimulation also has been investigated in our laboratory. Generally, the results of our experiments support the concept that differential cardiovascular adjustments in various states can be produced at least in part by selective patterns of sympathetic activation or inhibition.

METHODS

Experiments were performed in alpha-chloralose-anesthetized cats in which arterial baroreceptors had been denervated. Differential influences on simultaneously recorded activity of multifiber splenic and renal nerves were ascertained using standard electrophysiological techniques. In particular, splenic and renal responses were compared to determine whether patterned responses could be observed in components of sympathetic outflow to the abdominal viscera originating from the same or adjacent spinal segments. Reflex influences of spinal "sympathetic" afferent or vagal afferent neurons originating from the heart were investigated. These afferent neurons were excited chemically by epicardial superfusions or left atrial injections of bradykinin (1-10 μg). Lower thoracic splanchnic spinal afferent neurons were stimulated during visceral ischemia induced by occlusion of the celiac artery. The extent to which patterned responses originated from spinal cord organization was determined in some experiments after high cervical spinal cord transection. Mean responses were statistically compared by a least significant difference test or a Student-Newman-Keuls test following analysis of variance (Sokol and Rohlf, 1969). Further details of these methods are published elsewhere (Reimann and Weaver, 1980).

RESULTS

Reflexes Initiated from Cardiac Spinal Sympathetic Afferent Neurons

Cardiac afferent neurons traversing sympathetic nerves to enter the upper thoracic spinal cord initiate excitatory sympathetic reflexes when stimulated by myocardial ischemia (Malliani et al., 1969), increased myocardial tension (Pagani et al., 1974), or by chemicals such as bradykinin (Reimann and Weaver, 1980). The ability of these afferent neurons to initiate differential sympathetic responses was investigated in vagotomized cats. As illustrated in Figure 1, chemical stimulation of cardiac sympathetic afferent neurons by bradykinin caused greater excitation of splenic than renal nerve activity. At concentrations that evoked submaximal splenic nerve responses, renal nerve activity often was excited very little. The extent to which this preferential excitation of splenic nerves resulted from spinal neural organization was ascertained after high cervical spinal cord transection in these same cats. The differential excitation of splenic vs renal nerve activity was even more apparent in the spinalized state (Fig. 1), suggesting that this reflex specificity originated within spinal neural networks.

Reflexes Initiated from Splanchnic Spinal Afferent Neurons

Reflex responses to splanchnic spinal afferent stimulation during visceral ischemia were evaluated in vagotomized cats in which upper thoracic (T_1-T_6) sympathetic chains had been removed. Stimulation of the lower thoracic spinal afferent neurons was

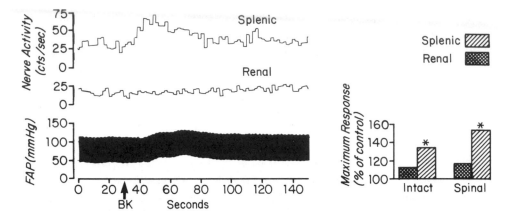

Fig. 1. Effect of chemical stimulation of cardiac sympathetic afferent nerves on splenic and renal sympathetic discharge and systemic arterial pressure. **Left:** top two traces are mean discharge rates of sympathetic activity monitored simultaneously with femoral arterial pressure (lower trace). Time in seconds is shown below tracings. Bradykinin (10 μg in 1 ml saline) was superfused over the heart at the time indicated BK. **Right:** mean maximum sympathetic responses of five cats to afferent stimulation by bradykinin before and 4 hours after high cervical spinal cord transection. Responses during 20-sec intervals are averaged. Asterisks indicate that splenic responses are significantly greater than renal responses (p < 0.05). Coefficients of variation are 10% in the intact state and 19% after transection.

accomplished by occlusion of the celiac artery for approximately 1 min to terminate blood flow to the spleen, liver and stomach. A typical response pattern to this visceral ischemia is illustrated in Figure 2. Occlusion of the celiac artery caused greater excitation of splenic than renal nerve activity. Splenic discharge increased by about 200% whereas renal nerve activity increased by only 50%. Mean simultaneously recorded responses in 11 cats are illustrated in Figure 3. Whereas both splenic and renal nerve responses were increased by occlusion of the celiac artery, splenic responses were significantly greater than renal responses. Thus, stimulation of lower thoracic spinal afferent neurons also can cause a differentiated excitation within these two components of splanchnic sympathetic outflow.

Summation of Opposing Reflexes

The most extreme example of "differential" influences on sympathetic outflow is the initiation of opposing reflexes in two nerves. Such opposition was demonstrated by responses to left atrial injections of bradykinin in cats in which upper thoracic sympathetic chains had been removed. This stimulus activated cardiac vagal afferent neurons which are said to have preferential inhibitory influences on renal sympathetic nerves

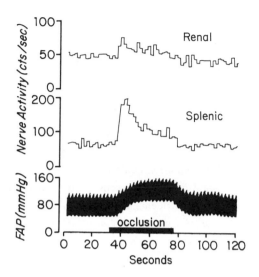

Fig. 2. Effect of splanchnic spinal afferent stimulation by celiac artery occlusion on renal and splenic sympathetic discharge. Format is similar to that of Fig. 1A. Period of occlusion is indicated by the bar beneath the time trace. Note that renal and splenic nerve activities are illustrated using different vertical scales.

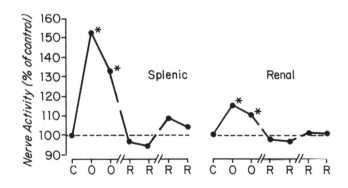

Fig. 3. Mean splenic and renal sympathetic responses of 11 cats to occlusion of the celiac artery. Average discharge rate is indicated during a 60-sec control period (C), during two continuous 20-sec intervals of occlusion (O), during two continuous 20-sec recovery periods (R) immediately after release of occlusion, and during 2 recovery periods sampled 2 min after release of occlusion. Asterisks indicate significant differences from control (p < 0.05). Coefficients of variations were 27% and 14% for respective comparisons of splenic and renal responses to control. Cross indicates that splenic responses during first 20 sec of occlusion were significantly greater than renal responses during entire occlusion (coefficient of variation: 18%).

(Mancia et al., 1975; Reimann and Weaver, 1980; Karim et al., 1972). In addition, as bradykinin reached the arterial circulation it seemed to stimulate the perivascular and muscle receptors that lead to sympathetic excitation (Guzman et al., 1962). The net effect of this complex stimulus on splenic and renal nerves is illustrated in Figure 4. The splenic nerves were consistently excited, whereas the renal nerve activity was either inhibited, slightly excited, or biphasically affected. Excitatory effects of stimulating lower thoracic or lumbar spinal afferent neurons were more pronounced in splenic than renal nerves. Splenic nerve excitation often was accompanied by inhibition of renal nerve activity in an individual cat. This inhibition could not be produced following vagotomy in the same cats. Thus cardiac vagal afferent neurons were responsible for the inhibitory responses and apparently had greater influences on renal than splenic nerve activity. The summation of these two reflex inputs to the nervous system led to a clearly differentiated, opposite response pattern in the renal and splenic components of splanchnic outflow.

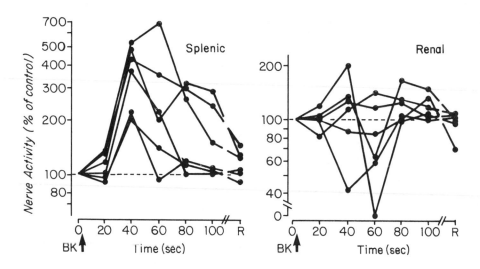

Fig. 4. Splenic and renal sympathetic nerve responses to intra-atrial injection of 10 μg bradykinin. Each line denotes the response of an individual cat. Average activity is illustrated during 20-sec intervals following injection of bradykinin (BK). The recovery period (R) is the average during a 60-sec interval.

DISCUSSION

The reflex responses observed in two components of splanchnic sympathetic outflow differed in magnitude and direction. These observations provide a basis for the suggestion that complex adjustments in blood flow to different tissues accompanying various behavioral states can be the consequence of complex neurogenic as well as local control mechanisms. Some differential patterns of sympathetic outflow seem to originate totally from spinal neural networks. The complex reflex patterns that were elicited within the splenic and renal sympathetic outflow suggest great potential discreteness of control within the sympathetic nervous system. These postganglionic neurons receive innervation from approximately the same spinal segments and often are located in the same ganglion.

The target organ responses to opposite reflexes occurring in different sympathetic nerves are clearly predictable. In contrast, the significance of unequal magnitudes of excitation among sympathetic nerves is more difficult to assess. For example, perhaps greater sympathetic excitation is required to cause splenic responses than is needed to affect renal function. This interpretation could indicate that the greater magnitude of splenic than renal nerve excitation is of little functional significance. However, splenic contraction can be initiated by electrical stimulation of splenic sympathetic nerves at frequencies as low as 0.5-2.0 Hz (Celander, 1954). This is the same frequency of stimulation of renal nerves used to evoke antinatriuresis and renin secretion (Slick et al., 1975; Zambraski and DiBona, 1976). Since the spleen seems to be as sensitive as the kidney to sympathetic activation, greater splenic than renal nerve excitation probably would lead to greater splenic than renal responses. Many cardiovascular adjustments to different behavioral needs may be regulated in part by discrete patterns of sympathetic control.

REFERENCES

Cannon, W.B. (1915) Bodily Changes in Pain, Hunger, Fear and Rage. An Account of Recent Researches into the Function of Emotional Excitement. D. Appleton and Co., New York.

Cannon, W.B. (1932) Wisdom of the Body. W.E. Norton and Co., Inc., New York.

Celander, O. (1954) The range of control exercised by the sympathico-adrenal system. Acta Physiol. Scand. 32, 68-75.

Folkow, B., Johansson, B. and Lofving, B. (1961) Aspects of functional differentiation of the sympatho-adrenergic control of the cardiovascular system. Med. Exp. 4, 321-328.

Guzman, F., Braun, C. and Lim, R.K.S. (1962) Visceral pain and the pseudo-affective response to intra-arterial injection of bradykinin and other algesic agents. Arch. Int. Pharmacodyn. 136, 353-384.

Karim, F., Kidd, C., Malpus, C.M. and Penna, P.E. (1972) The effects of stimulation of the left atrial receptors on sympathetic efferent nerve activity. J. Physiol. (Lond.) 227, 243-260.

Langley, J.N. (1892) On the origin from the spinal cord of the cervical and upper thoracic sympathetic fibers, with some observations on white and grey rami communicantes. Phil. Trans. B 183, 85-124.

Langley, J.N. (1899) On axon-reflexes in the preganglionic fibres of the sympathetic system. J. Physiol. (Lond.) 25, 365-398.

Malliani, A., Schwartz, P.J. and Zanchetti, A. (1969) A sympathetic reflex elicited by experimental coronary occlusion. Amer. J. Physiol. 217, 703-709.

Mancia, G., Shepherd, J.T. and Donald, D.E. (1975) Role of cardiac, pulmonary, and carotid mechanoreceptors in the control of hind-limb and renal circulation in dogs. Circulat. Res. 37, 200-208.

84

Ninomiya, I. and Irisawa, H. (1975) Non-uniformity of the sympathetic nerve activity in response to baroreceptor inputs. Brain Res. 87, 313-322.

Ninomiya, I., Nisimaru, N. and Irisawa, H. (1971) Sympathetic nerve activity to the spleen, kidney, and heart in response to baroreceptor input. Amer. J. Physiol. 221, 1346-1351.

Pagani, M., Schwartz, P., Banks, R., Lombardi, F. and Malliani, A. (1974) Reflex responses of sympathetic preganglionic neurones initiated by different cardiovascular receptors in spinal animals. Brain Res. 68, 215-225.

Reimann, K.A. and Weaver, L.C. (1980) Contrasting reflexes evoked by chemical activation of cardiac afferent nerves. Amer. J. Physiol. 239, H316-H325.

Slick, G.L., Aquilera, A.J., Zambraski, E.J., Dibona, G.F. and Kaloyanides, G.J. (1975) Renal neuroadrenergic transmission. Amer. J. Physiol. 229, 60-65.

Smith, O.A., Hohimer, A.R., Astley, C.A. and Taylor, D.J. (1979) Renal and hindlimb vascular control during acute emotion in the baboon. Amer. J. Physiol. 236, R198-R205.

Sokol, R.R. and Rohlf, F.J. (1969) Biometry. The Principles and Practice of Statistics in Biological Research. Freeman, San Francisco.

Zambraski, E.J. and DiBona, G.F. (1976) Angiotensin II in antinatriuresis of low-level renal nerve stimulation. Amer. J. Physiol. 231, 1105-1110.

Published 1982 by Elsevier Science Publishing Co., Inc.
Smith, Galosy, and Weiss, editors
CIRCULATION, NEUROBIOLOGY, AND BEHAVIOR

Neural Control of the Circulation in Exercise

LORING B. ROWELL

Departments of Physiology and Biophysics and of Medicine, University of Washington School of Medicine, Seattle, Washington

INTRODUCTION

Muscular exercise provides a striking example of highly integrated and precise neural control of the cardiovascular (CV) system. This finely adjusted control is operative over the full range of CV function. For example, in normal young humans cardiac output and heart rate are closely matched to metabolic rate in a highly reproducible manner over the full range of oxygen consumption, which can increase 10- to 20-fold. These increments are achieved by 3- to 4-fold increases in heart rate and systemic arterial-venous oxygen difference, the latter being augmented by a neurally controlled redistribution of blood flow from inactive to active regions (Rowell, 1974). Blood pressure rises despite the persistence of normal baroreflex sensitivity during exercise (Ludbrook et al., 1978).

The mechanism by which the tight coupling between circulatory and metabolic events is achieved has puzzled physiologists for nearly a century. What could be the stimulus or stimuli that govern the circulation during exercise? The earliest hypotheses expressed two fundamentally different ideas. The first was called "central command" or "cortical irradiation of motor impulses" (Krogh and Lindhard, 1913). Basically, the concept today is that centrally generated signals from the motor cortex and spinal motor centers activate in parallel both skeletal muscle and CV efferent systems. The second idea, first expressed for the respiratory system by Zuntz and Geppert (1886), was that a metabolic error signal emanates from chemosensitive nerves in skeletal muscle. Up to a point, the second idea has been somewhat easier than the first to deal with experimentally. What is required is some !'sensor" within the muscle that could detect small changes in the local chemical environment and thus serve to "monitor" the adequacy of muscle perfusion. Muscle would clearly be the ideal locus for such receptors since the CV response to exercise directs a major fraction of cardiac output to the working muscle. The studies reviewed by Kaufman et al. (this volume) reveal that a large portion of the smaller nerve fibers within skeletal muscle may act as local chemosensors.

Over the years, a number of other hypotheses have been offered to explain the CV and respiratory responses to exercise. Respiratory physiologists have, without much success, sought potential roles for arterial and central venous chemoreflexes (e.g., Whipp, 1978). Although muscle mechanoreceptors are commonly thought not to be involved in the "exercise reflex," it is premature to conclude that muscle mechanoreceptors have no important feedback to CV centers in exercising humans.

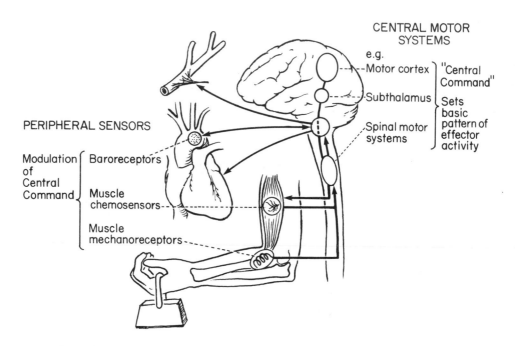

Fig. 1. Hypothesized interaction between centrally generated motor signals and reflexes from baroreceptors and receptors in skeletal muscle (see text).

Opinions vary concerning the potential role of baroreceptors. An early idea was that vasodilation of active muscle caused a fall in blood pressure, which would trigger a baroreflex. The rise in heart rate and cardiac output with exercise was thought to be caused by this reflex. However, what usually occurs is not a fall in blood pressure, but rather a rapid rise to levels exceeding resting values. Thus, circulatory control does not seem to be directed toward restoring blood pressure to some pre-exercise control level. At present, we lack any clear ideas about the importance of the baroreflex during exercise. Ludbrook et al. (1978) clearly showed that the sensitivity of the reflex is not reduced during exercise even though the heart rate response to a change in blood pressure is blunted. Somehow the operating point of the reflex seems to be changed to a higher level. If so, the question concerns the stimulus that resets this reflex. Actually, the baroreflex may have pivotal importance in the overall CV response to exercise, as will be discussed later.

The main focus of this chapter is on those two hypotheses that deal with central command and muscle chemosensors. A tendency has been to consider them separately; Figure 1 combines the two hypotheses into one. The basic idea stated in Figure 1 is that centrally generated motor signals, by acting through cortical and spinal motor systems, could set basic patterns of effector activity. This activity is in turn modulated by muscle chemosensors, baroreceptors and mechanoreceptors as appropriate error signals develop. The objective of this chapter is to put together some of the evidence that supports this conceptual scheme, recognizing at the same time, of course, that other schemes are equally plausible.

CENTRAL COMMAND

Until recently, evidence supporting the rather vague concept of a feed-forward control of the CV system called "central command" has come from humans. Recent evidence from other species and a more detailed treatment of the concept are presented in papers by Hobbs and Dormer elsewhere in this volume.

Clearly the central command hypothesis is a difficult one to test. Freyschuss (1970) showed a persistent pressor response in her subjects when they attempted static contraction of muscles that had been totally paralyzed by injection of succinylcholine. Centrally generated signals should have been present without any interference from reflexes within the muscle itself, since the muscle could not contract.

In an ingenious series of experiments, Goodwin et al. (1972) varied the motor command required to achieve a given isometric contraction force by exciting muscle spindle receptors with high-frequency (100 Hz) vibration. Such vibration of a contracting muscle facilitated its motoneurons and thus required a reduced motor command. The opposite occurred when vibration was applied to the antagonist muscle. Although the force generated by the muscle was kept constant, the heart rate and blood pressure responses were altered in accordance with the subject's perception of effort and with the predicted level of motor command.

The circulatory responses to a given level of static exercise were augmented when subjects were weakened by partial curarization (McCloskey, 1981). The inference is that the greater levels of motor command required to perform the work caused the additional rise in blood pressure and heart rate. However, these experiments did not rule out a reflex contribution from receptors within the muscle itself.

CHEMOREFLEXES FROM SKELETAL MUSCLE

Is there a muscle chemoreflex? Do chemosensitive nerves in skeletal muscle play any role in generating the CV responses to exercise? The first question is easier to answer and the neurophysiological evidence is presented by Kaufman et al. (this volume). Alam and Smirk (1937) took a simple approach in the first real test of the muscle chemosensor hypothesis. Their logic was that if metabolites produced within the exercising muscle can elicit CV responses, then entrapment of these substances within the muscle after cessation of exercise should provide a continuing stimulus to the CV system. They found that when the circulation to an exercising limb remained occluded after exercise stopped, blood pressure remained elevated (Fig. 2).

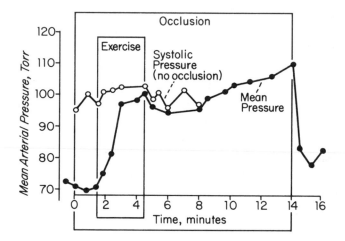

Fig. 2. Mean arterial pressure during and after dynamic exercise of the forearm with its circulation arrested. Pressure rose markedly during exercise and remained elevated as long as circulation was stopped. Mean pressures were calculated from the data of Alam and Smirk (1937). Dashed lines show systolic pressure only during forearm exercise without occlusion and indicate little or no rise in mean pressure. (From Rowell et al., 1971, with permission.)

Other evidence from humans also supports the hypothesis that skeletal muscle is involved in a pressor reflex. For example, the pressor response to static contractions is thought to result from mechanical compression of the blood vessels by contracting muscle (Lind et al., 1968); presumably, the resultant restriction in blood flow leads to muscle ischemia, which may be highly localized depending on the strength of contraction (Saltin et al., 1981). Patients with atherosclerosis obliterans show elevations in blood pressure when claudication occurs during exercise (Lorentsen, 1972). In this important clinical example, a reduction in perfusion of working muscle elicits a reflex that acts to increase muscle perfusion.

Recent studies showed some additional features of the pressor reflex from ischemic skeletal muscle. First, the pressor response can be graded in relation to the degree of muscle ischemia (Rowell et al., 1976). When the circulation to both legs was occluded immediately at the end of exercise, blood pressure remained at the exercise level as long as occlusion persisted. Progressive increments in blood pressure were achieved during this postexercise occlusion period if occlusion was applied 10, 20, or 30 sec before the end of exercise to generate progressively greater accumulation of muscle metabolites (Rowell et al., 1976). A second feature of the reflex is that the rise in blood pressure is directly proportional to the mass of muscle made ischemic (Freund et al., 1978). Third, the pressor reflex is buffered by a powerful baroreflex that acts mainly through the vasomotor system and produces a marked vasodilatation with little or no effect on heart rate (Rowell et al., 1978). Fourth, this reflex can be abolished in human subjects by differential blockade of sensory nerves (Freund et al., 1979). In these experiments, subjects performed mild (300 kpm/min) dynamic exercise (bicycle ergometer) in supine posture (Fig. 3). During the last 30 sec of exercise, circulation to both legs was arrested to augment muscle ischemia, and occlusion was maintained for 3 min after exercise.

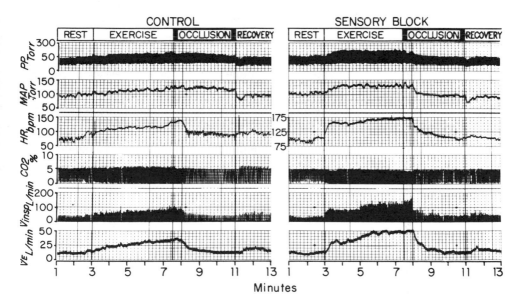

Fig. 3. Abolishment of ischemic muscle pressor response to maintained arterial occlusion after mild (50 W) dynamic exercise. Left: normal responses to exercise and occlusion of both legs during last 30 sec of exercise and 3 min postexercise. Right: responses from the same subject during the first bout of exercise after peridural anesthesia when motor weakness was still profound. Note loss of pressor response from 8 to 11 min and exaggerated circulatory responses (further details in text). (Reproduced from Freund et al., 1979, with permission.)

Before sensory nerve blockade, occlusion prevented the return of blood pressure to pre-exercise control levels. Parenthetically, the pressor response was relatively small in these experiments since the exercise had to be mild because of the motor weakness attending peridural anesthesia (Freund et al., 1979). Blockade of small sensory nerves (assessed by a battery of nerve function tests during the gradual recovery from complete motor and sensory blockade) abolished the pressor resonse to muscle ischemia.

CENTRAL COMMAND AND REFLEXES FROM SKELETAL MUSCLE

It is clear that CV adjustments to exercise cannot be expressed only in terms of reflex actions. How is one to explain the CV responses to mild dynamic exercise at a time when the muscle chemoreflex is inactivated? The CV responses to exercise shown in Figure 3 were exaggerated after nerve blockade and at a time when motor weakness was still profound. In this condition, exercise required greater effort so that motor command must have been augmented. As motor strength gradually returned toward normal, so did the CV responses to mild exercise, even though the pressor response to muscle ischemia remained blocked. One is tempted to argue that under these particular conditions of mild dynamic exercise, centrally generated motor signals elicited the CV responses since any muscle chemoreflex was absent. Two points are germane: first, regardless of what sensory nerve fibers were or were not blocked, the pressor response to muscle ischemia could be abolished without eliminating CV responses to either mild dynamic exercise or static exercise. In the case of static exercise, repeated attempts to perform maximum voluntary contractions of the quadriceps muscle after peridural anesthesia and during recovery of motor function always elicited a pressor response that was proportional to the force generated (Fig. 4). Thus, part of the pressor response to static contraction is not attributable to a reflex from ischemic muscle. The second point is that large fiber function, e.g., mechanoreceptor afferents, must have recovered along with normal motor function. Accordingly, a reflex elicited from mechanoreceptors could have contributed, along with central motor command, to the rise in blood pressure.

Observations analogous to those of Freund et al. (1979) were made by Alam and Smirk (1938) on a patient with an insentient leg (probably syringomyelia). Under ischemic conditions, exercise of either the normal or insentient limb produced the same pressor response (Fig. 5), but during postexercise occlusion no pressor response originated from the insentient limb. This observation suggests that motor command elicited the increase in blood pressure during exercise of the insentient limb; as soon as this command ceased after exercise, blood pressure fell. Again, the findings summarized above point toward two mechanisms of eliciting CV responses during exercise: a central one associated with motor command, and a peripheral one associated with a reflex of metabolic origin from skeletal muscle.

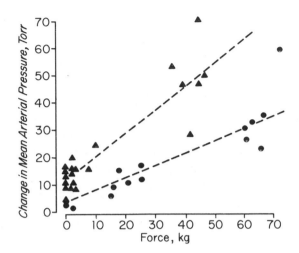

Fig. 4. Increments in mean arterial pressure (ΔMBP) in response to maximal isometric contractions of quadriceps muscles during recovery from peridural anesthesia (symbols denote two subjects). Repeated tests during the regression of motor nerve and other large fiber blockade showed that MBP progressively rose in proportion to the force generated while at the same time blockade of the ischemic muscle pressor response and of small nerve fibers persisted. (Reproduced from Freund et al., 1979, with permission.)

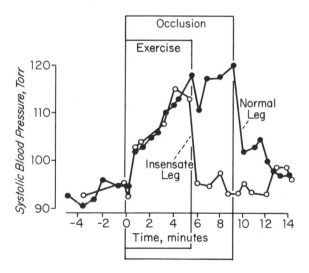

Fig. 5. Pressor responses to muscle ischemia in the normal (solid line) and insensate leg of a patient with a spinal cord lesion. The rise in systolic blood pressure was the same in both legs during ischemic exercise (circulation occluded), but there was no postexercise pressor response from the ischemic insensate leg. (Adapted from Alam and Smirk, 1938, and reproduced from Rowell et al., 1971, with permission.)

It is difficult to make sense of so many diverse findings. Variables include the severity and type of exercise and the degree to which normal circulation was disrupted. It seems clear that centrally generated motor signals are important. What is not clear is whether reflexes from muscle are important under conditions where blood flow to working muscle is uninterrupted. Clearly, total arrest of the circulation is an extreme stimulus that could elicit reflexes not normally attending exercise.

Figure 6 represents another way of expressing the muscle chemosensor hypothesis. The crucial point is this: if a muscle chemoreflex is playing an important role in controlling the circulation during exercise, then small perturbations in muscle blood flow should elicit reflexes that serve to restore blood flow and a particular concentration of metabolites within the muscle. The top of Figure 6 shows one specific hypothesis. Stepwise partial occlusion of the terminal aorta in an exercising dog should elicit stepwise increases in blood pressure, which in turn should serve to restore terminal aortic blood flow back toward normal exercise values. The degree to which terminal aortic flow recovers is one expression of the gain of the reflex. In this scheme, the muscle chemoreflex may be seen as being tonically active and always ready to correct small flow errors. A plot of systemic arterial blood pressure versus terminal aortic flow should show the relation depicted in the upper right panel.

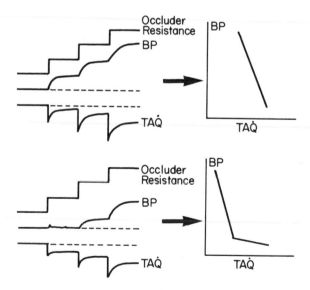

Fig. 6. A graphic illustration of the muscle chemosensor hypothesis. Upper panels predict that graded increments in resistance across an occluder on the terminal aorta (in an exercising dog) will elicit graded increments in systemic arterial blood pressure (BP), which will serve to restore terminal aortic flow (TAQ̇). Lower panels predict a threshold for this response so that BP will not rise until TAQ̇ decreases to some critical level (see text for details).

The lower half of Figure 6 shows an alternative hypothesis, namely, only when muscle blood flow is reduced below some critical level does a pressor reflex arise and serve to restore blood flow. That is, the muscle chemoreflex is not tonically active--it has a threshold. A plot of systemic blood pressure versus terminal aortic flow (lower right panel) would show a flat region in which no rise in blood pressure is associated with the initial reductions in terminal aortic flow.

Experiments employing the design depicted in Figure 6 have recently been done on dogs trained to run at different speeds and grades on a treadmill (Wyss et al., 1981). Dogs were chronically instrumented for measurement of aortic and terminal aortic blood flow, and systemic and femoral arterial blood pressures. When pressure was gradually increased in an occluder cuff placed on the terminal aorta, arterial blood pressure and terminal aortic flow both responded in the manner depicted in both panels of Figure 6. The first hypothesis applied only to moderate or heavier exercise where any reduction in muscle blood flow produced a sharp rise in blood pressure. The relation between systemic blood pressure and terminal aortic flow was essentially linear. The results suggest that a muscle chemoreflex may be tonically active during dynamic exercise of relatively moderate intensity.

The second hypothesis applied only to mild exercise where there was a distinct break or threshold in the relation between blood pressure and terminal aortic flow. Terminal aortic flow could be reduced substantially before a rise in blood pressure was elicited; thereafter, blood pressure rose markedly with each partial occlusion, the rise being four times greater than that attributable to the passive mechanical effects of occlusion. One could conclude from these results that the muscle chemoreflex is inoperative in mild dynamic exercise until some critical reduction in muscle blood flow is achieved. This suggests that during mild exercise, centrally generated signals elicit the CV responses (that is, if we can ignore mechanoreflexes).

Preliminary results suggest that the threshold for the pressor reflex is associated with a particular level of femoral venous PO_2 (Wyss, Scher, Rowell, unpublished observations). Figure 7 shows that when terminal aortic flow was reduced to a level where femoral venous PO_2 reached 15 Torr, blood pressure rose. As the severity of exercise increased and control values for femoral venous PO_2 came close to 15 Torr, less reduction in femoral blood flow was needed to elicit a pressor response. Finally, a level was reached where femoral venous PO_2 was normally 15 Torr during exercise and any change in terminal aortic flow elicited a pressor response. In this condition, muscle oxygen extraction or the metabolism:muscle blood flow ratio appears to be at a critical level so that any change in muscle blood flow elicits a local chemoreflex.

The role played by baroreflexes during exercise is far from clear. As mentioned previously, the sensitivity of the reflex is well maintained during exercise even when blood pressure is markedly elevated by muscle ischemia (Ludbrook et al., 1978; Rowell et al., 1973). These pressor reflexes are modulated by baroreflexes that appear to be "reset" to a higher operating point (by central command?). If pressure-raising reflexes from muscle are buffered by baroreflexes, then baroreceptor denervation should lead to marked alterations in blood pressure responses to exercise and muscle ischemia. Ardell et al. (1981) showed that blood pressure fell transiently when dogs with cervical sino-aortic denervation and acute vagus nerve block began to run on a treadmill. This denervation eliminates both arterial and cardiopulmonary baroreceptors. However, after 1 to 2 min (depending on the severity of exercise) blood pressure gradually recovered to a level close to that obtained by these same animals during exercise before denervation. The magnitude of decline and the rate at which blood pressure recovered increased with the severity of exercise. What caused blood pressure to recover? One hypothesis is that a transient hypoperfusion of muscle during the first minute of exercise elicited a muscle chemoreflex. The implication here is important. It appears that such a reflex can by itself serve to control blood pressure during exercise in the absence of a baroreflex.

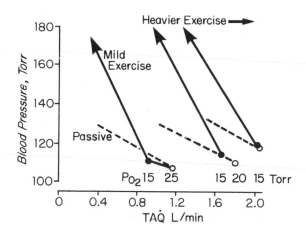

Fig. 7. Relation between systemic arterial blood pressure (BP) and terminal aortic flow (TAQ) at three levels of exercise. These preliminary results suggest that the threshold for the pressor response associated with decreased TAQ is associated with a particular femoral venous PO_2, in this case, 15 Torr. Other values for femoral venous PO_2 are control values during exercise before partial occlusion. Dashed lines show the calculated passive, mechanical effects of partial terminal aortic occlusion on BP.

Preliminary results from dogs suggest that the muscle chemoreflex can elicit greater pressor responses when buffering by baroreflexes is elminated, i.e., as though the full strength of the muscle chemoreflex were unveiled (Wyss et al., 1981). It appears that muscle chemoreflexes will correct imbalances between muscle blood flow and metabolism only within the limits permitted by the baroreflexes.

In conclusion, centrally generated motor signals, muscle chemoreflexes and the baroreflexes all appear to be important in establishing CV responses to exercise. Probably central command sets the basic patterns of effector activity. This activity must be modulated by these peripheral reflexes as appropriate error signals develop. The nature of the error signals probably depends on the severity of exercise.

ACKNOWLEDGMENTS

We gratefully acknowledge the assistance of Ms. Pam Stevens, Mr. David Wallace, and Mr. Pat Roberts.

The research from our laboratory was supported by National Heart, Lung and Blood Institute grant HL-16910. A part of this work was conducted through the Clinical Research Center of the University of Washington supported by National Institutes of Health grant RR-37.

REFERENCES

Alam, M. and Smirk, F.H. (1937) Observations in man upon a blood pressure raising reflex arising from the voluntary muscles. J. Physiol. (Lond.) 89, 372-383.

Alam, M. and Smirk, F.H. (1938) Unilateral loss of a blood pressure raising, pulse accelerating, reflex from voluntary muscle due to a lesion of the spinal cord. Clin. Sci. 3, 247-252.

Ardell, J.L., Scher, A.M. and Rowell, L.B. (1981) Effects of baroreceptor denervation on the cardiovascular response to dynamic exercise; in Arterial Baroreceptors and Hypertension, P. Sleight, ed. Oxford University Press, Oxford, pp. 311-317.

Freund, P.R., Hobbs, S.F. and Rowell, L.B. (1978) Cardiovascular responses to muscle ischemia in man--dependency on muscle mass. J. Appl. Physiol. 45, 762-767.

Freund, P.R., Rowell, L.B., Murphy, T.M., Hobbs, S.F. and Butler, S.H. (1979) Blockade of the pressor response to muscle ischemia by sensory nerve block in man. Amer. J. Physiol. 237, H433-H439.

Freyschuss, U. (1970) Cardiovascular adjustments to somatomotor activation. The elicitation of increments in heart rate, aortic pressure and venomotor tone with the initiation of muscle contraction. Acta Physiol. Scand. 343 (Suppl.), 1.

Goodwin, G.M., McCloskey, D.I. and Mitchell, J.H. (1972) Cardiovascular and respiratory responses to changes in central command during isometric exercise at constant muscle tension. J. Physiol. (Lond.) 226, 173-190, 1972.

Krogh, A. and Lindhard, J. (1913) The regulation of respiration and circulation during the initial stages of muscular work. J. Physiol. (Lond.) 47, 112-136.

Lind, A.R., McNicol, G.W., Bruce, R.A., MacDonald, H.R. and Donald, K.W. (1968) The cardiovascular responses to sustained contractions of a patient with unilateral syringomyelia. Clin. Sci. 35, 45-53.

Lorentsen, E. (1972) Systemic arterial blood pressure during exercise in patients with atherosclerosis obliterans of the lower limbs. Circulation 46, 257-263.

Ludbrook, J., Faris, I.B., Iannos, J., Jamieson, G.G. and Russell, W.J. (1978) Lack of effect of isometric handgrip exercise on the responses of the carotid sinus baroreceptor reflex in man. Clin. Sci. Molec. Med. 55, 189-194.

McCloskey, D.I. (1981) Centrally-generated commands and cardiovascular control in man. Clin. Exp. Hypertension 3, 369-378.

Rowell, L.B. (1974) Human cardiovascular adjustments to exercise and thermal stress. Physiol. Rev. 54, 75-159.

Rowell, L.B., Hermansen, L. and Blackmon, J.R. (1976) Human cardiovascular and respiratory responses to graded muscle ischemia. J. Appl. Physiol. 41, 693-701.

Saltin, B., Sjøgaard, G., Gaffney, F.A. and Rowell, L.B. (1981) Potassium, lactate, and water fluxes in human quadriceps muscle during static contractions. Circulat. Res. 48 (Suppl. 1), 118-124.

Whipp, B.J. (1978) The hyperpnea of dynamic muscular exercise. Exercise and Sport Sciences Reviews 5, 295-311.

Wyss, C.R., Ardell, J.L., Scher, A.M. and Rowell, L.B. (1981) Cardiovascular responses to graded terminal aortic restriction in exercising dogs. Fed. Proc. 40, 464.

Zuntz, N. and Geppert, J. (1886) Über die Natur der normalen Atemreize und den Ort ihrer Wirkung. Pflügers Arch. Ges Physiol. 38, 337.

Copyright 1982 by Elsevier Science Publishing Co.,Inc.
Smith, Galosy, and Weiss, editors
CIRCULATION, NEUROBIOLOGY, AND BEHAVIOR

Cardiovascular Control During Static Exercise: Central and Reflex Neural Mechanisms

MARC P. KAUFMAN, BARRY R. BOTTERMAN, WILLIAM J. GONYEA,
GARY A. IWAMOTO AND JERE H. MITCHELL
Departments of Internal Medicine, Physiology, and Cell Biology, and the Harry S. Moss
Heart Center, The University of Texas Health Science Center at Dallas, Texas

Although static exercise has been known for many years to increase blood pressure and heart rate, the mechanisms causing these cardiovascular (CV) adjustments are still not completely understood. At present, two theories, both based on neurogenic mechanisms, have attempted to explain the CV responses to static exercise (Fig. 1) (Johansson, 1895; Mitchell et al., 1977). The first theory, recently called "central command," suggests that neural impulses, arising from the motor cortex, activate medullary and spinal neuronal circuits that serve to increase CV function (Goodwin et al., 1972; Krogh and Lindhard, 1913/14). Many physiologists believe that central command is responsible for the immediate increase in heart rate observed during voluntarily performed static exercise (Shepherd et al., 1981). The second theory suggests that afferent endings in skeletal muscle, when stimulated by static exercise, reflexly increase CV function (Alam and Smirk, 1937, 1938; Coote et al., 1971; McCloskey and Mitchell,

CARDIOVASCULAR CONTROL DURING EXERCISE

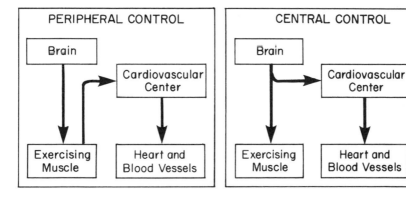

Fig. 1. Diagrammatic representation of the two mechanisms likely to be responsible for the cardiovascular responses caused by static exercise.

98

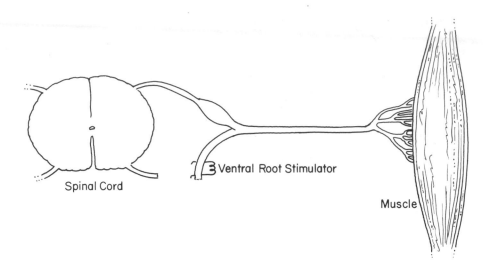

Fig. 2. Diagram of the preparation used to induce static exercise in dogs and cats. Electrical stimulation of the ventral roots (either L6 and L7 or L7 and S1) was used to contract the hindlimb. Afferent fibers with endings in the contracting skeletal muscle entered the spinal cord via the dorsal roots.

1972). Many believe that this reflex functions to match blood supply with demand in exercising skeletal muscle (Rowell et al., 1981; Shepherd et al., 1981). It should be emphasized strongly that these two theories are not mutually exclusive; there is substantial evidence that the neural mechanisms postulated by both theories contribute to the increase in CV function seen during static exercise (Coote et al., 1971; Goodwin et al., 1972; McCloskey and Mitchell, 1972; Mitchell and Wildenthal, 1974; Eldridge et al., 1981). We are currently investigating both of these mechanisms in our laboratory.

First, we will focus on the theory that reflex mechanisms, arising from afferent endings in exercising skeletal muscle, cause at least some of the CV increases evoked by static exercise (Alam and Smirk, 1937, 1938; Coote et al., 1971; McCloskey and Mitchell, 1972). To test the hypothesis that static exercise reflexly increases CV function, a preparation has been established (Coote et al., 1971; Crayton et al., 1979; Fisher and Nutter, 1974; McCloskey and Mitchell, 1972) that eliminates "central command" (Fig. 2). Thus, in anesthetized cats and dogs, the cut peripheral ends of the L7-S1 ventral roots, which contain the axons of alpha-motoneurons supplying hindlimb skeletal muscles, have been electrically stimulated. Because the hindlimb is fixed in one position, the ventral root-induced exercise is "static" in nature, i.e., the muscular contractions are almost isometric. The CV responses to static exercise are then measured in this preparation during rest and during static exercise.

The data obtained from this preparation have shown conclusively that static exercise, induced by ventral root stimulation, reflexly increases arterial blood pressure and heart rate. In addition, the data have suggested that muscle afferents of groups III and IV, but not groups I and II, were responsible for causing these reflex effects (McCloskey and Mitchell, 1972). The evidence supporting these findings was based on techniques that allowed the dorsal roots, which comprised the afferent limb of the exercise pressor reflex arc, to be both reversibly and differentially blocked. For example, in anesthetized cats, blockade of thickly myelinated afferents (i.e., groups I and II) with anodal current had no effect on the exercise pressor reflex (Fig. 3). However, blockade of thinly myelinated (group III) and unmyelinated (group IV) muscle afferents with lidocaine, applied topically to the dorsal roots, abolished the pressor reflex (Fig. 4). Occlusion of the arterial and venous supply of the hindlimb at the conclusion of the period of exercise was found to prolong the duration of the reflex pressor response, suggesting that a

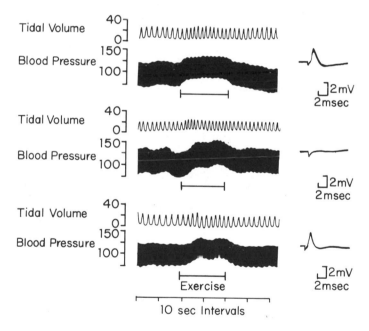

Fig. 3. The reflex increases in arterial pressure and minute volume of ventilation evoked by static exercise are not caused by stimulation of thickly myelinated muscle afferents. With each record of arterial pressure and integrated tidal volume, the compound action potential sampled from a slip of dorsal root central to the region of anodal blockade is shown. The compound action potential was evoked by a single pulse applied to the sciatic nerve. Top panel: a period of static exercise (signaled by the bracket) before anodal blockade of the L7-S1 dorsal roots. Middle panel: a period of static exercise 1 min after the application of anodal blockade just sufficient to block the A wave of the dorsal root compound action potential. Bottom panel: another period of exercise after turning off the anodal blockade.

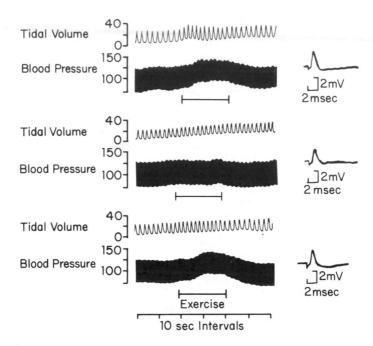

Fig. 4. The reflex increases in arterial pressure and minute volume of ventilation evoked by static exercise are caused by the stimulation of thinly myelinated and unmyelinated muscle afferents. Same cat as shown in Figure 3. In each panel, records of integrated tidal volume arterial pressure and dorsal root compound potentials are shown. Top panel: a period of exercise (signaled by the bracket) before topical application of lidocaine solution (0.125%) to the L7-S1 dorsal roots. Middle panel: period of exercise 3½ min after application of lidocaine solution. Note that this period of exercise evoked no change in either arterial pressure or ventilation, yet the A wave of the compound action potential was, for the most part, unaffected by the blockade. Bottom panel: another period of exercise after the lidocaine solution was washed away. Note the restoration of the arterial pressure and ventilatory responses to static exercise, proving that they are reflex in origin.

chemical substance, trapped in the exercised muscle, was stimulating the afferent endings responsible for the reflex pressor response.

In anesthetized cats, the reflex action of static exercise on the contractile state of the heart also has been studied (Mitchell et al., 1977). Electrical stimulation of the L7 and S1 ventral roots was shown to increase left ventricular dP/dt at a developed pressure of 25 mm Hg (Fig. 5), an index of myocardial contractility that has been found to be relatively independent of increases in aortic blood pressure (Wildenthal et al., 1969). Furthermore, left ventricular end-diastolic pressure during exercise did not differ from its control level, indicating that increases in left ventricular fiber length were not responsible for the exercise-induced increase in dP/dt. Finally, the increases in heart rate caused by ventral root stimulation were found to be much less than those needed to

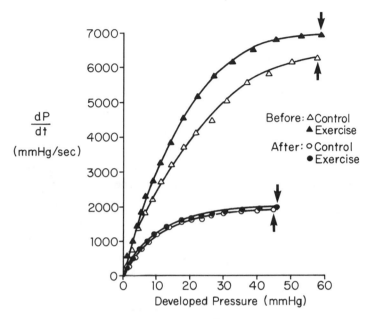

Fig. 5. Effect of propranolol (before and after) on the relation between left ventricular dP/dt and developed pressure of the left ventricle measured at rest (control) and during static exercise.

increase dP/dt via the Bowditch effect (Mitchell et al., 1963). Together, these findings raise the possibility that static exercise reflexly increases cardiac contractility, an effect that is mediated by the sympathetic nervous system.

If the sympathetic nervous system is responsible for causing an exercise-induced reflex increase in left ventricular contractility, a beta-adrenergic antagonist such as propranolol should prevent this reflex effect (Mitchell et al., 1977). This indeed was found to be the case (Fig. 5). In addition, the increase in heart rate evoked by static exercise was also prevented by propranolol. Moreover, the exercise-induced increases in heart rate and contractility were abolished by cutting the L7-S1 dorsal roots, demonstrating that these increases were reflex in origin. These experiments suggest that in anesthetized cats, static exercise evoked by stimulation of the ventral roots reflexly activates the sympathetic nervous system, which, in turn, increases cardiac contractility and rate. However, it remains to be determined whether these sympathetically induced actions on the heart are caused by catecholamine release from the adrenal gland or by norepinephrine release from postganglionic endings in the heart.

In a study by Crayton et al. (1979), the distribution of cardiac output during static exercise was determined. Blood flow to the various vascular beds in anesthetized dogs was measured with radioactive microspheres. Exercise was induced by electrical stimulation of the L6 and L7 ventral roots. Significant changes in blood flow were found in the vascular beds supplying the kidney (-18 ± 6%) and the contracting hindlimb muscles (+453 ± 154%). No change in flow was found in the vascular beds supplying the liver, spleen, brain, nonexercising hindlimb muscles, and myocardium. Moreover, static exercise was found to increase cardiac output, arterial pressure, and heart rate, although peripheral vascular resistance was unchanged. Cutting the L6 and L7 dorsal roots abolished both the decrease in flow to kidney and the increase in CV function, thereby establishing the reflex origin of these responses. However, the increase in flow to the exercising hindlimb muscle was unaffected by dorsal root section, which strongly suggests that this increase was caused by the increased metabolic demands of the contracting skeletal muscle.

In the study by Crayton et al. (1979), myocardial blood flow was unchanged during static exercise, even though this maneuver was found to increase the product of heart rate and systolic arterial pressure, an indicator of myocardial oxygen consumption. To explain this lack of effect on myocardial blood flow during static exercise, Aung-Din et al. (1981) examined in anesthetized dogs the effect of induced static exercise on myocardial blood flow before and after beta-adrenergic blockade with propranolol, a substance which, by preventing sympathetically mediated increases in cardiac contractility and rate, attenuated the increase in myocardial oxygen demand evoked by static exercise. In addition, propranolol was likely to prevent, or at least attenuate, any beta-adrenergic coronary vasodilation evoked by static exercise. Aung-Din et al. (1981) found that induced muscular contraction after beta-adrenergic blockade caused a decrease in myocardial blood flow, an effect that was abolished both by dorsal root section (L6 and L7) in one group of dogs and by alpha-adrenergic blockade in another group. These findings suggest that, during static exercise, blood flow to the heart is subjected to two competing influences. The first is a vasodilation caused by an increase in myocardial metabolism, although beta-adrenergic receptors may also contribute to this effect. When the first influence was blocked with propranolol, the second influence was unmasked; namely, an alpha-adrenergic vasoconstriction evoked reflexly by static exercise. Furthermore, these two competing influences appear to sum algebraically, which probably explains why Crayton et al. (1979) were unable to evoke changes in myocardial blood flow during ventral root stimulation.

Now that the CV adjustments that are reflexly evoked by static exercise have been described, we are beginning to investigate the central neural pathways and sites of integration of the reflex arc(s) causing these adjustments. We were, therefore, interested in a report by Ciriello and Calaresu (1977), who found that lesions of the lateral reticular nucleus abolished the reflex pressor response evoked by electrical stimulation of the central cut end of the cat's sciatic nerve. Hence, we were prompted to examine the role played by the lateral reticular nucleus in the reflex activation of the CV system by static exercise.

We found that the reflex increases in arterial blood pressure and heart rate, evoked by static exercise in anesthetized cats, were almost completely abolished by bilateral lesions of the lateral reticular nucleus (Fig. 6) (Iwamoto et al., in press). Moreover, the sympathetic nervous system of these cats was still functional after the lesions,

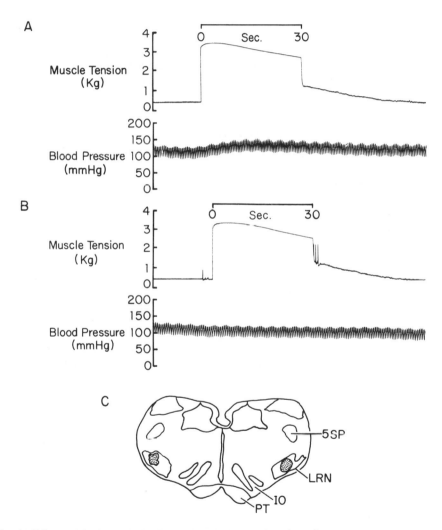

Fig. 6. Bilateral lesions of the lateral reticular nucleus (LRN) abolish the exercise pressor reflex. **A:** Before the lesions, static exercise induced by stimulation of the L7-S1 ventral roots increased arterial pressure. **B:** After the lesions, static exercise no longer evoked the exercise pressor reflex. **C:** Stippled area in LRN shows the extent of the lesions that abolish the exercise pressor reflex shown in **A.**

because electrical stimulation of pontine pressor sites markedly increased arterial pressure and heart rate, even though the reflex pressor response to static exercise was abolished in the same cats. Our findings suggest that the lateral reticular nucleus is part of the reflex arc that activates the CV system during static exercise. However, it remains to be determined if these lesions abolished the exercise pressor reflex by destroying cell bodies or fibers *en passage* in this medullary nucleus (Iwamoto et al., in press).

Our finding that intact lateral reticular nuclei were essential for the expression of the exercise pressor reflex suggested to us an animal preparation that might be useful for examining the central command theory of CV control during static exercise. To test this theory adequately, two requirements must be met. First, the animals must be awake and able to exercise voluntarily. Second, all reflex CV effects arising from exercising skeletal muscle must be eliminated.

Our laboratory has successfully met the first requirement. Conscious cats have been operantly conditioned to perform static exercise, as shown in Figure 7 (Diepstra et

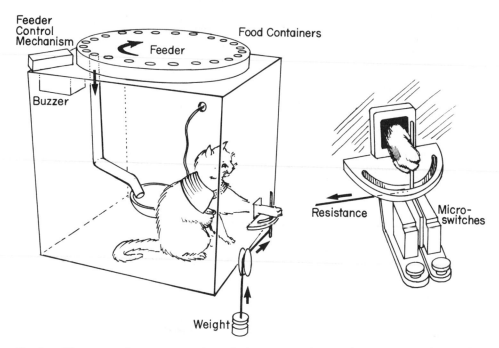

Fig. 7. Diagrammatic representation of the preparation used to measure the cardiovascular response to static exercise in the conscious cat. The cat was required to hold a weight that was attached via a pulley to a hinged bar. The hinged bar was set between two microswitches that provided an upper and lower limit that must be depressed. When the cat held the load for 15 sec, a feeding apparatus dispensed a food reward.

al., 1980). In addition, indwelling catheters have been implanted into the left ventricle and aorta of these cats, enabling us to measure left ventricular and aortic blood pressures. From these measurements, left ventricular dP/dt and heart rate have been calculated on-line. We have found that static exercise, when performed by the conscious cat, increases arterial blood pressure and left ventricular dP/dt (Fig. 8) (Gonyea et al., 1981).

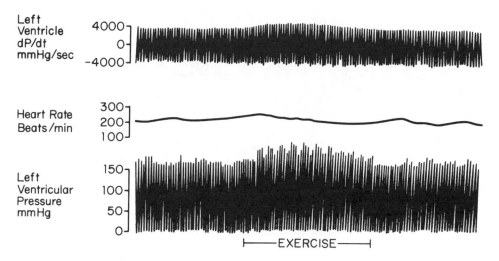

Fig. 8. Increases in left ventricular pressure and dP/dt during static exercise in the conscious cat. These effects were measured while the cat was holding a 700 g weight for 15 sec.

To meet the second requirement, we plan to make bilateral lesions of the lateral reticular nuclei. After the cats have recovered, they will be trained to perform static exercise. We hypothesize that any postlesion increase in CV function that these cats may show in response to exercise will be due solely to central command. This hypothesis can be easily verified by placing the cats under anesthesia and then stimulating the cut peripheral ends of the L7-S1 ventral roots, a maneuver that should evoke little, if any, CV effect.

In conclusion, we plan to continue our studies of both theories of CV control during static exercise. The central command theory will be studied in conscious cats trained to perform static exercise. The reflex theory will be studied in anesthetized cats by stimulating the cut peripheral ends of the ventral roots. Currently, we are characterizing the discharge properties of the groups III and IV muscle afferents causing the reflex CV increases evoked by static exercise (Kaufman et al., 1982a, b). In the future, we plan to unravel the neural pathways that are responsible for both the central and reflex mechanisms causing the CV responses to static exercise.

106

ACKNOWLEDGMENTS

Supported in part by the Harry S. Moss Heart Center, the Lawson and Rogers Lacy Research Fund in Cardiovascular Diseases, and by National Heart, Lung and Blood Institute grant P01-HL06296.

REFERENCES

Alam, M. and Smirk, F.M. (1937) Observations in man upon a blood pressure raising reflex arising from the voluntary muscles. J. Physiol. (Lond.) 89, 372-383.

Alam, M. and Smirk, F.M. (1938) Observations in man on a pulse-accelerating reflex from the voluntary muscles of the legs. J. Physiol. (Lond.) 92,167-177.

Aung-Din, R., Mitchell, J.H. and Longhurst, J.C. (1981) Reflex α-adrenergic coronary vasoconstriction during hindlimb static exercise in dogs. Circulat. Res. 48, 502-509.

Ciriello, J. and Calaresu, F.R. (1977) Lateral reticular nucleus: a site of somatic and cardiovascular integration in the cat. Amer. J. Physiol. 233, R100-R109.

Coote, J.H., Hilton, S.H. and Perez-Gonzalez, J.F. (1971) The reflex nature of the pressor response to muscular exercise. J. Physiol. (Lond.) 215, 789-804.

Crayton, S.C., Aung-Din, R., Fixler, D.E. and Mitchell, J.H. (1979) Distribution of cardiac output during induced isometric exercise in dogs. Amer. J. Physiol. 236, H218-H224.

Diepstra, G., Gonyea, W. and Mitchell, J.H. (1980) Cardiovascular response to static exercise during selective autonomic blockade in the conscious cat. Circulat. Res. 47, 530-535.

Eldridge, F.L., Millhorn, D.E. and Waldrop, T.G. (1981) Exercise hyperpnea and locomotion: parallel activation from the hypothalamus. Science 211, 844-846.

Fisher, M.L. and Nutter, D.O. (1974) Cardiovascular reflex adjustments to static muscular contractions in the canine hindlimb. Amer. J. Physiol. 226, 648-655.

Gonyea, W.J., Diepstra, G., Muntz, K.H. and Mitchell, J.H. (1981) Cardiovascular response to static exercise in the conscious cat. Circulat. Res. 48, 163-169.

Goodwin, G.M., McCloskey, D.I. and Mitchell, J.H. (1972) Cardiovascular and respiratory responses to changes in central command during isometric exercise at constant muscle tension. J. Physiol. (Lond.) 226, 173-190.

Iwamoto, G.A., Kaufman, M.P., Botterman, B.R. and Mitchell, J.H. (in press) Effects of lateral reticular nucleus lesions on the exercise pressor reflex. Circulat. Res.

Johansson, J.E. (1895) Ueber die Einwirkung der Muskelthätligkeit auf die Athmung und die Herzthätligkeit. Scand. Arch. Physiol. 5, 20-66.

Kaufman, M.P., Iwamoto, G.A., Longhurst, J.C. and Mitchell, J.H. (1982a) Effects of capsaicin and bradykinin on afferent fibers with endings in skeletal muscle. Circulat. Res. 50, 133-139.

Kaufman, M.P., Longhurst, J.C., Wallach, J.H., Rybicki, K.J. and Mitchell, J.H. (1982b). Effect of muscular contraction on thin fiber muscle afferents in cats. Fed. Proc. 41, 1604.

Krogh, A. and Lindhard, J. (1913/14) The regulation of respiration and circulation during the initial stages of muscular work. J. Physiol. (Lond.) 47, 112-136.

McCloskey, D.I. and Mitchell, J.H. (1972) Reflex cardiovascular and respiratory responses originating in exercising muscle. J. Physiol. (Lond.) 224, 173-186.

Mitchell, J.H., Reardon, W.C. and McCloskey, D.I. (1977) Reflex effects on circulation and respiration from contracting skeletal muscle. Amer. J. Physiol. 233, H374-H378.

Mitchell, J.H., Reardon, W.C., McCloskey, D.I. and Wildenthal, K. (1977) Possible role of muscle receptors in the cardiovascular response to static exercise. Ann. N.Y. Acad. Sci. 301, 232-242.

Mitchell, J.H., Wallace, A.G. and Skinner, N.S. (1963) Intrinsic effects of heart rate on left ventricular performance. Amer. J. Physiol. 205, 41-48.

Mitchell, J.H. and Wildenthal, K. (1974) Static (isometric) exercise and the heart: physiological and clinical considerations. Ann. Rev. Med. 25, 369-381.

Rowell, L.B., Freund, P.R. and Hobbs, S.F. (1981) Cardiovascular responses to muscle ischemia in humans. Circulat. Res. 48, 137-147.

Shepherd, J.T., Blomqvist, C.G., Lind, A.R., Mitchell, J.H. and Saltin, B. (1981) Static (isometric) exercise: retrospection and introspection. Circulat. Res. 48, 1179-1188.

Wildenthal, C.K., Mierzwiak, S. and Mitchell, J.H. (1969) Effect of sudden changes in aortic pressure on left ventricular dP/dt. Amer. J. Physiol. 216, 185-190.

Behavioral Stress and Cardiovascular Regulation: Neural Mechanisms

RICHARD A. GALOSY, ISAAC L. CRAWFORD AND MICHAEL E. THOMPSON
Pauline and Adolph Weinberger Laboratory of Cardiopulmonary Research and Departments of Internal Medicine and Cell Biology, Southwestern Medical School, University of Texas Health Sciences Center at Dallas, Dallas, Texas

INTRODUCTION

The influence of behavioral factors on physiological systems has been recognized for many years and anecdotal evidence has found its way into general language as represented in such phrases as "you are going to worry yourself sick." In recent years more emphasis has been placed on the scientific investigation of the relation between behavioral states and potentially pathological physiological conditions. These more recent investigations have provided results that strongly suggest behavioral factors may cause or exacerbate several disease states. Much current interest is focused on behavioral stress and although evidence indicates a role for stress in many diseases, relatively little is known about the physiological or biochemical mechanisms that mediate the relation between stress and disease.

The purpose of this chapter is to use selected previous and current research results in an attempt to formulate hypotheses related to the neural mechanisms responsible for the cardiovascular (CV) changes that accompany Sidman avoidance stress in dogs.

PERIPHERAL NEURAL MECHANISMS

An evaluation of the neural mechanisms of the peripheral nervous system that may be involved in the regulation of CV function in association with behavioral stress begins with a description of the CV changes observed during Sidman avoidance. Anderson and Brady (1971, 1972) initially reported that heart rate decreased and arterial blood pressure and pulse pressure increased during a pre-avoidance period in anticipation of Sidman avoidance. Once the avoidance procedure began, arterial blood pressure and pulse pressure remained elevated and heart rate rapidly increased above pre-avoidance levels. When the pre-avoidance period was lengthened, heart rate continued to decline and remained low while arterial blood pressure continued to rise and remained elevated for up to 15 hr (Anderson and Brady, 1973). Lawler et al. (1975), using a similar stress procedure, reported that in addition to the averaged daily session results reported by

Anderson and Brady, day-to-day fluctuations in arterial blood pressure were accompanied by changes in peripheral vascular resistance.

The results from the studies cited above have led to the hypothesis that increased arterial blood pressure and decreased heart rate during the pre-avoidance period are due to increased peripheral vascular resistance and parasympathetic activity to the heart, respectively. Increased heart rate and arterial blood pressure during the avoidance period are due to decreased parasympathetic activity to the heart and continued vaso-constriction, respectively. Day-to-day alterations in arterial blood pressure also seem to be a function of peripheral vascular mechanisms. From a neurophysiological point of view, it seems that heart rate is primarily controlled by changes in vagal activity, with arterial blood pressure primarily influenced by the sympathetic innervation to the peripheral vasculature. At this point there is little evidence regarding the role of the sympathetic innervation of the heart.

In an attempt to use CV parameters to elucidate the role of the sympathetic innervation of the heart during Sidman avoidance, we used the maximal rate of left ventricular pressure (Lvdp/dt) development as an index of sympathetic activity to the heart (Galosy et al., 1979). Compared with pre-avoidance levels, max Lvdp/dt increased significantly during the avoidance period as did heart rate and, to some extent, left ventricular systolic pressure on all days of the experiment, suggesting that a significant increase in sympathetic activity to the heart occurred during the avoidance period. Comparing day-to-day changes in heart rate, max Lvdp/dt and left ventricular systolic pressure, we found that pre-avoidance heart rate gradually increased while max Lvdp/dt and left ventricular systolic pressure remained relatively low but variable.

Based on the studies cited above, which used CV parameters as indices of the underlying neural mechanisms, one might hypothesize that within a daily avoidance session pre-avoidance is characterized by decreasing heart rates due to increased parasympathetic activity to the heart and increasing arterial blood pressure due to increased sympathetic activity to the peripheral vasculature. During the avoidance period, increased heart rates are due to a combination of decreased parasympathetic and increased sympathetic activity to the heart, with continued sympathetic peripheral vasoconstriction responsible for elevated arterial blood pressure. Such alterations on the same day seem to be superimposed on tonic elevations in heart rate mediated via decreased parasympathetic activity and arterial blood pressure levels mediated via sympathetic activity to the peripheral vasculature during pre-avoidance periods. Heart rate increases during avoidance seem to be due to a combination of increased sympathetic and decreased parasympathetic activity to the heart, with sympathetic activity to the peripheral vasculature continuing to be responsible for blood pressure elevations.

These hypotheses are attractive, but are based on indirect evidence associated with the hemodynamic changes that accompany the stressful task. More direct evidence has been provided from studies using pharmacological blocking agents (Anderson and Brady, 1976; Anderson et al., 1976). Using the beta blocking agent propranolol, Anderson and Brady (1976) showed that during an average daily stress procedure, pre-avoidance decreases in heart rate and increases in blood pressure were unaffected by the blockade. During the avoidance period, however, heart rate elevations were partially attenuated while the blood pressure changes were unaffected by the blockade (Fig. 1). In a similar study using the alpha blocking agent phenoxybenzamine (Anderson et al., 1976), pre-

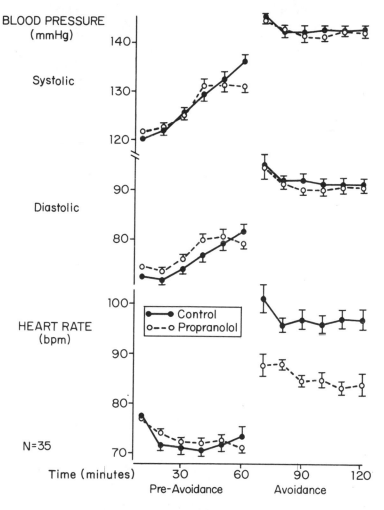

Fig. 1. Effect of beta-adrenergic blockade on arterial blood pressure and heart rate in dogs experiencing Sidman avoidance. (From Anderson and Brady, 1976, with permission.)

avoidance changes in heart rate and arterial blood pressure and avoidance changes in heart rate were unaffected, while the elevation in arterial blood pressure during the avoidance period was blocked by the pharmacological intervention (Fig. 2). These results confirm the hypothesis regarding the neural mechanisms operating during the avoidance period, but require some modification of the pre-avoidance mechanisms. Heart rate during pre-avoidance seems to be dominated by parasympathetic mechanisms, while arterial blood pressure levels are unaffected by either of the blocking agents. If peripheral vascular mechanisms are responsible for pre-avoidance blood pressure levels, something other than alpha adrenergic factors must be involved. Anderson et al. (1976) suggested that cholinergically mediated shifts in blood flow could account for the pre-avoidance blood pressure changes.

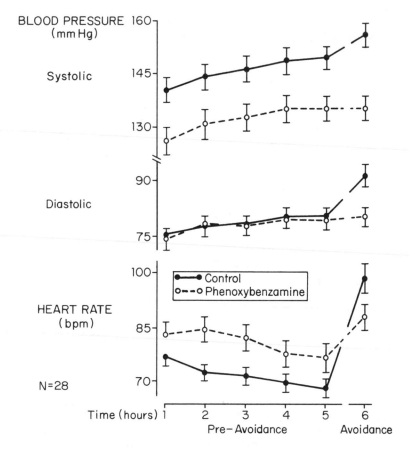

Fig. 2. Effect of alpha-adrenergic blockade on arterial blood pressure and heart rate in dogs experiencing Sidman avoidance. (From Anderson et al., 1976, with permission.)

In an attempt to understand some of the specific pathways that have been hypothesized to control CV function during Sidman avoidance, we conducted a study to determine the effect of transection of a specific sympathetic pathway to the heart on CV dynamics during the avoidance procedure (Galosy and Clarke, 1980). Transection of the left dorsal and ventral ansa subclavian nerves eliminated both the left ventricular systolic pressure and max Lvdp/dt changes during the pre-avoidance and avoidance periods (Figs. 3 and 4). Tonic levels of heart rate were unaffected, while the increased heart rate during avoidance was eliminated (Fig. 5).

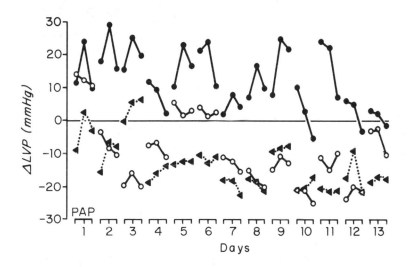

Fig. 3. Left ventricular systolic pressure (Lvp) differences from baseline for intact stressed (●), denervated stressed (▲) and nonstressed control (o) dogs during pre-avoidance (P), avoidance (A) and post-avoidance (P) periods. (From Galosy and Clarke, 1980, with permission.)

In summary, all of the data presented seem to support the following hypotheses. During pre-avoidance periods, heart rate is influenced primarily by parasympathetic activity to the heart and blood pressure is influenced by peripheral vascular mechanisms, possibly through a cholinergic system. On the other hand, although alpha-adrenergic mechanisms to the peripheral vasculature control blood pressure during avoidance, this control is partially dependent on afferent neural activity from the heart coursing in the left dorsal and ventral ansa subclavian nerves. Heart rate changes during avoidance seem to be a function of both sympathetic and parasympathetic innervations to the heart. Obviously these hypotheses are based on just a few studies and require considerable verification; however, they suggest several testable mechanisms that provide a sound basis for

114

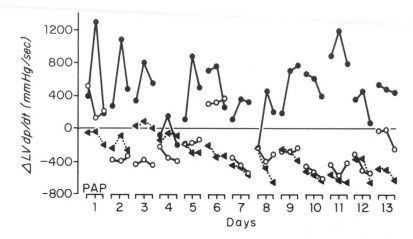

Fig. 4. Maximal rate of left ventricular pressure development (Lvdp/dt) difference from baseline for intact stressed (•), denervated stressed (▲) and nonstressed control (o) dogs during pre-avoidance (P), avoidance (A) and post-avoidance (P) periods. (From Galosy and Clarke, 1980, with permission.)

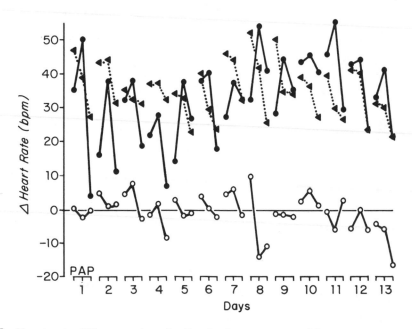

Fig. 5. Heart rate differences from basline for intact stressed (•), denervated stressed (▲) and nonstressed control (o) dogs during pre-avoidance (P), avoidance (A) and post-avoidance (P) periods. (From Galosy and Clarke, 1980, with permission.)

further investigations of the peripheral neural mechanisms responsible for CV changes that accompany Sidman avoidance stress.

CENTRAL NERVOUS SYSTEM

Our understanding of the central nervous system (CNS) mechanisms that control CV function is progressing very rapidly (see Galosy et al., 1981). However, unlike the situation for the peripheral nervous system, there are no published studies of CNS regulation of CV function during Sidman avoidance stress. In our laboratory, we have tried to relieve this unfortunate situation via two approaches.

The first approach was to use the "kindling procedure" to influence neuronal function of the amygdala. To induce kindling, we placed chronic stimulating-recording electrodes in the amygdala and presented a sequential series of stimulations beginning at low intensities. After each short (3 sec) stimulation, EEG activity was recorded from the stimulation site to determine whether afterdischarges had occurred. Using this procedure, we determined the stimulation threshold for producing afterdischarges, and set subsequent stimulation intensities at 70% of the threshold. Repeated stimulations at the subthreshold intensity were presented at 24-hr intervals until afterdischarges occurred and eventually produced generalized convulsions. The procedure was terminated after six convulsive episodes, at which time the animal was determined to be "kindled." Kindling has been reported to produce permanent changes in neuronal excitability, the mechanisms of which are not clearly understood (Wada, 1981); however, the procedure does provide a unique technique for studying the potential involvement of CNS nuclei and pathways in control of CV function.

We combined kindling of the left amygdala with Sidman avoidance in an attempt to elucidate the role of the amygdala and associated pathways in the control of CV function during Sidman avoidance. The results from this study are shown for heart rate and left ventricular pressure in Figures 6 and 7. Three groups of dogs were evaluated: kindled stressed (KS), nonkindled stressed (NKS), and nonkindled nonstressed (NKNS). Because of baseline differences between the groups, they were analyzed and are presented as differences from baseline values. Analysis of variance revealed significant differences between groups as well as between days and pre-avoidance, avoidance and post-avoidance periods. These differences are reflected in the figures as elevations in heart rate and left ventricular systolic pressure in the KS and NKS groups compared with the NKNS group. In addition, the KS group exhibited higher heart rates and left ventricular systolic pressures than the NKS group during the majority of the periods on each of the dogs. These results suggest that prior kindling of the left amygdala significantly altered the amygdala or other brain sites influenced by the spread of afterdischarges. At the very least, these data indicate that the amygdala and its associated pathways are involved in regulating CV

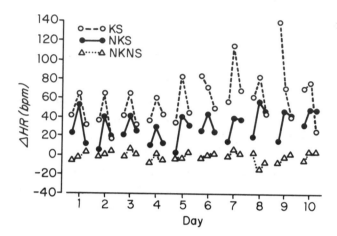

Fig. 6. Heart rate differences from baseline for kindled stressed (KS), nonkindled stressed (NKS) and nonkindled, nonstressed (NKNS) dogs during pre-avoidance, avoidance and post-avoidance periods.

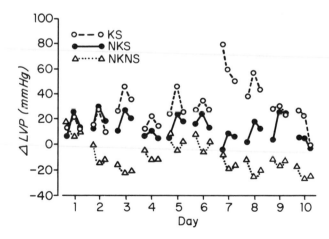

Fig. 7. Left ventricular systolic pressure differences from baseline for kindled stressed (KS), nonkindled stressed (NKS) and nonkindled, nonstressed (NKNS) dogs during pre-avoidance, avoidance and post-avoidance periods.

function during Sidman avoidance directly or via other nuclei that are influenced by amygdaloid activity.

Our second approach to studying CNS control of CV function during Sidman avoidance was to assess neurochemical changes accompanying the stress procedure. High-pressure liquid chromatographic techniques were used to assay seven specific forebrain nuclei for levels of serotonin (5-HT), 5-hydroxyindoleacetic acid (5-HIAA), dopamine (DA), homovanillic acid (HVA) and norepinephrine (NE) in stressed and nonstressed dogs (Table 1). Analysis of these data resulted in a significant increase only for 5-HIAA in the pyriform cortex of nonstressed dogs although, for example, concentrations of DA in the amygdala and hippocampus of the stressed dogs was about twice that seen in nonstressed animals. These results led us to hypothesize that there is no single neurochemical variable and/or forebrain region in which changes would accurately differentiate between the stressed and nonstressed animals. It may be that a combination of forebrain regions or neurochemical variables may more accurately differentiate the groups. We have begun an evaluation of the above hypothesis using multiple discriminant analysis to predict group inclusion retrospectively using a subset of neurochemistry and/or forebrain regions.

In our first discriminant analysis, we used all neurochemical variables and brain regions in an iterative procedure to determine the optimal subset of variables that would maximally predict group inclusion. This analysis yielded seven variables that discriminated between the two groups with 100% accuracy: HVA--pyriform cortex; DA--right amygdala; 5-HIAA--frontal cortex, pyriform cortex, and right hippocampus; 5-HT--frontal cortex and pyriform cortex.

Although it predicted group inclusion with 100% accuracy and had a very high correlation coefficient, this discriminant function was not statistically significant owing to the large number of variables relative to the small number of subjects. The results could be misleading. To evaluate these variables further, we conducted a second discriminant analysis using only the seven variables listed above. The results showed that six of the seven variables were required to discriminate between the stressed and nonstressed animals with 100% accuracy, and resulted in a statistically significant (p<0.01) discriminant function. The only exception was the first variable, HVA--pyriform cortex. This latter result suggests that the above combination of six neurochemical variables and forebrain regions may uniquely describe the difference between stressed and nonstressed dogs.

Based on the above analysis, it would appear that 5-HT and its metabolite 5-HIAA may be an important neurotransmitter system involved in differentiating stressed and nonstressed animals, since they were present in five of the six variable combinations. Based on this observation, we conducted a second set of discriminant analyses, each using a single neurochemical variable across the brain regions where it was measured. Five of

TABLE 1

MEAN ± STANDARD ERROR OF THE MEAN OF NEUROCHEMICAL VARIABLES
FOR EACH FOREBRAIN REGION IN STRESSED (S) AND NONSTRESSED (NS) DOGS

	HVA		5-HT		DA		NE		5-HIAA	
	S	NS	S	NS	S	NS	S	NS	S	NS
Frontal x	442	491	268	177	ND	ND	2655	2029	448	357
Cortex SEM	63	67	57	63	ND	ND	322	239	113	35
Cingulate x	1768	558	304	272	ND	ND	1641	1478	182	126
Cortex SEM	1537	333	117	44	ND	ND	287	200	73	21
Caudate x	17624	26037	1262	1260	OS	OS	2662	2386	877	1118
Nucleus SEM	2476	3159	192	202	OS	OS	425	285	102	196
Pyriform x	908	982	916	1267	ND	ND	1113	1283	883	1483*
Cortex SEM	387	178	59	312	ND	ND	234	320	96	199
Right x	1494	744	12548	12596	495	209	2004	1701	4133	5239
Amygdala SEM	425	97	2000	1364	160	18	438	100	686	1175
Right x	ND	ND	342	305	244	72	1684	1376	644	837
Hippocampus SEM	ND	ND	57	49	113	6	139	82	103	84
Septum x	2275	4057	960	1507	556	772	2155	1255	337	615
SEM	557	1928	249	850	178	471	960	438	33	156
Ventromedial x	1401	477	1114	738	275	265	3494	1242	588	742
Hypothalamus SEM	879	84	157	110	73	176	1086	267	174	165

ND = Nondetectable (not enough tissue available for assay).
OS = Off scale (value off scale on upper end).
All values expressed as ng/gm tissue wet weight.
*p<0.05

the eight brain regions having 5-HT (frontal cortex, cingulate cortex, caudate, pyriform cortex and ventromedial hypothalamus), and five of the eight brain regions having 5-HIAA (cingulate cortex, pyriform cortex, right hippocampus, septum and ventromedial hypothalamus) were found to discriminate between stressed and nonstressed animals significantly ($p < 0.01$) with 100% accuracy. No combination of the other neurochemical variables significantly discriminated between the stressed and nonstressed animals. These latter results further support the possibility that the 5-HT neurotransmitter may have the strongest involvement in the relation between the CV system and the behavioral stress investigated in our studies.

CONCLUSION

The studies reviewed and the data presented in this chapter indicate that the peripheral autonomic innervation of the CV system plays an important role in the control of CV function during a Sidman avoidance stress task. Specifically, both the parasympathetic and sympathetic efferent innervations of the heart influence heart rate changes that accompany the stressful task. The relative contributions of each of the innervations seem to depend on whether the animal is anticipating or experiencing the stress. Blood pressure control seems to be primarily dependent on peripheral vascular mechanisms: anticipatory changes seem to depend on cholinergically mediated shifts in regional blood flow, whereas changes during stress depend on alpha-adrenergically mediated shifts in peripheral vascular resistance. In addition, the changes in peripheral vascular resistance are in part influenced by afferent activity from the heart coursing in peripheral cardiac nerves.

Few previous studies have investigated CNS mechanisms controlling CV function during Sidman avoidance stress. Recent data from our laboratory suggest that the amygdala and associated pathways may play an important role in regulating the CV system during a specific behavioral stress. In addition, analyses of putative neurotransmitters and their metabolites in forebrain nuclei suggest that the serotonin system may be of importance in regulating CV function during stress.

It seems clear that the elucidation of peripheral neural mechanisms is progressing well, but that more emphasis must be placed on the investigation of CNS mechanisms responsible for CV regulation during behavioral stress.

ACKNOWLEDGMENTS

We thank Mr. Lewis Clarke, Ms. Virginia Johnson and Mr. John Smith, who provided helpful suggestions, data collection and analysis, and Ms. Helen Patterson and Ms. Alicia Benitez for typing and proofreading. Preparation of this manuscript was supported in part by NIH grant HL24127 and VA-MRIS 1603.

REFERENCES

Anderson, D.E. and Brady, J.V. (1971) Preavoidance blood pressure elevations accompanied by heart rate decreases in the dog. Science 172, 595-597.

Anderson, D.E. and Brady, J.V. (1972) Differential preparatory cardiovascular responses to amine and operative behavioral conditioning. Condit. Refl. 7, 82-96.

Anderson, D.E. and Brady, J.V. (1973) Prolonged preavoidance effects upon blood pressure and heart rate in the dog. Psychosom. Med. 35, 4-12.

Anderson, D.E. and Brady, J.V. (1976) Cardiovascular responses to avoidance conditioning in the dog; effects of beta adrenergic blockade. Psychosom. Med. 38, 181-189.

Anderson, D.E., Yingling, J.E. and Brady, J.V. (1976) Cardiovascular responses to avoidance conditioning in the dog: effects of alpha adrenergic blockade. Pav. J. Biol. Sci. 11, 150-161.

Galosy, R.A. and Clarke, L.K. (1980) The effect of left dorsal and ventral ansa subclavian transection on cardiac changes during behavioral stress in dogs. Physiol. Behav. 25, 195-203.

Galosy, R.A., Clarke, L.K. and Mitchell, J.H. (1979) Cardiac changes during behavioral stress in dogs. Amer. J. Physiol. 236, 750-758.

Galosy, R.A., Clarke, L.K., Vasko, M.R. and Crawford, I.L. (1981) Neurophysiology and neuropharmacology of cardiovascular regulation and stress. Neurosci. Biobehav. Res. 5, 137-175.

Lawler, J.R., Obrist, P.A. and Lawler, K.E. (1975) Cardiovascular function during pre-avoidance, avoidance and post-avoidance periods in dogs. Psychophysiology 12, 4-11.

Wada, J.A., ed. (1981) Kindling II. Raven Press, New York, pp. 1-361.

Published 1982 by Elsevier Science Publishing Co., Inc.
Smith, Galosy, and Weiss, editors
CIRCULATION, NEUROBIOLOGY, AND BEHAVIOR

Stress and Cardiomyopathy

K. C. CORLEY
Department of Physiology, Medical College of Virginia, Richmond, Virginia

Even though the mortality attributed to cardiovascular (CV) disorders has decreased in recent years, CV disease remains the leading cause of death in the United States (Cohen and Cabot, 1979). While many factors contribute to this mortality, stress has been demonstrated to be involved with all the major types of CV disease (Henry and Stephens, 1977). Numerous reports have shown that CV disorders in humans are associated with traumatic life events (Cebelin and Hirsch, 1980; Engel, 1971; Parkes et al., 1969). Because these studies, of necessity, must be retrospective, accurate analysis of the relation between events and pathology is almost impossible. Thus, only animal models of these phenomena can accurately assess the relation between environmental stressors and pathophysiology. Since myocardial pathology and dysfunction can be elicited by brief exposure to environmental stressors, these disturbances necessarily have few antecedent events. Therefore, a relation with stressors of myocardial pathology and dysfunction should be more easily described than that of other disturbances, i.e., stress-induced atherosclerosis or chronic hypertension, which require repeated exposure to stressors for development of symptoms. Although many factors may predispose an organism to stress-induced myopathy or arrhythmias, the initiating mechanisms should be identifiable. The rapidity of the occurrence of these phenomena suggests neurogenic involvement, particularly the autonomic nervous system.

Intense autonomic nervous system activity has been demonstrated to induce myocardial pathology and dysfunction. While histochemical alterations and modification of subcellular organelles associated with cardiomyopathy have been described (Jonsson and Johanson, 1974), light microscopic changes identified as myofibrillar degeneration (Reichenbach and Benditt, 1968) and coagulative myocytolysis (Baroldi, 1975) have been studied more often. The earliest changes are a hypercontraction of myofibrils and cross-band formations, which are selectively stained by fuchsin. The fuchsinophilia marks either the entire cell or a specific portion, giving a banded appearance (Fig. 1A, B). Necrosis is also observed as clear evidence of tissue damage with myocytolysis and leukocytic infiltration (Fig. 1C). Although some of these early changes may be reversible (Selye, 1958), permanent damage is indicated by myocardial fibrosis which is elaborated in experiments terminated more than 7 days after the stress (Fig. 1C). While this cardiopathy is concentrated in the subendocardium of the left ventricle, the changes are widespread, and the affected muscle fibers or fiber segments are surrounded by apparently normal tissue.

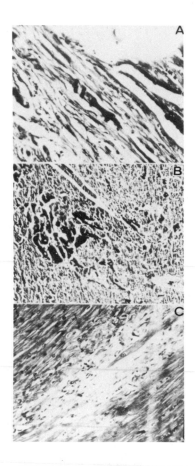

Fig. 1. Myocardial lesions observed with Masson trichrome stain in 5-μm sections from left ventricle of experimental monkeys. **A:** fuchsinophilia in segmental transverse bar configuration (338X). **B:** fuchsinophilia involving discrete staining of the cross-sectional and longitudinal portions of individual myocardial cells (250X). **C:** infarct-like lesion showing myofibrillary disintegration, cellular infiltration and fibrosis (250X). (After Corley et al., 1973b.)

Myocardial pathology and dysfunction have been associated with sympathetic innervation and related to norepinephrine (NE). Sustained infusions of NE have been shown to induce both morphological and hemodynamic alterations (Moss and Schenk, 1970). While hemodynamic alterations were blocked by alpha-adrenergic receptor blockade, the morphological changes were prevented by beta-adrenergic receptor blockade. Because the myopathy occurred in the absence of the hemodynamic alterations, it was induced by activation of beta-adrenergic receptors alone, and the hemodynamic alterations were not necessary for the NE-induced lesions. Furthermore, the hemodynamic alterations in the absence of the cardiopathy indicated that they were not caused by the lesions.

Although acetylcholine-induced cardiomyopathy has been reported, direct parasympathetic involvement is not the only explanation. Subendocardial degeneration and fibrosis were associated with chronic infusion of acetylcholine (Hall et al., 1936), and with chronic electrical stimulation of the vagus (Groover and Stout, 1965; Manning et al., 1937). Horswell (1941), however, failed to find any significant acetylcholine-induced myocardial pathology. Corley et al. (1973a) also attempted to induce cardiopathy by vagal stimulation. Because vagal stimulation could elicit a reflex enhancement of sympathetic activity, the preparation was spinalized, and cardiac beta-adrenergic receptors blocked. Although vagal stimulation produced sustained bradycardia, myocardial pathology was not observed. Thus, parasympathetic stimulation *per se* was not found to induce myocardial pathology. The most likely explanation for these contradictory reports is an indirect activation of the sympathetic myocardial innervation.

Other points on the neuraxis that mediate sympathetic input to the myocardium have also been found to induce myocardial pathology and arrhythmias. Acute cervical spinal cord injury has been shown to elicit electrocardiographic (EKG) changes and hypertension, as well as myofibrillar degeneration (Greenhoot and Mauck, 1972; Greenhoot et al., 1972). Similar hemodynamic and morphological changes have been induced by electrical stimulation of the brain stem (Chen et al., 1974; Greenhoot and Reinchenbach, 1969) and lateral hypothalamus (Melville et al., 1963, 1969). EKG abnormalities of ST segment and T waves associated with increased intracranial pressure have also been shown to be indicative of cardiomyopathy in animals (Burch et al., 1967; Eichbaum et al., 1965; Hawkins and Clower, 1971) and in man (Cannon, 1957, Shuster, 1960). Since the myocardial pathology is similar to that induced by NE and the changes can be blocked by autonomic blockade, these cardiomyopathies are attributed to the sympathetic release of NE in the myocardium.

Enhanced sympathetic activity induced by central nervous system (CNS) stimulation has also been related to myocardial dysfunction and sudden cardiac death. Ventricular fibrillation, which frequently precedes cardiac death in humans, can be influenced by sympathetic inputs. Susceptibility to ventricular fibrillation increases during NE infusion (Rabinowitz et al., 1976) and decreases with a reduction in sympathetic tone (Lown et al., 1977). Ventricular fibrillation threshold can also be reduced by posterior hypothalamic stimulation (Verrier et al., 1975). Because other hemodynamic changes were blocked by vagotomy and adrenalectomy without affecting the fibrillation threshold changes, the reduction in ventricular fibrillation threshold was not directly related to other CV alterations induced by the stimulation. Since these changes were also prevented by beta-adrenergic receptor blockade, the reduction in ventricular fibrillation threshold was attributed to the direct sympathetic release of NE in myocardium which was induced by the hypothalamic stimulation.

Myocardial dysfunction and arrest may also result from a decrease or cessation of autonomic input to the myocardium. Stimulation of the cingulate gyrus has been shown to produce sinus bradycardia, ventricular arrest, and atrial flutter and fibrillation (Mauck, 1973). Since vagotomy abolished these arrhythmias, the dysfunction was attributed to enhanced parasympathetic input to the myocardium. Septal stimulation has also been shown to decrease ventricular contraction, heart rate and blood pressure (Manning et al., 1963). While vagotomy did not affect these responses, decreased ventricular contraction and heart rate were abolished by either surgical denervation of the myocardium or beta-adrenergic receptor blockers. Since hypotension was blocked only by alpha-adrenergic blockers, which did not affect the reduction in contraction and heart rate, these CV changes were attributed to an inhibition of sympathetic tone and were not secondary to the pressure change. Therefore, CNS-mediated myocardial dysfunction and possibly sudden cardiac death may involve an autonomic imbalance that may be associated with sympathetic activation, parasympathetic activation, or sympathetic inhibition.

Research has also demonstrated that the infusion of pharmacological agents or electrical stimulation of the CNS is not necessary to induce myocardial pathology and dysfunction. Cardiomyopathy can be elicited by exposure to noxious stimuli, i.e., electrical shock (Hirsch and Zylberszac, 1947; Johannson et al., 1974) or presentation to rats of a cat-rat fight recording (Raab et al., 1964). Intense psychosocial stimulation over 6 months can result in not only myocardial pathology but also atherosclerotic degeneration and kidney damage in mice (Henry et al., 1971). Crowding over two weeks can induce cardiomyopathy as well as pulmonary and liver problems in rabbits (Weber and Van der Walt, 1973). While the extent of myocardial damage was not sufficient to be a primary contributor, animals also succumbed to the environmental stressors in these experiments.

Other experiments also suggest that environmental stressors can be involved in sudden cardiac death. Rats exposed to a swimming task succumbed within 5-10 min (Richter, 1957). Although a bradycardia occurred immediately before death, stress-induced, vagal-mediated cardiac arrest has been challenged as the mechanism of death. The alternative explanation is that the rats drowned while they were searching the tank bottom for an escape route (Hughes et al., 1978).

Myocardial dysfunction has also been associated with electrical shock. Dogs were more susceptible to ventricular fibrillation in an environment where they had previously experienced shock than in an environment where they had not (Lown et al., 1973). Because these pathophysiological phenomena could be reduced or prevented by manipulation of autonomic input to the myocardium, activation of CNS autonomic mechanisms is necessary for their occurrence. While cardiomyopathy was related to sympathetic release of NE on myocardial beta-receptors, myocardial dysfunction involved either sympathetic or parasympathetic activation, which induced an autonomic imbalance or electrical instability that resulted in sudden cardiac death.

Psychological factors in humans associated with life events have been shown to be important contributors to myocardial pathology and dysfunction. Myocardial infarction in many individuals has been related to an increase in life stress before the onset of dysfunction (Rahe et al., 1974; Theorell and Rahe, 1975). Voodoo deaths seem to be related to a victim's belief that an influential person has the power to control their life or death (Cannon, 1957; Wintrob, 1972). Widowhood has been found to increase the incidence of death related to CV disease (Parkes et al., 1969). All of these situations, which provoke the pathophysiology, are associated with a threat to continued life that is more imagined than real.

While psychological factors are difficult to study in animal experiments, they can be manipulated, and behavioral effects of an electrical shock can be separated from the physical effects. Unsignaled shock avoidance is a behavioral situation that uses shock to establish avoidance responding (Sidman, 1953). While shock in primate experiments is initially necessary to establish the avoidance responding, few shocks are necessary to sustain a constant state of vigilance and regular responding over long periods. Exposure to long sessions of unsignaled shock avoidance has been shown to induce a variety of disorders. Sessions of 6-hr "on" avoidance alternated with 6-hr "off" avoidance have induced lethal gastrointestinal lesions in rhesus macaques (Porter et al., 1958). Hypertension, however, occurred when rhesus macaques were exposed to 12-hr "on-off" avoidance (Forsyth, 1968, 1969). Unsignaled shock avoidance induces psychosomatic disorders in monkeys and the type of pathology seems to be related to the "on-off" characteristics of the schedule.

Additional evidence of psychological factors was found in studies of the incidence of gastrointestinal ulcers in "yoked-pair" studies. In these studies, a monkey trained on an avoidance schedule was connected in series with a yoked partner, which received each shock delivered to the avoidance monkey. The yoked monkey had no way to control shock occurrence. Both avoidance and yoked animals developed gastrointestinal lesions. While the ulcers were more extensive in the avoidance than the yoked monkeys (Porter et al., 1958), in similar studies using rats there was a higher incidence in the yoked partner than in the avoidance animal (Weiss, 1972). This discrepancy may be due to the avoidance performance itself. Response contingencies associated with avoidance behavior were more stressful in the avoidance monkey, and the unpredictability of shock occurrence was more stressful in the yoked rat. Although stress-induced pathology associated with unsignaled shock avoidance may be induced by both the avoidance and yoked situations, these results indicate that psychological factors are more important for the occurrence of stress-induced pathology than electrical shock itself.

Unsignaled shock avoidance has also been shown to produce myocardial pathology and dysfunction in the squirrel monkey. Exposure to shock avoidance for 1 hr a day for over two years resulted in elevated serum cholesterol, 17-ketosteroids, coronary artery atherosclerosis, and ST and T wave changes in the EKG (Lang, 1967). We found additional pathology and dysfunction when the avoidance paradigm was modified (Corley et al., 1973b). Squirrel monkeys trained in unsignaled shock avoidance and then exposed to 8-hr "on-off" avoidance showed cardiomyopathy and arrhythmias. Myocardial fuchsinophilia and fibrosis (Fig. 1) were significantly greater in avoidance monkeys than in other animals that were only restrained for a comparable period (Table 1). While restraint monkeys exhibited only EKG rate changes, ST and T wave changes were the most common rhythm disturbance in the avoidance monkeys (Fig. 2). Heart rate changes included an initial tachycardia followed by a bradycardia, which usually stabilized at about 200 bpm. A profound rate decrease with a rate drop from 200 to below 100 in 5-10 min was noted in two monkeys during the "off" avoidance period. Physical debilitation accompanied this slowing and was characterized by a loss of motor tone and a failure to respond to sensory stimuli. While one monkey was immediately sacrificed, the bradycardia progressed to cardiac arrest in the other monkey. Thus, both myocardial pathology and dysfunction were induced in squirrel monkeys by training in unsignaled shock avoidance followed by 8-hr "on-off" avoidance. Because the morphological changes were similar to those previously induced by the effects of NE on myocardial beta-receptors, the cardiomyopathy was attributed to enhanced sympathetic activity. Since ventricular asystole was observed, myocardial dysfunction with cardiac arrest also seemed to involve parasympathetic activity.

We studied the effects of this shock stress in yoked pairs of squirrel monkeys, to determine whether the myocardial pathology and dysfunction could be related to the response contingencies associated with the avoidance situation rather than shock itself (Corley et al., 1975). Shock stress for each pair, however, had to be terminated earlier than planned owing to the previously described physical debilitation and/or ventricular

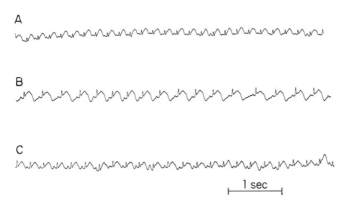

A

B

C

|—— 1 sec ——|

Fig. 2. EKG obtained from experimental monkey during a 1-hr shock avoidance session. A: the beginning of the session shows a normal heart rate of 270 bpm. B: an irregular heart rate from 137 to 198 bpm with marked ST elevation and T wave changes, which are indicative of myocardial pathology and dysfunction, occurred during the middle of the session. C: EKG returns towards normal with heart rate from 224 to 240 bpm, and a reduction in the number of ST and T wave abnormalities observed by the end of the session. The EKG was normal again by the next training session.

TABLE 1

FUCHSINOPHILIA AND FIBROSIS ASSOCIATED WITH RESTRAINT ALONE AND WITH 8-HR "ON-OFF" AVOIDANCE AFTER TRAINING

Condition	N	Ratings[a]					X^{2b}
		0	1	2	3	4	
Restraint	8	2	4	2	0	0	
Avoidance	9	0	0	4	4	1	$(p<0.001)$ 12.21

[a]Ratings: 0, no change; 1, isolated fuchsinophilia (or fibrosis); 2, widespread fuchsinophilia (or fibrosis) or focal fuchsinophilia and fibrosis; 3, isolated fuchsinophilia (or fibrosis) combined with widespread fibrosis (or fuchsinophilia); 4, widespread fuchsinophilia and fibrosis.

[b]X^2 is the Kolmogorov-Smirnov two-sample test of differences from restraint alone.

asystole. While only one avoidance monkey required the stress to be stopped, five yoked monkeys succumbed before their partners showed any adverse effects of the stress. Blood pressure recorded during severe bradycardia remained adequate until asystole occurred (Fig. 3). Thus, vasopressor syncope did not seem to be involved in the stress-induced cardiac arrest. Pathology was again restricted to the myocardium, but no significant differences were found among restraint, avoidance and yoked stress situations (Table 2). Because the experiment was terminated early, the stress in the avoidance situation was not sufficient to induce the myocardial pathology previously observed. Although the relation of cardiomyopathy to shock remained unclear, these data suggested that stress-induced cardiac arrest was more related to the inability to cope with shock stress in the yoked situation than contending with response contingencies in the avoidance situation.

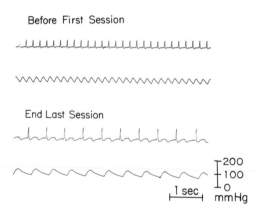

Before First Session

End Last Session

200
100
0

1 sec   mmHg

Fig. 3. EKG and systemic blood pressure recorded from a monkey before first and last sessions of 8-hr "on-off" stress. CV measures before the first session were 294 bpm and 110/75 mm Hg. Heart rate at the end of the last session dropped to 100 bpm, and blood pressure was decreased to 100/57 mm Hg. Physical debilitation accompanied this bradycardia, which was followed by ventricular asystole.

TABLE 2

FUCHSINOPHILIA AND FIBROSIS ASSOCIATED WITH RESTRAINT ALONE AND WITH 8-HR "ON-OFF" SHOCK STRESS IN YOKED PAIRS WITH TRAINED AVOIDANCE MONKEYS

Condition	N	Ratings[a]				
		0	1	2	3	4
Restraint	5	1	2	2	0	0
Avoidance	6	2	0	2	1	1
Yoked	6	1	2	2	1	1

[a]Ratings as in Table 1.

In another study, we modified the stress procedure so that the occurrence of myocardial pathology was enhanced in the avoidance situation, and the incidence of cardiac arrest was reduced in the yoked situation (Corley et al., 1977). Avoidance stress was intensified by exposing the avoidance monkeys to a single 24-hr stress session of unsignaled shock avoidance without prior adaptation or training in the experimental environment. While the yoked monkeys were randomly assigned to the avoidance or yoked situation, they were matched, as much as possible, with respect to body weight and aggressive behavior so that the potential contribution of these dispositional factors to the myocardial pathology and dysfunction was controlled. Since stress was limited to the single session, only fuchsinophilia and necrosis were elaborated. Although fuchsinophilia in both avoidance and yoked situations was greater than that observed with no stress (Table 3), comparison within yoked pairs revealed that fuchsinophilia was more extensive in the avoidance than yoked monkeys--Wilcoxon matched-pairs signed-ranks test $T (8) = 0$; $p<0.01$. Necrosis was also more evident in the avoidance than yoked situation (Table 3). While most monkeys were sacrificed at various time intervals after the stress, three avoidance and one yoked monkey succumbed to the stress. Because myocardial pathology and dysfunction in this study were more evident in the avoidance than the yoked situation, response contingencies associated with shock avoidance behavior in this stress paradigm were demonstrated to be more pathogenic than shock *per se*.

TABLE 3

FUCHSINOPHILIA AND NECROSIS ASSOCIATED WITH A SINGLE
24-HR SHOCK STRESS IN YOKED PAIRS WITHOUT PRIOR TRAINING
OF THE AVOIDANCE MONKEY

Condition	N	Fuchsinophilia						Necrosis					
		Ratings[a]					X^{2b}	Ratings[a]					X^{2b}
		0	1	2	3	4		0	1	2	3	4	
No stress	10	6	4	0	0	0		9	1	0	0	0	
Avoidance	11	0	3	2	4	2	12.26 ($p<0.01$)	3	6	1	1	0	8.32 ($p<0.05$)
Yoked	11	1	4	4	2	0	7.42 ($p<0.05$)	6	2	2	1	0	2.57

[a]Ratings: 0, no change; 1, small focal areas of diffuse changes involving less than 25% of the myocardium; 2, single large area with 25-30% of the myocardium affected; 3, 50-75% of the myocardium affected by diffuse changes; 4, several large areas or more than 75% of the myocardium affected.

[b]X^2 is Kolmogorov-Smirnov two-sample test of differences from no stress.

We have also studied autonomic involvement in this pathophysiology (Corley et al., 1979). The incidence of myocardial pathology and dysfunction was investigated after the selective removal of either parasympathetic (vagotomy) or sympathetic (propranolol) input to the myocardium. Bilateral cervical vagotomy alone induced myocardial pathology. After a single 24-hr shock stress session, the hearts of vagotomized monkeys displayed fibrosis as well as significant fuchosinophilia and necrosis (Table 4). Since fibrosis cannot be elaborated rapidly enough to occur as a result of the 24-hr shock stress, it and some of the other pathology were attributed to enhanced sympathetic activity associated with vagotomy. While both fuchsinophilia and necrosis were significantly different from those in nonstressed animals, vagotomy confounded any differences between the avoidance and yoked situations (Table 4). The ability of propranolol to block these lesions was evidence that the action of NE on myocardial beta-adrenergic receptors was involved in this pathology (Table 4).

TABLE 4

FUCHSINOPHILIA, NECROSIS AND FIBROSIS ASSOCIATED WITH NO STRESS AND WITH 24-HR SHOCK STRESS IN VAGOTOMIZED AND PROPRANOLOL-INJECTED ANIMALS WITHOUT PRIOR TRAINING[a]

Condition	N	Fuchsinophilia		Necrosis		Fibrosis	
		Ratings	X^2	Ratings	X^2	Ratings	X^2
		0 1 2 3 4		0 1 2 3 4		0 1 2 3 4	
No Stress	10	6 4 0 0 0		9 1 0 0 0		10 0 0 0 0	
Vagotomy:							
Avoidance	6	0 1 4 1 0	10.33^b	0 2 1 1 2	12.15^b	3 2 1 0 0	3.76
Yoked	6	0 1 4 0 1	10.33^b	0 2 3 1 0	12.15^b	4 1 0 0 1	1.67
Propranolol:							
Avoidance	6	2 1 2 1 0	3.75	3 3 0 0 0	2.40	5 1 0 0 0	0.42

[a]Ratings and X^2 as in Table 3.
[b]$p < 0.01$

Autonomic manipulations, however, were not found to prevent stress-induced dysfunction. Reduction of parasympathetic activity by atropine had mixed effects (Corley and Mauck, 1974). While atropine sometimes reversed heart rate decreases, at other times the bradycardia was unaffected and ventricular asystole followed. Furthermore, stress-induced cardiac arrest was observed in vagotomized monkeys (Fig. 4) (Corley et al., 1979). Since a monkey that had received propranolol also succumbed, an autonomic imbalance associated with the removal of either autonomic input was suggested to be involved. Thus, either electrical instability induced by increased sympathetic activity after vagotomy or enhanced parasympathetic activity after beta-adrenergic receptor blockade may induce cardiac arrest.

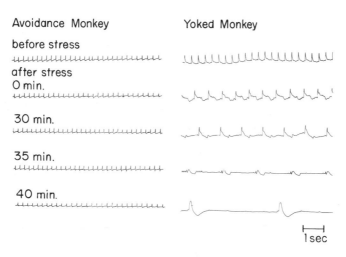

Fig. 4. EKG from a pair of vagotomized monkeys before and during a stress session. While the heart rate and rhythm of the avoidance monkey remained stable at 300-312 bpm throughout stress, the yoked monkey exhibited severe bradycardia and arrhythmias. The yoked monkey's heart rate was 220 bpm before stress, and during the 10th hour of stress it slowed to 108 bpm at 0 min, 69 bpm at 30 min, 54 bpm at 35 min, and 13 bpm at 40 min. Dysfunction at the beginning of the 10th hour was indicated by an elevation of the ST segment during the initial 30 min, and then a complete heart block occurred immediately before cardiac arrest.

In summary, environmental stress through the activation of neural autonomic pathways was shown to be capable of inducing myocardial pathology and dysfunction. This pathophysiology is similar whether elicited by direct activation of the neuraxis or by behavioral stress. While environmental stimuli could induce myocardial pathology and dysfunction, psychological factors associated with these stimuli were also important in the incidence of these phenomena. Study of the stress effects of unsignaled shock avoidance with yoked pairs permitted analysis of these psychological factors. Although myocardial pathology was previously observed in avoidance monkeys subjected to sessions of 8-hr "on-off" avoidance, yoked monkeys succumbed before significant pathology was found in their avoidance partners. When this stress was modified to a continuous 24-hr session without training of the avoidance monkey, myocardial pathology and dysfunction were most evident in avoidance monkeys. Analysis of the autonomic contribution to this pathophysiology suggested that the cardiomyopathy results from the action of NE on beta-adrenergic receptors of the myocardium, and myocardial dysfunction was associated with an autonomic imbalance of inputs to the myocardium.   Thus, environmental stress in squirrel monkeys can be induced through the autonomic innervation with occurrence of myocardial pathology and/or dysfunction depending on psychological factors associated with the ability to cope with the stress.

REFERENCES

Baroldi, G. (1975) Different morphological types of myocardial cell death in man; in Recent Advances in Studies on Cardiac Structure and Metabolism, Vol. 6. Pathophysiology and Morphology of Myocardial Cell Alterations, A. Fleckenstein and G. Rona, eds. University Park Press, Baltimore, pp. 383-397.

Burch, G.E., Sun, S.C., Colcolough, H.L., Pasquale, H.P. and Sohal, R.S. (1967) Acute myocardial lesions following experimentally-induced intracranial hemorrhage in mice. Arch. Path. 84, 517-521.

Cannon, W.B. (1957) "Voodoo" death. Psychosom. Med. 19, 182-190.

Cebelin, M.S. and Hirsch, C.S. (1980) Human stress cardiomyopathy: myocardial lesions in victims of homicidal assaults without internal injuries. Hum. Path. 11, 123-132.

Chen, H.J., Sun, S.C., Chai, C.Y., Kau, S.L. and Kau, C. (1974) Encephalogenic cardiomyopathy after stimulation of the brain stem of monkeys. Amer. J. Cardiol. 33, 845-852.

Cohen, D.H. and Cabot, J.B. (1979) Toward a cardiovascular neurobiology.   Trends Neurosci. 2, 273-276.

Corley, K.C. and Mauck, H.P. (1974) Autonomic nervous system involvement in cardiac dysfunction. Soc. Neurosci. Abstr. 4, 177.

Corley, K.C., Mauck, H.P. and Shiel, F.O'M. (1975) Cardiac responses associated with "yoked-chair" shock avoidance in squirrel monkeys. Psychophysiology 12, 439-444.

Corley, K.C., Mauck, H.P., Shiel, F.O'M., Barber, J.H., Clark, L.S. and Blocher, C.R. (1979) Myocardial dysfunction and pathology associated with environmental stress in squirrel monkey: effect of vagotomy and propranolol. Psychophysiology 16, 554-560.

Corley, K.C., Shiel, F.O'M. and Mauck, H.P. (1973a) The effect of vagal stimulation on the myocardium in the cat. Proc. Soc. Exp. Biol. Med. 144, 909-911.

Corley, K.C., Shiel, F.O'M, Mauck, H.P., Clark, L.S. and Barber, J.H. (1977) Myocardial degeneration and cardiac arrest in squirrel monkey: physiological and psychological correlates. Psychophysiology 14, 322-328.

Corley, K.C., Shiel, F.O'M., Mauck, H.P. and Greenhoot, J.H. (1973b) Electrocardiographic and cardiac morphological changes associated with environmental stress in squirrel monkeys. Psychosom. Med. 35, 361-364.

Eichbaum, F.W., Gazetta, B., Bissetti, P.C. and Pereira, C.B. (1965) Electrocardiographic disturbances following acute increase of intracranial pressure experiments in dogs. Z. Ges. Exp. Med. 139, 721-734.

Engel, G.L. (1971) Sudden and rapid death during psychological stress: folklore or folk wisdom? Ann. Intern. Med. 74, 771-782.

Forsyth, R.P. (1968) Blood pressure and avoidance conditioning: a study of 15-day trials in rhesus monkey. Psychosom. Med. 30, 125-235.

Forsyth, R.P. (1969) Blood pressure responses to long-term avoidance schedules in the restrained rhesus monkey. Psychosom. Med. 31, 300-309.

Greenhoot, J.H. and Mauck, H.P. (1972) The effect of cervical cord injury on cardiac rhythm and conduction. Amer. Heart. J. 83, 659-662.

Greenhoot, J.H., Shiel, F.O'M. and Mauck, H.P. (1972) Experimental spinal cord injury. Arch. Neurol. 26, 524-529.

Greenhoot, J.H. and Reichenbach, D.D. (1969) Cardiac injury and subarachnoid hemorrhage. J. Neurosurg. 30, 521-531.

Groover, M.E. and Stout, C. (1965) Neurogenic myocardial necrosis. Angiology 16, 180-186.

Hall, G.E., Ettinger, G.H. and Banting, F.G. (1936) An experimental production of coronary thrombosis and myocardial failure. Canad. Med. Ass. J. 34, 9-15.

Hawkins, W.E. and Clower, B.R. (1971) Myocardial damage after head trauma and simulated intracranial hemorrhage in mice: the role of the autonomic nervous system. Cardiovasc. Res. 5, 524-529.

Henry, J.P., Ely, D.L., Stephens, P.M., Ratcliffe, H.L., Santisteban, G.A. and Shapiro, A.P. (1971) The role of psychosocial factors in the development of arteriosclerosis in mice. Atherosclerosis 14, 203-218.

Henry, J.P. and Stephens, P.M. (1977) Stress, Health and the Social Environment. Springer-Verlag, New York.

Hirsch, S. and Zylberszac, S. (1947) Cardiac infarcts induced by excitation and over exertion of rats. Exp. Med. Surg. 5, 383-390.

Horswell, R.G. (1941) Observations on the production of myocardial disease with acetyl-choline. Amer. Heart J. 22, 116-121.

Hughes, C.W., Stein, E.A., and Lynch, J.J. (1978) Hopelessness-induced sudden death in rats. J. Nerv. Ment. Dis. 166, 387-401.

Johannson, G., Jonsson, L., Lanneck, N., Blomgren, L., Lindberg, P. and Poupa, O. (1974) Severe stress-cardiopathy in pigs. Amer. Heart J. 87, 451-457.

Jonsson, L. and Johanson, G. (1974) Cardiac muscle cell damage induced by restraint stress. Virchows Arch. B Cell Path. 17, 1-12.

Lang, C.M. (1967) Effects of psychic stress on atherosclerosis in the squirrel monkey. Proc. Soc. Exp. Biol. Med. 126, 30-34.

Lown, B., Verrier, R.L. and Corbalan, R. (1973) Psychological stress and threshold for repetitive ventricular response. Science 182, 834-836.

Lown, B., Verrier, R.L. and Rabinowitz, S.H. (1977) Neural and psychological mechanisms and problems of sudden cardiac death. Amer. J. Cardiol. 39, 890-902.

Manning, G.W., Hall, G.E. and Banting, F.G. (1937) Vagal stimulation and the production of myocardial damage. Canad. Med. Ass. J. 37, 314-318.

Manning, J.W., Charbon, G.A. and Cotten, M.DeV. (1963) Inhibition of tonic cardiac sympathetic activity by stimulation of brain septal region. Amer. J. Physiol. 205, 1221-1226.

Mauck, H.P. (1973) Neural effects on cardiac rate and rhythm. MCV Quarterly 9, 11-12.

Melville, K.I., Blum, B., Shister, H.E. and Silver, M.D. (1963) Cardiac ischemic changes and arrhythmias induced by hypothalamic stimulation. Amer. J. Cardiol. 12, 781-791.

Melville, K.I., Garvey, H.L., Shister, H.E. and Knaack, J. (1969) Central nervous system stimulation and cardiac ischemic changes in monkeys. Ann. N.Y. Acad. Sci. 156, 241-260.

Moss, A.J. and Schenk, E.A. (1970) Cardiovascular effects of sustained norepinephrine infusions in dogs. Circulat. Res. 27, 1013-1022.

Parkes, C.M., Benjamin, B. and Fitzgerald, R.G. (1969) Broken heart: a statistical study of increased mortality among widowers. Brit. Med. J. 1, 740-743.

Porter, R.W., Brady, J.V., Conrad, D., Mason, J.W., Galambos, R. and Rioch, D.McK. (1958) Some experimental observations on gastrointestinal lesions in behaviorally conditioned monkeys. Psychosom. Med. 20, 379-394.

Raab, W., Chaplin, J.P. and Bajusz, E. (1964) Myocardial necroses produced in domesticated rats and wild rats by sensory and emotional stresses. Proc. Soc. Exp. Biol. Med. 116, 665-669.

Rabinowitz, S.H., Verrier, R.L. and Lown, B. (1976) Muscarinic effects of vagosympathetic trunk stimulation on the repetitive extrasystole (RE) threshold. Circulation 53, 622-627.

Rahe, R.H., Romo, M., Bennett, L. and Siltanen, P. (1974) Recent life changes, myocardial infarction and abrupt coronary death. Arch. Intern. Med. 113, 221-228.

Reichenbach, D.D. and Benditt, E.P. (1968) Myofibrilla degeneration: a response of the myocardial cell to injury. Arch. Path. 85, 189-199.

Richter, C.P. (1957) On phenomenon of sudden death in animals and man. Psychosom. Med. 38, 191-198.

Selye, H. (1958) The Chemical Prevention of Cardiac Necroses. Ronald Press, New York.

Shuster, S. (1960) The electrocardiogram in subarachnoid hemorrhage. Brit. Heart J. 22, 316-320.

Sidman, M. (1953) Avoidance conditioning with brief shock and no exteroceptive warning signal. Science 118, 157-158.

Theorell, T. and Rahe, R.H. (1975) Life change events, ballistocardiography and coronary death. J. Hum. Stress 1, 18-24.

Verrier, R.L., Calvert, A. and Lown, B. (1975) Effect of posterior hypothalamic stimulation on ventricular fibrillation threshold. Amer. J. Physiol. 228, 923-927.

Weber, H.W. and Van der Walt, J.J. (1973) Cardiomyopathy in crowded rabbits: a preliminary report. S. Afr. Med. J. 47, 1591-1595.

Weiss, J.M. (1972) Somatic effects of predictable and unpredictable shock. Sci. Amer. 226, 104-113.

Wintrob, R. (1972) Hexes, roots, snake eggs? MD vs. occult. Med. Opinion 1, 54-57.

Ingestive Behavior and the Circulation

JOHN B. SIMPSON
Department of Psychology, University of Washington, Seattle, Washington

It has long been known that there is a relation between ingestive behavior and the cardiovascular (CV) system. For example, long-term hydromineral and caloric intake can be related to circulatory alterations, such as the relations between sodium intake or obesity and hypertension. On the other hand, the actual behaviors of eating and drinking produce changes in various circulatory parameters. As is the case with other behaviors, the patterns of circulatory changes seen during eating or drinking are specific to the behavior. Further, if one examines drinking behavior in response to dehydration, one finds that it is altogether appropriate for circulatory adjustments to accompany alterations in water intake and excretion. Such adjustments, however, function as interim measures only; the animal must replenish depleted fluid reserves with behavioral means in order to restore both circulatory and fluid homeostasis. This paper will review some of the relations between the circulation and ingestive behavior, and the case will be made that the dehydrated animal offers an excellent model for illustration of the synergy between various behavioral and physiological mechanisms directed at maintaining homeostasis.

The concept that distinct patterns of CV changes accompany different behaviors is illustrated in Figure 1, which shows different patterns of circulatory alterations seen during eating behavior or during exercise in conscious baboons. Moderate exercise for 4 min is accompanied by a substantial tachycardia along with a large increase in mean blood pressure and terminal aortic blood flow, while renal blood flow decreases. In addition, terminal aortic resistance decreases while renal resistance increases. These circulatory changes during moderate exercise are substantial, and contrast with the pattern of alterations seen during eating. During the ingestive behavior, mean aortic pressure and heart rate increase slightly, as do terminal aortic resistance and, to a lesser extent, renal resistance. Terminal aortic flow decreases, while renal flow appears unchanged. These data illustrate that different patterns of circulatory events accompany different behaviors, and that ingestion is related to distinctive circulatory alterations.

In the rat, water ingestion following a moderate (3-hr) water deprivation is accompanied by an increase in mean aortic pressure (Fig. 2). This pressor effect is time-locked to the onset of drinking, and in general outlasts the ingestion of water by less than

136

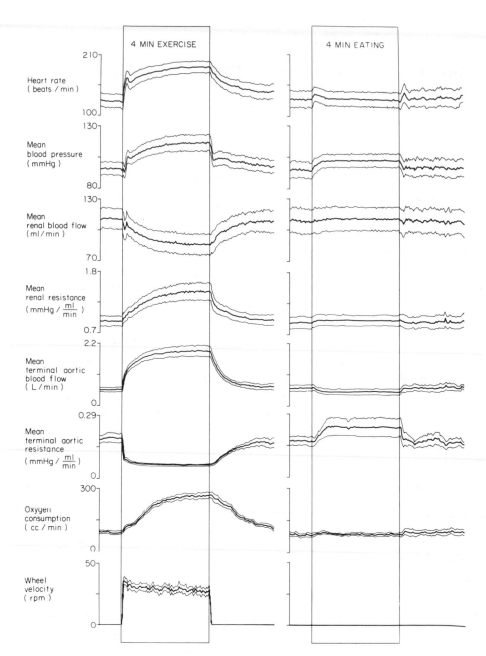

Fig. 1. Changes in CV parameters shown in conscious baboons during the behaviors of wheel-turning exercise or eating. Values are shown as means ± S.E.M. (From Smith et al., 1980, with permission.)

1 min. The amplitude of this effect is 12 mm Hg or less, and is maximal by 20 sec following the initiation of the behavior (Fig. 2).

If a rat is driven to drink by an intracranial injection of the hormone angiotensin II (A II), a pressor effect again accompanies this behavior (Fig. 2). However, this pressor effect is substantially greater than that seen following water ingestion per se, and it begins before the behavior and outlasts the behavior by several minutes. Increased secretion of renin by the kidney, which in turn leads to increased blood titers of A II, is one mechanism by which the dehydrated animal compensates for decreased fluid volume. Indeed, if the causes of drinking in the dehydrated animal are considered, it becomes clear that there are important homeostatic relations between fluid intake, fluid excretion, and the circulation. The remainder of this paper will focus on the interactions between some of the neural systems that control body fluid balance and some that adjust the circulation during dehydration.

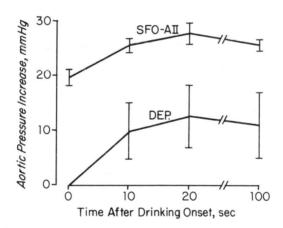

Fig. 2. Increases in mean aortic pressure as a function of time after onset of drinking behavior provoked by 3-hr water deprivation (DEP) or injection of A II into the SFO in rats. Values are means ± S.E.M.

It is now apparent that mammals drink for a variety of reasons, and their drinking falls into two categories: "primary" drinking, which is caused by dehydration, and "secondary" drinking, which occurs in the absence of any identified perturbation in fluid balance. Primary drinking will result following dehydration of either the cellular or the extracellular body fluid compartment. Either type of dehydration alone is sufficient to provoke water ingestion, and the interaction between the two classes of dehydration drinking is such that their effects on drinking are additive. Water deprivation will result in dehydration of both fluid compartments, and the water intake following dehydration will reflect both cellular and extracellular drinking.

Dehydration of the cellular fluid compartment produces water intake that typically is termed "cellular dehydration drinking" or "osmotic drinking." It is produced experimentally by increasing the effective osmolality of the interstitial fluid, thereby causing an osmotic shift of water from the intracellular to the extracellular compartment. The pioneering work of Verney (1947) introduced the concept of "forebrain osmoreceptors," neurons that function as mechanoreceptors that are sensitive to their own size. A decrease in cellular volume due to osmotic water loss is the adequate stimulus for these sensory receptors. Activation of osmoreceptors leads to antidiuresis (Verney, 1947), natriuresis (Thornborough et al., 1973), a pressor response (Johnson et al., 1978), and water intake (Holmes and Gregersen, 1950).

It appears that osmoreceptors are located within the basal forebrain. Blass and Epstein in the rat (1971) and Peck and Novin in the rabbit (1971) indicated that the lateral preoptic area most likely contained the osmoreceptors responsible for thirst. Hatton and colleagues (1976) found evidence of osmoreceptors in the nucleus circularis of the rostral hypothalamus. Andersson (1971) has suggested that in the goat the osmoreceptors are really ventricular sodium receptors, although this does not seem to be true in other species (Blass, 1974; Thrasher et al., 1980b). Finally, recent data suggest that osmoreceptors stimulated by intracarotid infusions of hypertonic solutions reside within the circumventricular organs (Thrasher et al., 1980a). Investigators agree that the osmoreceptors are located within the basal forebrain, and that these cells likely are not the magnocellular neurons of the supraoptic or paraventricular nuclei.

Loss of water from the extracellular fluid compartment also produces a constellation of cardiovascular, endocrine and behavioral adjustments directed at restoration of fluid imbalance. The receptors that monitor hypovolemia and lead to drinking following extracellular dehydration seem to be located in two separate areas. First, vascular afferents may be shown to monitor volume depletion, and contribute to homeostasis by causing circulatory alterations, secretion of vasopressin, and water intake. Recent data have indicated that destruction of the right atrial appendage in the sheep prevents the drinking caused by hypovolemia but does not affect the drinking caused by cellular dehydration (Zimmerman et al., 1981). These same receptors may contribute to vasopressin secretion during hypovolemia (Henry et al., 1968).

The second source of afferent information about hypovolemia is the renal secretion of renin. This secretion is the principal rate-determining step in the activity of the renin-angiotensin system, a hormonal system whose diverse effects can be understood as synergistic in defense of the extracellular fluid volume. The proteolytic enzyme, renin, acts in the circulation on renin substrate (angiotensinogen) to release the decapeptide, angiotensin I. Angiotensin I in turn is cleaved to form the octapeptide, angiotensin II (A II), through which most of the effects of the renin-angiotensin system are mediated (Reid et al., 1978).

The renin-angiotensin system has effects that may be divided conveniently into those that occur within the periphery and those that occur within the central nervous system (CNS). The major peripheral effects of this hormonal system include a potent pressor effect via action on vascular smooth muscle, thus helping to maintain blood flow to critical tissue beds in the hypovolemic animal. A II also modulates synaptic transmission within the sympathetic nervous system, and it is the principal modulator of the secretion of sodium-retaining aldosterone from the adrenal cortex.

A II acts on the CNS to provoke a variety of diverse actions that have in common the maintenance of blood flow in the hypovolemic animal and the restoration of depleted extracellular fluid stores. Thus it is now understood that A II acts centrally to cause a pressor effect that is independent of its action on the peripheral vasculature (Bickerton and Buckley, 1971). The central pressor effect of A II is mediated via both sympathetic discharge and secretion of vasopressin. Next, A II provokes pituitary secretion both of adrenocorticotropic hormone (Maran and Yates, 1977) and vasopressin (Keil et al., 1975). The former pituitary effect, via glucocorticoid secretion, sensitizes the vasculature to the pressor effects of catecholamines. Vasopressin secretion, besides producing a pressor effect, acts to prevent additional water loss from the kidney. Vasopressin and aldosterone, then, act in synergy to prevent further fluid depletion by minimizing water and sodium losses through urine formation.

We also know that A II acts centrally to provoke two effects that are the appropriate behavioral analogs of the effects of vasopressin and aldosterone at the kidney. Thus, A II acts centrally to provoke ingestion of both water (Epstein et al., 1970) and sodium (Bryant et al., 1980; Avrith and Fitzsimons, 1980). These behavioral effects are the only practical means by which water and salt balance may be restored in the hypovolemic animal.

There has been considerable interest in recent years in the location of receptors within the CNS for the actions of circulating A II (Phillips, 1978; Brody and Johnson, 1980; Simpson, 1981). However, A II does not cross the blood-brain barrier. This paradox is resolved by the presence within the brain of a collection of structures, the circumventricular organs, which lack the blood-brain barrier and hence are accessible to circulating polar peptides such as A II. These structures are located at several periventricular loci within the forebrain and hindbrain. They possess dense vascularization and fenestrated capillaries, and they border the cerebrospinal fluid of the third and fourth cerebral ventricles (Weindl, 1973). Included within the circumventricular organs are the area postrema of the medulla, the subfornical organ, organum vasculosum laminae terminalis, median eminence, and neurohypophysis of the forebrain. Several of these unique central structures have been identified as sites of action of A II for its effects on fluid balance (see Simpson, 1981, for review).

The subfornical organ (SFO) is located in the dorsal portion of the third ventricle, adjacent to the foramina of Monro (see Dellman and Simpson, 1978, for review). The neurons there are accessible to circulating A II, and they are richly interconnected with other forebrain loci (Miselis et al., 1979) that are thought to play a role in fluid homeostasis (Brody and Johnson, 1980). Circulating A II binds to the SFO (van Houten et al., 1980), and it appears that the peptide acts there to provoke the appropriate synergistic behavioral, circulatory and endocrine effects in the hypovolemic animal.

Our research strategy has been to study the central actions of A II at the SFO from two points of view: (1) that several effects of one peptide may emanate from a common receptor tissue, and (2) that the central effects of A II are synergistic. We have now determined that A II acts at the SFO not only to provoke drinking, but to produce a pressor effect and vasopressin secretion as well.

Previous work had indicated that the SFO was important for the A II effects on drinking (Simpson and Routtenberg, 1973; Simpson et al., 1978). A more recent study has observed the effects of A II injected into the SFO on drinking and blood pressure simultaneously (Mangiapane and Simpson, 1980a).

Rats were prepared with an intracranial cannula terminating in the SFO or in adjacent tissue. At one to two weeks following this surgery, each animal was fitted with an aortic catheter for direct measurement of mean aortic pressure. For the actual running of the experiment, animals were connected via polyethylene tubing for measurement of blood pressure and for remote intracranial injection via the chronic cannula. All tests were made in animals in which restraint was minimal, and in which blood pressure had stabilized before the intracranial injection was delivered. Injections consisted of Ile^5-angiotensin II delivered in 0.2 μl isotonic saline in doses of 10^{-16} to 10^{-11} moles.

The results of that study indicated that highly correlated increases in blood pressure and drinking were provoked by injection of angiotensin at the SFO (Fig. 3). Several observations deserve comment. The onset of the pressor response in all cases preceded the onset of drinking behavior (Fig. 4). For example, the onset of the pressor response following the 10^{-12} mole dose was 6.4 ± 3.0 sec, whereas the onset of drinking in these rats was 45.4 ± 6.3 sec. The lowest doses of A II tested provoked short-latency pressor responses in the animals in the absence, in some cases, of a drinking response. The threshold dose for the pressor response appeared to be lower than that for the drinking response. Both pressor and dipsogenic effects were antagonized by pretreatment with the competitive A II antagonist, saralasin. Finally, the pressor response was not secondary to the drinking because (1) the onset of the pressor effect always preceded the onset of drinking, if it occurred, (2) withholding drinking water reduced but did not eliminate the pressor response, and (3) chloralose anesthesia likewise reduced but did not eliminate the pressor response to A II in the SFO. These data clearly indicate that both pressor and dipsogenic effects of A II are provoked at a single locus of application.

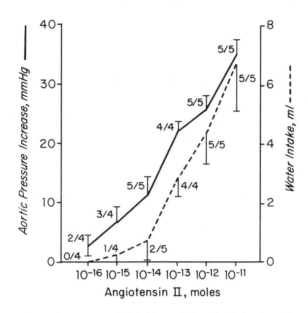

Fig. 3. Aortic pressure increase and drinking elicited by injection of various doses of A II into the SFO of rats. Denominator at each point is number of rats injected, and numerator is number that responded. Values are means ± S.E.M. (From Mangiapane and Simpson, 1980a, with permission.)

The central actions of angiotensin on drinking, blood pressure, and vasopressin secretion are synergistic, as noted above. If, then, these effects are means to a common homeostatic end, it would seem plausible that all three might emanate from a common locus of action. We have recently found that injection of A II into the subfornical organ will provoke increases in plasma vasopressin as well as drinking and the pressor response.

Animals were prepared with a single intracranial cannula terminating within the SFO or elsewhere within the forebrain (Simpson et al., 1979), and were tested twice for drinking following injection of 5 ng of A II. Then, 60 sec after a third injection, trunk blood was collected for measurement of plasma vasopressin by radioimmunoassay. Drinking water was not offered during the last test. Vasopressin levels increased following A II application at the SFO (17.4 ± 5.8 pg/ml vs. control of 2.4 ± 1.2 pg/ml). In these same animals, drinking had been elicited by prior A II injections (7.11 ml). Action of circulating A II at the SFO, then, provokes pressor, dipsogenic, and antidiuretic effects.

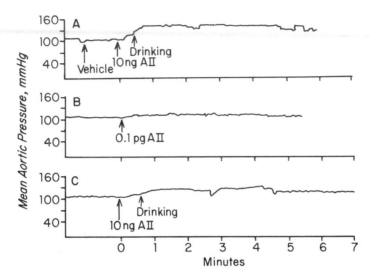

Fig. 4. Individual records from rats injected in the SFO (A, B) or adjacent third ventricle (C) showing relations between mean aortic pressure and the onset of drinking. Doses of A II are shown on records. (From Mangiapane and Simpson, 1980a, with permission.)

It thus seems that the animal simultaneously uses behavioral and physiological strategies for fluid balance and circulatory control, and that these effects may be produced by action of the hormone at one locus.

Another way of viewing the synergy between the central circulatory and fluid balance effects of A II is to study the effect of specific destruction of presumed receptor sites. As indicated above, the SFO is a locus at which three of the central actions of A II are provoked by injection of the hormone. The first experiment employing the lesion technique is illustrated in Figure 5 (Simpson et al., 1978). Animals were prepared with jugular catheters through which various doses of A II were infused. In addition, each animal received either a specific and localized lesion that destroyed the SFO, a control lesion of equivalent volume in adjacent tissue, or operative control procedures. In animals subjected to the operative control condition, intravenous infusion of A II at 8-128 ng/min provoked dose-dependent increases in water intake. Lesions adjacent to but not including the SFO did not prevent drinking to the A II infusion. In contrast, however, lesions of the SFO resulted in a complete elimination of the dipsogenic effect of intravenous A II. Subsequent studies found that this effect was permanent because animals still failed to respond to intravenous A II three months after receiving the SFO lesion. This effect also occurs in mongrel dogs (Thrasher et al., in press) and in opossums (Findlay et al., 1980). The effect of this lesion in rats and dogs is relatively specific to A II, because drinking in response to cellular dehydration is normal or slightly reduced (Simpson et al., 1978) and 24-hr daily water intakes are normal in the animals with SFO lesions (Simpson and Routtenberg, 1972).

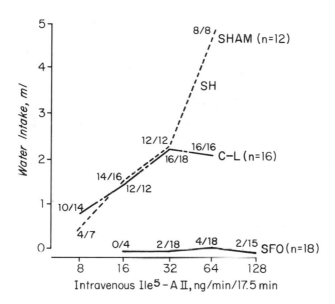

Fig. 5. Water intake as a function of dose of intravenous A II in rats with lesions of the subfornical organ (SFO), tissue adjacent to the subfornical organ (C-L), or operative controls (SHAM). Denominator at each point indicates number of animals infused, and numerator indicates number of rats that drank. (From Simpson et al., 1978, with permission.)

More recent studies have focused on the effects of the SFO lesion on the pressor effects of intravenous A II (Mangiapane and Simpson, 1980b). Lesions of this locus reduce the pressor effect of infusions of the peptide (Table 1). However, whereas the dipsogenic effect of similar doses of systemic A II is completely eliminated by the lesion, the pressor effect is only reduced. It should be recalled, however, that A II produced its pressor effect both by direct vascular action and by effects mediated indirectly by the CNS. These data may indicate the magnitude of the CNS contribution to the total pressor effect produced by elevations in blood-borne A II. The SFO lesions described here did not affect the pressor effect of intravenous phenylephrine, suggesting that vascular reactivity is not altered. In addition, the mean aortic pressure of resting rats is unaffected by this lesion. These data, then, indicate that lesions of the SFO affect not only a behavioral effect of A II, but a circulatory effect as well.

TABLE 1

INCREASES IN MEAN ARTERIAL PRESSURE (±S.E.M.) INDUCED BY
VARIOUS DOSES OF A II BEFORE AND AFTER LESIONS OF THE SFO
OR ADJACENT TISSUE (CONTROL) IN RATS

Dose of A II (i.v., ng/10 μl/min)		Control	SFO
6	prelesion	29.2 ± 2.1	28.2 ± 2.1
	postlesion	28.1 ± 3.4	16.7 ± 3.0
12	prelesion	43.6 ± 2.0	40.1 ± 2.4
	postlesion	41.6 ± 3.7	29.6 ± 3.1
24	prelesion	51.6 ± 1.9	51.6 ± 2.5
	postlesion	51.2 ± 2.9	43.1 ± 3.2

Source: Mangiapane and Simpson, 1980b.

Let us consider one final study of the effects of SFO lesions on central A II actions (Mangiapane et al., in press). Intraventricular injections of A II cause increases in plasma vasopressin (Keil et al., 1975). Having found that the drinking and pressor responses of A II are reduced or eliminated by lesions of the SFO, we studied the effects of this lesion on vasopressin secretion following intraventricular administrations of A II. The lesion reduced the magnitude of the vasopressin secretion following intraventricular injection of 5 ng of peptide. This is in parallel with the effects of SFO lesions on the other central actions of A II concerning circulation and behavior.

Other agents that have been identified by biochemical or immunocytochemical means as being endogenous to the SFO also have been studied in the rat prepared for simultaneous measurement of blood pressure and water intake. Like A II, agents that provoke drinking also cause an increase in blood pressure that is not secondary to the elicited behavior. Thus, acetylcholine (or the cholinomimetic, carbachol), vasopressin, and serotonin provoke drinking that is preceded in time by a pressor effect. These effects are correlated. Conversely, application of norepinephrine, oxytocin, or dopamine to the SFO causes neither drinking nor a pressor effect. If these effects are viewed as synergistic in the dehydrated animal, then it is appropriate that the agents that act at the SFO to cause drinking should also act there to cause a synergistic pressor response. This has been precisely our experience.

As noted in other contributions in this volume, it is now clear that patterned activity distinctive to different behaviors is the case in autonomic activity. Eating and drinking are accompanied by changes in the circulation. When the animal's responses to dehydration are considered, it appears that there is considerable synergy between the behavioral and physiological responses made in adjustment to the fluid deficit.   In particular, if the central actions of A II are noted, it is clear that the animal uses a variety of strategies in order to replenish the extracellular volume deficits signaled by the hormone. Animals use a coordinated series of responses--behavioral, cardiovascular, and endocrine--as means to a common homeostatic end. The role that behavior plays in cardiovascular function is becoming increasingly clear, especially in dehydration.

ACKNOWLEDGMENTS

Personal research described here was supported by NIH grants HL21799 and HL21800.

REFERENCES

Andersson, B. (1971) Thirst--and brain control of water balance. Amer. Sci. 59, 408-415.

Avrith, D.B. and Fitzsimons, J.T. (1980) Increased sodium appetite in the rat induced by intracranial administration of components of the renin-angiotensin system. J. Physiol. (Lond.) 301, 349-364.

Bickerton, R.K. and Buckley, J.P. (1961) Evidence for a central mechanism in angiotensin-induced hypertension. Proc. Soc. Exp. Biol. Med. 106, 834-836.

Blass, E.M. (1974) Evidence for basal forebrain thirst osmoreceptors in rats. Brain Res. 82, 69-76.

Blass, E.M. and Epstein, A.N. (1971) A lateral preoptic osmosensitive zone for thirst in the rat. J. Comp. Physiol. Psychol. 76, 378-394.

Brody, M.J. and Johnson, A.K. (1980) Role of the anteroventral third ventricle (AV3V) region in fluid and electrolyte balance, arterial pressure regulation, and hypertension; in Frontiers in Neuroendocrinology, Vol. 6, W.F. Ganong and L. Martin, eds. Raven Press, New York.

Bryant, R.W., Epstein, A.N., Fitzsimons, J.T. and Fluharty, S.J. (1980) Arousal of a specific and persistent sodium appetite in the rat with continuous intracerebro-ventricular infusion of angiotensin II. J. Physiol. (Lond.) 301, 365-382.

Dellmann, H.D. and Simpson, J.B. (1979) The subfornical organ. Int. Rev. Cytol. 58, 333-421.

Epstein, A.N., Fitzsimons, J.T. and Rolls, B.J. (1970) Drinking induced by injection of angiotensin into the brain of the rat. J. Physiol. (Lond.) 210, 457-474.

Findlay, A.L.R., Elfont, R.M. and Epstein, A.N. (1980) The site of the dipsogenic action of angiotensin II in the North American opossum. Brain Res. 180, 85-94.

Hatton, G.T. (1976) Nucleus circularis. is it an osmoreceptor in the brain? Brain Res. Bull. 1, 123-131.

Henry, J.P., Gupta, P.D., Meehan, J.P., Sinclair, R. and Share, L. (1968) The role of afferents from the low-pressure system in the release of antidiuretic hormone during nonhypotensive hemorrhage. Canad. J. Physiol. Pharmacol. 46, 287-295.

Holmes, J.H. and Gregersen, M.I. (1950) Observations on drinking induced by hypertonic solutions. Amer. J. Physiol. 162, 326-337.

Johnson, A.K., Hoffman, W.E. and Buggy, J. (1978) Attenuated pressor responses to intracranially injected stimuli and altered antidiuretic activity following preoptic-hypothalamic periventricular ablation. Brain Res. 157, 161-166.

Keil, L.C., Summy-Long, J. and Severs, W.B. (1975) Release of vasopressin by angiotensin II. Endocrinology 96, 1063-1065.

Mangiapane, M.L. and Simpson, J.B. (1980a) Subfornical organ: forebrain site of pressor and dipsogenic action of angiotensin II. Amer. J. Physiol. 239, R382-R389.

Mangiapane, M.L. and Simpson, J.B. (1980b) Subfornical organ lesions reduce the pressor effect of intravenous angiotensin. Neuroendocrinology 31, 380-384.

Mangiapane, M.L., Thrasher, T.N., Keil, L.C., Simpson, J.B. and Ganong, W.F. (in press) Subfornical organ lesions impair the vasopressin response to hyperosmolality or angiotensin II. Fed. Proc.

Maran, J.W. and Yates, F.E. (1977) Cortisol secretion during intrapituitary infusion of angiotensin II in conscious dogs. Amer. J. Physiol. 233, E273-E285.

Miselis, R.R., Shapiro, R.E. and Hand, P.J. (1979) Subfornical organ efferents to neural systems for control of body water. Science 205, 1022-1024.

Peck, J.W. and Novin, D. (1971) Evidence that osmoreceptors mediating drinking in rabbits are in the lateral preoptic area. J. Comp. Physiol. Psychol. 74, 134-147.

Phillips, M.I. (1978) Angiotensin in the brain. Neuroendocrinology 25, 354-377.

Reid, I.A., Morris, B.J. and Ganong, W.F. (1978) The renin-angiotensin system. Ann. Rev. Physiol. 40, 377-410.

Simpson, J.B. (1981) The circumventricular organs and the central actions of angiotensin. Neuroendocrinology 32, 248-256.

Simpson, J.B., Epstein, A.N. and Camardo, J.S., Jr. (1978) The localization of dipsogenic receptors for angiotenin II in the subfornical organ. J. Comp. Physiol. Psychol. 92, 581-608.

Simpson, J.B., Reed, M., Keil, L.C., Thrasher, T.N. and Ramsay, D.J. (1979) Drinking, vasopressin secretion, and ACTH secretion induced by intracranial angiotensin. Soc. Neurosci. Abstr. 5, 459.

Simpson, J.B. and Routtenberg, A. (1972) The subfornical organ and carbachol-induced drinking. Brain Res. 45, 135-157.

Simpson, J.B. and Routtenberg, A. (1973) Subfornical organ: site of drinking elicitation by angiotensin II. Science 181, 1172-1175.

Smith, O.A., Astley, C.A., Hohimer, A.R. and Stephenson, R.B. (1980) Behavioral and cerebral control of cardiovascular function; in Recent Topics in Physiology, Neural Control of Circulation, M.J. Hughes and C.D. Barnes, eds. Academic Press, New York.

Thornborough, J.R., Passo, S.S. and Rothballer, A.B. (1973) Receptors in cerebral circulation affecting sodium excretion in the cat. Amer. J. Physiol. 225, 138-141.

Thrasher, T.N., Brown, C.J., Keil, L.C. and Ramsay, D.J. (1980a) Thirst and vasopressin release in the dog: an osmoreceptor or sodium receptor mechanism? Amer. J. Physiol. 238, R333-R339.

Thrasher, T.N., Jones, R.G., Keil, J.C., Brown, C.J. and Ramsay, D.J. (1980b) Drinking and vasopressin release during ventricular infusions of hypertonic solutions. Amer. J. Physiol. 238, R340-R345.

Thrasher, T.N., Simpson, J.B. and Ramsay, D.J. (in press) Lesions of the subfornical organ block angiotensin-induced drinking in the dog. Neuroendocrinology.

van Houten, M., Schiffrin, E.L., Mann, J.F.E., Posner, B.I. and Boucher, R. (1980) Radioautographic localization of specific binding sites for blood-borne angiotensin II in the rat brain. Brain Res. 186, 480-485.

Verney, E.B. (1947) The antidiuretic hormone and the factors which determine its release. Proc. Roy. Soc. B, 135, 25-106.

Weindl, A. (1973) Neuroendocrine aspects of circumventricular organs; in Frontiers in Neuroendocrinology, W.F. Ganong and L. Martini, eds. Oxford University Press, New York, pp. 3-32.

Zimmerman, M.B., Blaine, E.H. and Stricker, E.M. (1981) Water intake in hypovolemic sheep: effects of crushing the left atrial appendage. Science 211, 489-491.

Central Neural Mechanisms Linking
Behavior and Cardiovascular Responses

Basal Autonomic Tone and Intrinsic Rhythmicity

GERARD L. GEBBER, SUSAN M. BARMAN, SHAUN F. MORRISON
AND JEFFREY L. ARDELL
Department of Pharmacology and Toxicology, Michigan State University, East Lansing, Michigan

INTRODUCTION

One of the least understood aspects of autonomic neurophysiology concerns the manner in which the basal discharges in sympathetic nerves are generated. Our approach to this problem has been to study the neural circuitry involved in generating the 2-6 c/s rhythm (normally entrained to the cardiac cycle by the baroreceptor reflexes) in sympathetic nerve discharge (SND) of the cat. The 2-6 c/s rhythm is ubiquitous to SND under a wide variety of experimental conditions including hypocapnia, asphyxia and extremes of body temperature. The rhythm persists in SND after baroreceptor denervation (Barman and Gebber, 1980; Gebber and Barman, 1981; Taylor and Gebber, 1975) and is not eliminated by decerebration at the midcollicular level (Barman and Gebber, 1980). The 2-6 c/s rhythm in SND, however, is eliminated by acute transection of the neuraxis at the medullo-spinal junction (McCall and Gebber, 1975). On this basis, we have suggested that the ubiquitous 2-6 c/s rhythm is representative of the fundamental organization of the brain stem sympathetic generator (Barman and Gebber, 1980; Gebber, 1980). If this assumption is accepted, it becomes important to determine how the rhythm (and thus a significant proportion of the basal discharges in sympathetic nerves) is generated.

BRAIN STEM SYMPATHETIC GENERATOR

Several possibilities arise concerning the mechanisms responsible for the 2-6 c/s rhythm in SND. The rhythm may be generated by a group of brain stem neurons with inherent pacemaker activity. Alternatively, it may be a consequence of network interactions. For instance, the rising phase of the 2-6 c/s burst of SND (recorded as a slow wave using a wide preamplifier bandpass) may result from the synchronous discharges of one group of brain stem neurons while the falling phase may be due to active inhibition produced by the synchronous discharges of a second group of brain stem neurons. Such neuronal networks may interact directly to form a rhythm generator. Additional neuronal networks may be involved in switching from the excitatory to the inhibitory (and vice versa) phase of SND. Consideration of these possibilities requires the identification of the neuronal types that comprise the brain stem sympathetic generator. We have approached this problem by using the method of spike-triggered averaging (Barman and Gebber, 1981a,b; Gebber and Barman, 1981; Morrison and Gebber, in press). That is, the spikes of single brain stem neurons (recorded extracellularly with metal microelectrodes) are used to trigger the computation of an average of accompanying changes in the activity of a sympathetic nerve bundle (usually the inferior cardiac postganglionic sympathetic nerve). This method has allowed us to locate single neurons in the dorsolateral medullary reticular formation (Barman and Gebber, 1981a) and caudal raphe nuclei (Morrison and Gebber, in press) with naturally occurring discharges synchronized to the cardiac-related rhythm in SND.

A problem arises concerning which of the brain stem neurons with cardiac-related activity are indeed contained in networks responsible for basal SND. The problem is that a number of functionally distinct brain stem systems share baroreceptor input. For instance, the baroreceptor reflexes influence cortical activity (Baust and Heinemann, 1967), respiratory function (Richter and Seller, 1975), and somatomotor reflexes (Coote and MacLeod, 1974) in addition to autonomic nerve activity. Thus, the cardiac-related rhythm in SND may be temporally related to that in the discharges of a number of functionally distinct types of brain stem neurons. We have approached this problem by searching the brain stem for neurons with sympathetic nerve-related activity in baroreceptor-denervated cats (Barman and Gebber, 1981b; Gebber and Barman, 1981; Morrison and Gebber, in press). This approach has enabled us to locate brain stem neurons with 2-6 c/s activity locked to that in inferior cardiac SND, but not to the cardiac cycle. Such neurons (located in dorsolateral medullary reticular formation and caudal raphe nuclei) fall into two categories--those with activity locked to the rising phase of the 2-6 c/s slow wave in SND, and those with activity locked to the falling phase of inferior cardiac sympathetic nerve activity.

Whereas our results in baroreceptor-denervated cats were encouraging, we were still left with the problem of how to identify elements of the brain stem sympathetic network under more natural circumstances, i.e., under the condition in which the baroreceptor homeostatic reflex mechanism is not interrupted. Regarding this point, we have recently developed a test that allowed us to distinguish brain stem sympathetic neurons in the baroreceptor-innervated cat from other neuronal types that also exhibit a cardiac-related discharge pattern. The test is based on the fact that it is possible to shift the phase relations between the pulse synchronous components of baroreceptor nerve activity and SND by changing heart rate with ventricular pacing (Gebber, 1976). Thus, it was reasoned that the temporal relations between brain stem sympathetic unit discharges and the activity of peripheral sympathetic nerves should not be affected during changes in heart rate that shift the phase relations between baroreceptor nerve activity and SND.

As a corollary, we predicted that the temporal relations between SND and the discharges of other types of brain stem neurons exhibiting cardiac-related activity (such as interneurons in the afferent limb of the baroreceptor reflex arc) should be altered during changes in heart rate. As detailed in our recent study (Morrison and Gebber, in press), we were successful in distinguishing between such neuronal types.

Identification of the cell types that comprise the brain stem sympathetic network is only the first step in understanding how the 2-6 c/s rhythm is generated. The second step is to define the network interactions that underlie the genesis of oscillatory activity and thus a major component of the basal discharges in sympathetic nerves. The phenomena that require explanation include (1) synchronization of the discharges of those neurons responsible for the rising (i.e., excitatory) phase of the 2-6 c/s sympathetic nerve slow wave, (2) synchronization of activity of those neurons responsible for the falling (i.e., inhibitory) phase of the slow wave, and (3) switching from the excitatory to the inhibitory phase and vice versa. We have recently begun to study the underlying mechanisms responsible for these phenomena using crosscorrelation analysis to examine the short-term interactions (millisecond time scale) between brain stem sympathetic neurons. Neuronal interactions that occur on a short time scale (indicative of mono- and/or oligosynaptic connections) ultimately result in periodic firing of sympathetic nerves on a longer time scale (hundreds of milliseconds in the case of the 2-6 c/s rhythm).

A working model of those brain stem circuits involved in the genesis of the 2-6 c/s rhythm in SND and its entrainment to the cardiac cycle by the baroreceptor reflexes is shown in Figure 1. Five unit types were defined in experiments in which spike-triggered averaging and post-R wave interval analysis were used to identify brain stem sympathetic neurons. S_eR neurons are units with cardiac-related activity whose discharges are synchronized to a point on the rising phase of the 2-6 c/s slow wave in SND. S_iR neurons are the same as S_eR neurons, except that unit discharge is synchronized to a point on the falling phase of the 2-6 c/s slow wave in SND. SE neurons are units with activity related to SND and that receive input from forebrain (FB) regions as evidenced by synchronization of their discharges to EEG rhythms. As discussed by Gebber and Barman (1981), such neurons are believed to provide inputs to S_eR and S_iR neurons. B neurons are interneurons in afferent limb of the baroreceptor reflex arc. Unlike S_eR and S_iR units, whose discharges remain locked to SND during changes in ventricular rate that shift the phase relations between the pulse synchronous components of baroreceptor nerve activity and SND, B neuron discharges remain locked to baroreceptor nerve activity. Off-switch (O.S.) neurons are unique in that they seem to receive excitatory inputs both from the baroreceptors and from elements of the efferent network responsible for the 2-6 c/s rhythm in SND (Morrison and Gebber, unpublished observations). Such neurons may be contained in a recurrent inhibitory loop that acts to switch the phase of SND from excitation to inhibition.

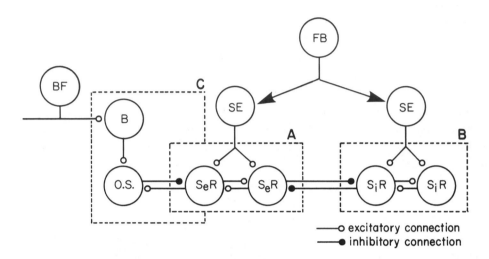

Fig. 1. Working model of brain stem sympathetic generator. B, interneuron in afferent limb of baroreceptor reflex; BF, baroreceptor fiber; FB, forebrain; O.S., off-switch neuron that may help terminate the rising (i.e., excitatory) phase of 2-6 c/s slow wave in SND; S_eR and S_iR, neurons with spontaneous activity related to SND and R wave of ECG. Discharges of S_eR neurons are synchronized to points on the rising phase of sympathetic nerve slow wave. Discharges of S_iR neurons are synchronized to points on the falling (i.e., inhibitory) phase of slow wave in SND. SE, units with activity related to SND and cortical rhythms; Circuit A, responsible for synchronization of discharges of S_eR units; Circuit B, responsible for synchronization of discharges of S_iR units; Circuit C contains a recurrent inhibitory loop that may be responsible for termination of the excitatory phase of SND. Interactions between circuits A and B may also participate in switching from the rising to falling phase (and vice versa) of sympathetic nerve slow wave. Open circles, excitatory connections; closed circles, inhibitory connections. Proposed neuronal interconnections are described in the text.

The model contains a number of hypothetical circuits that are currently being scrutinized using unit → unit crosscorrelation analysis. Circuit A is for the synchronization of the discharges of S_eR neurons in order to form the rising phase of the 2-6 c/s slow wave in SND. Synchronization may occur via direct excitatory synaptic connections between S_eR neurons (one-way or reciprocal) and/or via the sharing of common input (perhaps from SE neurons). Circuit B is for the synchronization of the discharges of S_iR neurons responsible for the falling phase of SND. Potential mechanisms for synchronization in circuit B are the same as in circuit A. One-way or reciprocal inhibition between S_eR and S_iR neurons in circuits A and B are considered as possible mechanisms for phase switching, as is the recurrent inhibitory loop in circuit C. The candidate for the off-switch neuron in circuit C is the type of unit that is excited both by baroreceptor input and by elements (presumably S_eR) of the sympathetic generator. The probability of discharge of these neurons gradually increases during the development of the rising phase of the sympathetic nerve slow wave, presumably due to excitatory input from S_eR neurons. S_eR unit discharge is terminated when O.S. unit activity reaches a critically high level. Baroreceptor inputs also excite the O.S. neuron, and thus may influence the timing of S_eR unit cutoff (i.e., phase switching). Regarding this point, the duration of the rising phase of the sympathetic nerve slow wave is prolonged when the interval between successive baroreceptor nerve cycles is lengthened by slowing ventricular rate (Morrison and Gebber, in press). The reader surely will recognize that the recurrent inhibitory loop in circuit C is analogous to that which has been postulated (Cohen, 1979) to play a role in inspiratory cutoff (i.e., loop containing inspiratory neurons of the I_α and I_β types).

SPINAL SYMPATHETIC GENERATOR

It is well established that acute transection of the cervical spinal cord leads to a profound fall in blood pressure which can be attributed to a marked reduction in the basal level of activity in sympathetic nerves (Alexander, 1946; Bernard, 1863). Although residual SND is asynchronous in nature under normocapnic conditions in the acute spinal preparation (McCall and Gebber, 1975), the characteristics of SND in the chronic spinal animal have yet to be defined. This problem is important since blood pressure and SND begin to recover toward normal levels within a week after cervical spinal transection (Brooks, 1933, 1935). Thus, we undertook a study of the characteristics of basal SND in cats in which the spinal cord had been sectioned 9-37 days earlier at the level of the sixth cervical segment, below phrenic nerve outflow but above preganglionic sympathetic nerve ouflow (Ardell et al., 1981). Our primary aim was to determine whether thoraco-lumbar networks in chronic spinal cats are capable of rhythm generation and/or synchronization of the discharges of populations of sympathetic fibers. Recordings were made from the central ends of the sectioned external carotid and renal sympathetic nerves in chloralose-anesthetized preparations.

In contrast to the asynchronous nature of SND in acute spinal cats, SND in chronic spinal preparations exhibited slow wave activity in the 2-6 c/s frequency band (as determined from power spectra). This activity pattern was similar to that observed immediately following baroreceptor denervation in cats with an intact neuraxis, in that intervals between slow waves were variable. The similarity of SND in baroreceptor-denervated and chronic spinal cats ended here. As reported by Barman and Gebber (1980), conversion of the aperiodic 2-6 c/s activity pattern in SND to a true rhythm (i.e., essentially constant interval between slow waves) can be accomplished immediately after baroreceptor denervation during short periods of asphyxia. In contrast, asphyxia failed to convert the aperiodic 2-6 c/s pattern in SND to a true rhythm in chronic spinal cats. Moreover, and in contrast to the results obtained by Barman and Gebber (1980) in baroreceptor-denervated cats with an intact neuraxis, 2-6 c/s slow waves in SND of the chronic spinal animal generally could not be synchronized to shocks applied to somatic afferent nerves. These results indicate that while the isolated spinal cord is capable of aperiodic synchronization of SND, generation of a true rhythm requires the integrity of bulbospinal connections.

The question whether brain stem sympathetic networks in isolation from the spinal cord are capable of rhythm generation required additional investigation. As already indicated, the phase relations between baroreceptor nerve activity and SND in cats with intact baroreceptor reflexes can be shifted by changing heart rate (Gebber, 1976). Such shifts are indicative of the ability of the baroreceptor reflexes to entrain a sympathetic nerve rhythm of central origin to the cardiac cycle. As previously noted, we have located neurons in the cat medulla whose discharges remain locked to inferior cardiac SND during changes in heart rate that shift the phase relations between SND and the arterial pulse wave (a monitor of baroreceptor nerve activity). Obviously, it is not possible to demonstrate relations between brain stem unit discharge and inferior cardiac SND after cervical spinal transection. Nevertheless, we have routinely found brain stem neurons in spinal cats with cardiac-related activity. That such activity was the result of entrainment of a brain stem oscillator by the baroreceptor reflexes was indicated by the results obtained with ventricular pacing. The point of peak probability of cardiac-related unit discharge shifted relative to the arterial pulse wave when ventricular rate was changed. Such shifts occurred in the same direction and were of similar magnitude as those for brain stem neurons whose discharges remained locked to SND during ventricular pacing in animals with an intact neuraxis. Although indirect, these data support the view that brain stem sympathetic networks are inherently capable of rhythm generation in the absence of afferent information transmitted over spinal-bulbar pathways. Thus, the tenet that the circuits responsible for generation of the 2-6 c/s rhythm (normally cardiac-related) in SND are self-contained in the brain stem remains viable.

SUMMARY

A basic problem in autonomic neurophysiology is to understand how the basal discharges in sympathetic nerves (and, thus, the neurogenic component for the support of blood pressure) are generated. It is generally agreed that basal SND arises primarily in brain stem circuits. We have worked under the assumption that the 2-6 c/s rhythm (normally cardiac-related) in SND is representative of the fundamental organization of the brain stem generator. Modeling of the generator requires the identification of those neuronal types that comprise the oscillator as well as studies on the synaptic interactions of such neurons. Our efforts along these lines have been summarized in this article. In addition, recent work is described on the ability of spinal networks to generate an aperiodic yet synchronized pattern of SND that presumably accounts for the recovery of blood pressure occurring several weeks after the surgical interruption of bulbo-spinal connections.

ACKNOWLEDGEMENTS

This study was supported by grants HL13187 and NS06693 from the National Institutes of Health.

REFERENCES

Alexander, R.S. (1946) Tonic and reflex functions of medullary sympathetic cardiovascular centers. J. Neurophysiol. 9, 205-217.

Ardell, J.L., Barman, S.M. and Gebber, G.L. (1981) Sympathetic nerve discharge (SND) in chronic spinal cats. Soc. Neurosci. Abstr. 7, 365.

Barman, S.M. and Gebber, G.L. (1980) Sympathetic nerve rhythm of brain stem origin. Amer. J. Physiol. 239 (Regulat. Integrat. Comp. Physiol. 8), R42-R47.

Barman, S.M. and Gebber, G.L. (1981) Brain stem neuronal types with activity patterns related to sympathetic nerve discharge. Amer. J. Physiol. 240 (Regulat. Integrat. Comp. Physiol. 9), R335-R347.

Barman, S.M. and Gebber, G.L. (1981) Problems associated with the identification of brain stem neurons responsible for sympathetic nerve discharge. J. Autonom. Nerv. Syst. 3, 369-377.

Baust, W. and Heinemann, H. (1967) The role of the baroreceptors and of blood pressure in the regulation of sleep and wakefulness. Exp. Brain Res. 3, 12-24.

Bernard, C. (1863) Lecons sur la Physiologie et la Pathologie du Systeme Nerveux. Paris: Balliere, vol. 1.

Brooks, C. McC. (1933) Reflex activation of the sympathetic system in the spinal cat. Amer. J. Physiol. 106, 251-266.

Brooks, C. McC. (1935) The reaction of chronic spinal animals to hemorrhage. Amer. J. Physiol. 114, 30-39.

Cohen, M.I. (1979) Neurogenesis of respiratory rhythm in the mammal. Physiol. Rev. 59, 1105-1173.

Coote, J.H. and MacLeod, V.H. (1974) Evidence for the involvement in the baroreceptor reflex of a descending pathway. J. Physiol. (Lond.) 241, 477-496.

Gebber, G.L. (1976) Basis for phase relations between baroreceptor and sympathetic nervous discharge. Amer. J. Physiol. 230, 263-270.

Gebber, G.L. (1980) Central oscillators responsible for sympathetic nerve discharge. Amer. J. Physiol. 239 (Heart Circ. Physiol. 8), H143-H155.

Gebber, G.L. and Barman, S.M. (1981) Sympathetic-related activity of brain stem neurons in baroreceptor-denervated cats. Amer. J. Physiol. 240 (Regulat. Integrat. Comp. Physiol. 9), R348-R355.

McCall, R.B. and Gebber, G.L. (1975) Brain stem and spinal synchronization of sympathetic nervous discharge. Brain Res. 89: 139-143.

Morrison, S.F., and Gebber, G.L. Classification of raphe neurons with cardiac-related activity. Amer. J. Physiol. (Regulat. Integrat. Comp. Physiol.), in press.

Richter, D.W., and Seller, H. (1975) Baroreceptor effects on medullary respiratory neurones of the cat. Brain Res. 86, 168-171.

Taylor, D.G. and Gebber, G.L. (1975) Baroreceptor mechanisms controlling sympathetic nervous rhythms of central origin. Amer. J. Physiol. 228: 1002-1013.

Published 1982 by Elsevier Science Publishing Co., Inc.
Smith, Galosy, and Weiss, editors
CIRCULATION, NEUROBIOLOGY, AND BEHAVIOR

Effect of Ambient and Conditioned Stimuli on Arterial Pressure After Central Disruption of the Baroreflexes

MARC A. NATHAN AND R. ALLAN BUCHHOLZ
Department of Pharmacology, University of Texas Health Science Center at San Antonio, San Antonio, Texas

INTRODUCTION

Traditionally, the arterial baroreflexes have been considered the primary mechanism in maintaining the arterial blood pressure at normotensive levels (Heymans and Neil, 1958). Accordingly, disruption of baroreflex function by peripheral denervation of arterial baroreceptors should result in a sustained elevation of arterial pressure. Until recently, this outcome was generally seen after denervation. However, several conflicting reports have shown variable increases in the mean level of arterial pressure ranging from less than 1 mm Hg to over 40 mm Hg (Krieger, 1964; Ferrario et al., 1969; Cowley et al., 1973; McRitchie et al., 1976; Alexander et al., 1980; Cowley et al., 1980; Norman et al., 1981; Ito and Scher, 1981). Differences in results between the various studies may be due to the method and completeness of denervating the baroreceptors, impact of environmental stimuli, method of measuring the arterial pressure, length of the measurement period, and the species tested. However, most of these studies did show that the lability of arterial pressure is increased following peripheral denervation. Moreover, a few investigators reported that the lability is frequently associated with emotional excitement and other behaviors (Ferrario et al., 1969; Cowley et al., 1973).

Several years ago we placed electrolytic lesions in the cat solitary complex as a means of disrupting baroreflex function. We reasoned that more complete disruption of the baroreflexes might be obtained in this manner since the afferent fibers synapse in a relatively confined area of the solitary complex comprising mainly the medial, dorsal, dorsolateral, and commissural nuclei of the solitary complex (Berger, 1980; Kalia and Welles, 1980; Panneton and Loewy, 1980; Ciriello et al., 1981; Davies and Kalia, 1981). Complete peripheral denervation is difficult, if not impossible, because of the widespread distribution of the baroreceptors and their afferent fibers (Ito and Scher, 1974). We found that placement of the lesions in the solitary complex successfully disrupted baroreflex function (Nathan and Reis, 1977). Furthermore, the average level of the mean arterial pressure (MAP) in the lesion group was 34 mm Hg higher than that of the control group, although the level of MAP seemed to depend on the environmental conditions in which the cats were tested. The largest elevations were obtained when the cats were tested in cages placed in an open, busy laboratory. Measurements made from the same cats at night, when the laboratory was relatively quiet, resulted in a mean difference between the lesion and control groups of only 19 mm Hg. Perhaps even more striking was the finding that, while the lability of arterial pressure in the lesion group was more than four times greater than that observed in the control animals, there were no differences between the two groups at night. Since publication of our findings, others have reported comparable increases in arterial pressure in the dog after placement of electrolytic lesions in the solitary complex (Laubie and Schmitt, 1979; Carey et al., 1979).

Another interesting finding in cats with lesions of the solitary complex was the occurrence of exaggerated cardiovascular (CV) responses either to the incidental presentation of environmental stimuli or in association with the spontaneous occurrence of various behaviors. For example, the usually small elevations of arterial pressure associated with grooming or orienting were substantially enhanced: transient elevations of arterial pressure of up to 100 mm Hg were commonly seen. These exaggerated responses suggested that it might be possible to raise the arterial pressure to rather high levels if environmental stimuli were systematically presented, particularly if these stimuli signaled the occurrence of a stressful event. We believed that classical conditioning might accomplish this goal, and that the repeated, neurally mediated elevations of arterial pressure produced by the classical conditioning procedure might lead to vascular changes which, in turn, would produce a chronic elevation of arterial pressure. Thus, we would have an animal model of behaviorally conditioned, neurogenic hypertension. The contribution of alterations in vascular smooth muscle to the maintenance of hypertension has been highlighted in several investigations (Sivertsson and Olander, 1968; Folkow et al., 1973; Bevan et al., 1976). In addition, we hoped to determine whether the degree of change in baroreflex function caused by the lesions is associated with the magnitude of the conditioned pressor response or with possible permanent elevation of arterial pressure after the completion of the conditioning procedure. A preliminary report of this effort has appeared elsewhere (Nathan et al., 1978).

METHODS
Animals and General Procedures

Seventeen vaccinated, adult cats of both sexes were used in these experiments. Nine of these were instrumented for the recording of CV activity and then received lesions or sham lesions in a second operation. The other eight cats received instrumentation and lesions in a single operation. Twelve cats had lesions in the solitary complex, while the other five received sham lesions. The effects of the lesions on the MAP were assessed during a postconditioning period.

Instrumentation

The cats were prepared for general anesthesia with i.m. injections of Ketamine HCl (25 mg/kg) and atropine sulphate (0.05 mg/kg). Tracheal intubation was followed by administration of halothane (1-3% in 50% oxygen-50% nitrogen or 100% oxygen) delivered by mechanical ventilation (Mark 7, Bird Co.).

Body temperature was maintained at $37^{\circ}C$ ($\pm 0.5^{\circ}C$) by a rectal probe connected to a thermostatically regulated electric heating pad. The cats were maintained on normal saline or lactated Ringers throughout the surgery. All surgical procedures were performed under aseptic conditions.

Either the right or left common carotid artery and external jugular vein were exposed by splitting the sternocleidomastoid muscle and retracting the digastric muscle. In some cats, polyvinylchloride (PVC) cannulas (0.022 inches, I.D.) were inserted into the common carotid artery and external jugular vein. In other cats, Teflon tubing (0.015 inches, I.D.) bonded to the PVC tubing was used. Only the Teflon portion of the cannula was inserted into the vessel. The tip of the arterial cannulas rested either in the brachiocephalic artery, aortic arch, or thoracic aorta. The venous cannulas were always positioned just distal to the right atrium.

After insertion into the vessels and fixation to surrounding muscle, the cannulas were passed subcutaneously to an incision at the top of the head, then threaded through 13-gauge stainless steel tubes cut to a length of 1.5 cm. The tubes were oriented vertically to the top of the head and cemented to the skull with dental acrylic. Two stainless steel disc electrodes (1 cm diameter) were implanted subcutaneously over the flanks on either side of the midline. The wires from the electrodes were threaded subcutaneously to the head incision and then soldered to a connector (Augat, Inc.). The connector in turn was cemented to the skull.

At the completion of the surgery all cats were given 5% dextrose and water or lactated Ringers (i.v.) until they were eating and drinking normally. Cats scheduled for instrumentation only were returned to their home cages at this time. The arterial and venous cannulas were threaded through flexible metal springs. One end of each spring was fitted over the metal tube that had been cemented to the skull, and a plug was inserted into the free end of the venous cannula. The free end of the arterial cannula and the spring enlosing it were attached to a hydraulic swivel (Model 192-03, BRS/LVE or 375 series, Instech) which was mounted in a plastic enclosure attached to the cage ceiling. The springs prevented the cannulas from kinking during the cat's movements. The other end of the swivel was connected by PVC tubing to a pump (Model A.Z., Razel) so that the arterial cannula could be kept patent by constant infusion of heparinized saline (50 U/ml at 1 ml/hr). During recording periods the tubing from the swivel was attached to a strain gauge transducer (Bentley, Model 800). The venous cannula was kept patent by daily flushing. Pulsatile arterial pressure was displayed on one channel of a stripchart recorder (Beckman, Type RM or 611). The pulsatile arterial pressure was averaged by a resistance-capacitance circuit (time constant = 0.53 sec) and displayed on a second channel of the recorder. A correction factor was used to compensate for the difference in the height of the transducer and the level of the heart. The peak of the pulsatile pressure was used to trigger a cardiotachometer (Beckman 9857) and the heart rate was simultaneously displayed on a third channel of the recorder. All CV functions were recorded online by a computer (DEC 11/34) via an analog to digital converter set at a sampling rate of 200 Hz.

Placement of Lesions

Cats that had lesions placed in a second operation were anesthetized with alpha-chloralose (60-80 mg/kg, i.v.), intubated, and mechanically ventilated. They were placed in a stereotaxic frame with the head flexed (usually about 25°) to permit entry to the brain stem through the foramen magnum. The atlantooccipital membrane was incised after visualization by midline separation and retraction of the posterior neck muscles. Approximately 2-4 mm of the supraoccipital bone was removed to facilitate exposure of the region of the obex. The field was then viewed with an operating microscope, the overlying arachnoid dissected free, and the posterior vermis of the cerebellum was gently retracted rostrally.

Two procedures were followed for placement of the lesions. The first was used in cats that were anesthetized with chloralose. First, the cardiomotor component of the baroreflexes was elicited by administration of various pressor agents. Then an electrode connected to a stimulator (Pulsar 6 bp, Frederick Haer & Co.) was inserted into the solitary complex. Penetrations, separated by 0.5 mm, were made 0.0-1.5 mm anterior of the obex, 1.1-1.75 mm to the right and left of the midline, and 1.3-1.5 mm below the surface of the brain stem. During each penetration the electrode was lowered in 0.1- to 0.2-mm steps. The electrode consisted of stainless steel or tungsten wire (0.18 mm diameter) insulated with Teflon to within 0.2 mm of the tip. An indifferent electrode consisted of a clip attached to a retractor that separated the neck muscles. Points were selected for placement of lesions that, when stimulated for 10-20 sec (10-100 Hz, 0.1 msec pulse width, 0.05-2.0 mA), produced a bradycardia or depressor response, or both. Next the electrode was connected to a lesion maker (Grass Instruments, model LM 5) and anodal current of 2-5 mA was passed for 2-5 sec. After placement of the lesion, the point was restimulated and another lesion was made if the CV response was still present. Periodically the baroreflexes were retested, and the procedure was repeated for each penetration until the baroreflexes were abolished. The second procedure was used in cats that were anesthetized with halothane. Selection of lesion sites was guided only by reference to the stereotaxic coordinates, since baroreflex activity and the CV responses to electrical stimulation of the solitary complex are markedly blunted with halothane anesthesia.

Sham lesions were made at the same stereotaxic points by inserting and withdrawing the electrode. No current was passed during the penetrations.

Classical Conditioning

Classical conditioning of all cats began 2-3 weeks after the preconditioning period ended. All recordings were made with the cats placed in sound-shielded chambers. The conditioning procedure was conducted for a total of 30 sessions distributed 5-7 per week. Two tones of different frequencies (2222 and 1136 Hz, referenced to a C-weighted scale) were presented randomly during each session. Each tone was presented ten times. The high-frequency tones terminated with delivery of an electrical shock (50 Hz square wave, 10-36 V for 1 sec), set to elicit an increase in arterial pressure of 40-50 mm Hg while causing minimal discomfort. The low-frequency tone was never followed by electrical shock. The duration of the tones was 10 sec for sessions 1-10; 30 sec for sessions 11-20; and 60 sec for sessions 21-30. The intertone interval varied randomly between 60 and 150 sec.

To adjust for baseline variations in CV activity, each conditioned response was computed as the change relative to the average response level recorded for the 10 sec just before presentation of the tone. The number of data samples was reduced to 60 values by dividing the tone period into 1-sec intervals and computing the average CV response that occurred during each interval. Each conditioned response for purposes of statistical comparison was reduced to the average response increase that occurred during the entire duration of the tone. Thus, the average response increase was calculated as the mean of the 60 values. For purposes of graphic presentation of the responses, the corresponding interval values from each cat were pooled according to group, and the average interval was computed. This procedure was repeated for each 1-sec measurement period.

Pre- and Postconditioning Period

One-hour recordings of MAP were made during the preconditioning period (6-32 days after placement of the lesions and 1-3 days before conditioning began) and during the postconditioning period (3-20 days following the last conditioning session). The recordings were made while the cats lay quietly in the sound-shielded chambers. The frequency histograms were constructed from the MAP of each cardiac cycle of the recording period. From these values, frequency tallies were made of the number of times that a particular value occurred during the recording period. To compare frequency histograms from different animals, the frequencies were converted to percent of occurrence during the recording period. The mean and standard deviation of the frequency histograms were used as indexes of the mean level and lability of MAP during the entire recording period.

Baroreflex Analysis

The cardiac component of the baroreflexes was assessed during the pre- and postconditioning periods by measuring the lengthening of interbeat interval as a function of rising systolic arterial pressure following administration of either norepinephrine (0.5 μg/kg) or phenylephrine (4.0-8.0 μg/kg). The slope of the plot of interbeat interval as a function of rising systolic arterial pressure was calculated by the method of least squares using the equation for a parabolic curve (Nathan and Reis, 1980). Each slope was then divided by the number of cardiac cycles occurring between the onset of the rise in systolic pressure and the lengthening of interbeat interval to take into account the response latency. This final measure was used as an index of baroreflex sensitivity.

Statistical Comparisons

All statistical comparisons were made using either a paired or unpaired Student's t-test and Pearson product-moment correlation coefficients. Differences were considered significant at $p < 0.05$ (one-tailed tests).

RESULTS

Effect of Lesions of the Solitary Complex on Baroreflex Function

In agreement with our earlier findings (Nathan and Reis, 1977; Nathan et al., 1978), there was a significant difference ($p < 0.005$) between the baroreflex sensitivity of the lesion group (0.054 ± 0.127) and that of the control group (1.786 ± 1.012) during the preconditioning period. The differences were still highly significant ($p < 0.005$) during the postconditioning period, 30-45 days after placement of lesions or sham lesions. The baroreflex sensitivity of the lesion group at the completion of conditioning had risen to 0.210 ± 0.106 and that of the control group to 2.227 ± 0.686. However, these increases were not significant.

Enhancement of Conditioned Pressor Responses After Disruption of Baroreflex Function

Large differences in the conditioned increases of MAP were found between the lesion and control groups during the final conditioning session (Fig. 1). The comparisons were made by using the change in MAP relative to baseline, because the baseline pressures varied over a wide range (54-106 mm Hg). There were no significant differences in the mean baseline levels of the two groups. The latency of the increase in MAP from the onset of the tone in both groups was similar (2-3 sec). However, the rate of increase of MAP in the lesion group was much more rapid and generally more sustained. The steepest rise occurred during the first 20 sec of tone presentation. By the 20th second the MAP had increased 34 mm Hg, while during the same time period an increase of only 5 mm Hg was observed in the control group (p<0.01). After the first 20 sec, the MAP of the lesion group continued to rise, although not so steeply, and it reached a maximum of only 15 mm Hg (p<0.01). The most striking difference between the two groups was shown by the average increase of MAP during presentation of the tone. The MAP of the lesion group increased an average of 35 mm Hg, a value more than five times larger than the average increase of 7 mm Hg recorded from the control group (p <0.001). Although the absolute level of the response to electrical shock was higher in the lesion group than in the control group, the response increases were nearly identical when measured relative to the level of MAP recorded at the end of the tone.

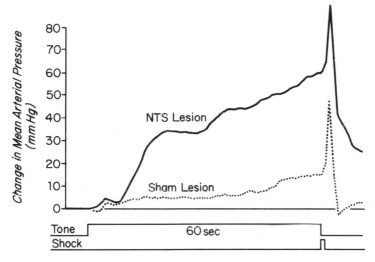

Fig. 1. Averaged conditioned increases of mean arterial pressure in the group with lesions of the solitary complex (NTS lesion group, n = 4) and the sham lesion group (n = 4) during session 30. Deflection of the signal pen at the bottom of the figure indicates onset, duration, and termination of the tone and electrical shock. (From Nathan et al., 1978, with permission.)

Relation of Baroreflex Function to Conditioned Pressor Responses

Although there was a highly significant difference in baroreflex sensitivity between the lesion and control groups, the effect of the lesions on baroreflex sensitivity was not uniform. Baroreflex sensitivity even in the control group and in cats whose prelesion values were available ranged from a low of 0.611 to a high of 6.150. Thus, this spectrum of baroreflex sensitivities offered the opportunity to study the possible relation between baroreflex function and conditioned pressor responses, as well as the mean level and lability of MAP during the pre- and postconditioning periods. We found a significant inverse correlation between baroreflex sensitivity and the magnitude of the conditioned pressor responses (Table 1). The correlations were computed from responses obtained during the 30th conditioning session and baroreflex tests collected on the next day. Selection of three animals showing low (-0.085), medium (0.214) and high baroreflex sensitivity (2.913) and their corresponding conditioned responses graphically depicts this relationship (Fig. 2).

TABLE 1

CORRELATIONS OF BAROREFLEX SENSITIVITY, MEAN ARTERIAL PRESSURE (MAP), AND ITS STANDARD DEVIATION DURING PRECONDITIONING, CONDITIONING (LAST SESSION), AND POSTCONDITIONING PERIODS

	Preconditioning		Conditioning (Last Session)	Postconditioning	
	MAP (mm HG)	S.D. (mm Hg)	ΔMAP (mm Hg)	MAP (mm Hg)	S.D. (mm HG)
Baroreflex sensitivity	-0.242 (13)	-0.280 (13)	-0.714 (10)	-0.311 (14)	-0.643
P	NS	NS	$\leqslant 0.01$	NS	0.01
Standard Deviation	0.337 (13)	--	0.565 (10)	0.131 (14)	--
P	NS	--	$\leqslant 0.050$	NS	--

All statistics were computed from the last frequency histograms collected during the preconditioning period, the average of the conditioned responses recorded during the 30th conditioning session, or the last frequency histograms collected during the post-conditioning period 3-20 days after conditioning ended. ΔMAP is change in MAP during presentation of the tones relative to pre-tone baseline. Samples of conditioned responses are shown in Fig. 1. All values are Pearson product-moment correlation coefficients; the number of pairs used to calculate the coefficients is in parentheses. Correlations are based on pooled responses of the lesion and control groups. P, significance level; NS, not significant.

Effect of Conditioning on the Mean Level and Lability of Arterial Pressure

The effect of the classical conditioning procedure on the mean level and lability of MAP extended into the postconditioning period. These findings are based on the means and standard deviations (index of lability) of frequency histograms constructed from the data collected 3-20 days after the last conditioning session (Table 2). There were no differences between these groups before the conditioning began. However, we found a significant average difference in MAP of 17.5 mm Hg between the lesion and control groups after conditioning. The difference emerged as a consequence of conditioning because the MAP of the control group tended to decrease while that of the lesion group increased significantly. The same general findings were seen when the lability of MAP was examined. The lability was significantly greater in the lesion group compared with that in the control group after the completion of conditioning. However, the difference emerged because lability diminished in the control group while remaining essentially unchanged in the lesion group.

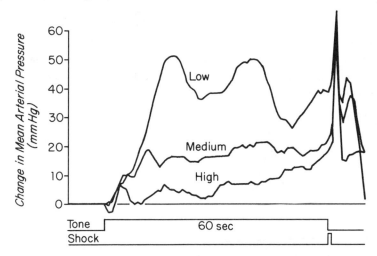

Fig. 2. Averaged increases of mean arterial pressure during session 30 from cats selected as representative of the low, medium and high baroreflex sensitivities. Deflection of the signal pen at the bottom of the figure indicates onset, duration, and termination of the tone (conditioned stimulus). Electrical shock (US) occurred at the termination of the tone.

TABLE 2

EFFECT OF LESIONS OF THE SOLITARY COMPLEX ON MEAN ARTERIAL PRESSURE AND ITS STANDARD DEVIATIONS BEFORE AND AFTER CONDITIONING

	Mean Arterial Pressure (mm Hg)		
	Preconditioning	Postconditioning	P
Lesion	82.5 ± 2.83 (12)	93.0 ± 2.83 (12)	<0.01
Control	86.2 ± 7.84 (5)	75.5 ± 5.03 (5)	NS
P	NS	<0.05	

	Standard Deviation of Arterial Pressure (mm Hg)		
	Preconditioning	Postconditioning	P
Lesion	11.3 ± 1.23 (12)	13.0 ± 1.46 (12)	NS
Control	11.3 ± 2.03 (5)	6.8 ± 0.68 (5)	<0.05
P	NS	<0.01	

All statistics were computed from the last frequency histograms collected before conditioning started (preconditioning period) and 3-20 days after conditioning ended (postconditioning period). Samples of the frequency histograms after conditioning ended are shown in Fig. 3. All values are expressed as means ± S.E.; the number of cats in each group is in parentheses. P, significance level; NS, not significant.

Relation of Baroreflex Function, Mean Level and Lability of Arterial Pressure During the Pre- and Postconditioning Periods

There was no relation between baroreflex sensitivity, mean level or lability of MAP during the preconditioning period, but there was a significant inverse correlation between baroreflex sensitivity and lability during the postconditioning period (Table 1). In Figure 3, the broad bases of the frequency histograms of the cats with low and medium baroreflex sensitivity reflect the greater lability of MAP in these animals compared with the lesser lability and thus narrower base and prominent peak of the frequency histogram of the cat with high baroreflex sensitivity.

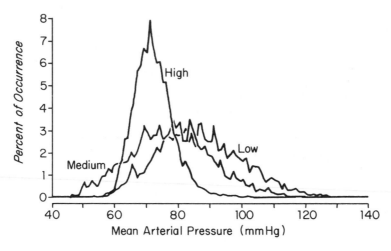

Fig. 3.   Frequency histograms of mean arterial pressure taken 3-20 days after the completion of conditioning.   The data were collected from the same cats whose conditioned responses are shown in Fig. 2.

DISCUSSION

The conditioned pressor responses obtained in cats with lesions of the solitary complex are substantially larger than those previously reported from classical conditioning studies and, with a few exceptions, the responses exceeded those in which operant conditioning procedures were used (Harris and Brady, 1974). The procedures of operant and classical conditioning are quite different and perhaps can be compared only on the basis of total conditioning time required to produce comparable increases of arterial pressure. Generally more time is required for operant conditioning of increases in arterial pressure, and some of these procedures are complicated compared with classical conditioning. The most successful operant studies, which produced increases in pressure that were comparable to ours, required animals to raise their arterial pressures in order to obtain rewards or avoid punishments (Harris and Brady, 1974; Harris and Turkkan, 1981).

These studies required 3-6 months of conditioning while our conditioning period lasted only 30-45 days. Therefore, significant reduction in baroreflex sensitivity by placement of lesions in the solitary complex increases the efficacy of conditioning unusually large increases in MAP and suggests that the baroreflexes exert an important inhibitory role on the conditioned increases of arterial pressure.

Alternative explanations for the inhibition of conditioned increases in MAP should also be considered. First, the lesions may destroy pathways that normally exert an inhibitory influence on sympathetic vasomotor activity, and thus contribute to the potentiated conditioned pressor responses we observed. Our results cannot be explained solely on the basis of this possibility, however, because baroreflex sensitivity correlated so highly with the magnitude of the conditioned pressure responses. Second, the lesions may have somehow altered the cats' emotional states, making them more reactive to the presentation of the tones. This did not seem to be the case, however, as the increase in MAP after delivery of the shock was comparable in the lesion and control groups.

Many investigators have reported elevations and lability of arterial pressure after sinoaortic denervation (Krieger, 1964; Ferrario et al., 1969; McRitchie et al., 1976; Alexander et al., 1981), while a few have shown findings more similar to ours (Cowley et al., 1980; Norman et al., 1981). The uncontrolled environments in which the animals were tested in many of these studies probably contributed to the elevation and lability of arterial pressure. Our animals, on the other hand, were tested in sound-shielded chambers that minimized environmental stimuli. They were well adapted to the chambers, and generally rested quietly during the recording periods. That there were no observed differences between the lesion and control groups in the mean level or lability of MAP during the preconditioning period in a controlled environment supports our earlier findings that the mean level of MAP, and particularly the lability of MAP, apparently were affected by the impact of environmental stimuli (Nathan and Reis, 1977). Thus, much of the disagreement in the literature regarding elevation of arterial pressure after abolishment of baroreflex function probably results from the relatively uncontrolled environmental conditions, as Norman et al. (1981) and Cowley et al. (1980) have suggested. However, these findings may be species-specific. We recently discovered that rats with lesions of the solitary complex are normotensive but display marked lability of MAP regardless of the environmental conditions under which they are tested (unpublished observations).

Baroreflex sensitivity bore no relation to MAP or the lability of MAP during the preconditioning period, probably because of the low level of environmental stimulation and inactivity of the cats. Thus, it is possible that arterial pressure can be easily regulated, even in animals deprived of normal baroreflex function, in situations of low environmental stimulation and behavioral inactivity. This possibility is supported by the observation that a significant relation between baroreflex sensitivity and the magnitude of the increases in arterial pressure emerges only when conditioned pressor responses are elicited by presentation of the tones associated with electrical shock.

Baroreflex sensitivity is not correlated with the mean level of MAP during the postconditioning period, although the MAP is significantly elevated. Thus, some other mechanism, perhaps alterations in vascular smooth muscle, may be responsible for the continued elevation of MAP. Another possibility is that stimuli inherent to the sound-shielded chambers, and thus associated with delivery of shock during the conditioning period, could be responsible for the elevated pressure. It is doubtful that the baroreceptors have reset to a higher level of pressure since there were no changes in pre- to postconditioning baroreflex sensitivity.

Baroreflex sensitivity and lability were inversely correlated during the postconditioning period. The MAP of the control group showed a pre- to postconditioning decrease in lability, suggesting that the normally functioning baroreflexes of the control group so effectively limit the responsiveness of pressure to stimuli inherent to the chamber that lability is actually reduced. In contrast, the lesion group showed slightly increased lability, probably because of reduced baroreflex sensitivity and consequently increased vascular responsiveness to the same stimuli. If this is the case, then this finding supports the possibility that the baroreflexes do not establish the mean level of arterial presure but simply limit the excursions of arterial pressure from the mean level. Furthermore, the magnitude of these excursions or lability is dependent on the impact of environmental stimuli.

In summary, several tentative conclusions can be drawn. First, the baroreflexes actively oppose conditioned pressor responses in cats. Second, the MAP can be significantly elevated even after a short period of conditioning in animals deprived of normal baroreflex function. The mechanisms underlying the maintenance of the elevation in pressure are not understood at this time. Third, under conditions of low ambient environmental stimulation, the mean level and lability of arterial pressure are entirely normal, suggesting that the heightened lability and elevation of arterial pressure in cats with decreased baroreflex sensitivity is a function of the amount of environmental stimulation and behavioral activity. As a final caveat, although the second and third possibilities are considered to be tenable, the issue of whether baroreflex activity establishes the mean level of arterial pressure is far from closed. It might be possible to demonstrate a significant elevation of arterial pressure in a controlled environment if a study were conducted in which the baroreflex function was totally abolished in a sufficient number of animals. However, the five animals in which we were able to abolish baroreflex function totally did **not** display the five highest pressures within the lesion group.

ACKNOWLEDGMENT

Supported by grants HL24529 and HL00558 from the National Institutes of Health.

REFERENCES

Alexander, N., Velasquez, M.T., Decuir, M. and Maronde, R.F. (1980) Indices of sympathetic activity in the sinoaortic-denervated hypertensive rat. Amer. J. Physiol. 238, H521-H526.

Berger, A.J. (1980) The distribution of the cat's carotid sinus nerve afferent and efferent cell bodies using the horseradish peroxidase technique. Brain Res. 190, 309-320.

Bevan, R.D., Van Martheus, E. and Bevan, J.A. (1976) Hyperplasia of vascular smooth muscle in experimental hypertension in the rabbit. Circulat. Res. 38 (Suppl. 2), 59-62.

Carey, R.M., Dacey, R.G., Jane, J.A., Winn, H.R., Ayers, C.R. and Tyson, G.W. (1979) Production of sustained hypertension by lesions in the nucleus tractus solitarii of the American foxhound. Hypertension 1, 246-254.

Ciriello, J., Hrycyshyn, A.W. and Calaresu, F.R. (1981) Horseradish peroxidase study of brain stem projections of carotid sinus and aortic depressor nerves in the cat. J. Autonom. Nerv. Syst. 4, 43-61.

Cowley, A.W. Jr., Liard, J.F. and Guyton, A.C. (1973) Role of baroreceptor reflex in daily control of arterial blood pressure and other variables in dogs. Circulat. Res. 32, 564-576.

Cowley, A.W. Jr.,* Quillen, E.N. and Barber, B.J. (1980) Further evidence for lack of baroreceptor control of long-term level of arterial pressure; in Arterial Baroreceptors and Hypertension, P. Sleight, ed. Oxford University Press, Oxford, pp. 391-399.

Davies, R.O. and Kalia, M. (1981) Carotid sinus nerve projections to the brain stem in the cat. Brain Res. Bull. 6, 531-541.

Ferrario, C.M., McCubbin, J.W. and Page, I.H. (1969) Hemodynamic characteristics of chronic experimental neurogenic hypertension in unanesthetized dogs. Circulat. Res. 24, 911-922.

Folkow, B., Hallback, M., Lundgren, R., Sivertsson, R. and Weiss, L. (1973) Importance of adaptive changes in vascular design for establishment of primary hypertension, studied in man and in spontaneously hypertensive rats. Circulat. Res. 32-33 (Suppl. 1), 2-16.

Harris, A.H. and Brady, J.V. (1974) Animal learning--visceral and autonomic conditioning. Ann. Rev. Psychol. 25, 107-133.

Harris, A.H. and Turkkan, J.S. (1981) Generalization of conditioned blood pressure elevations: schedule and stimulus control effects. Physiol. Behav. 26, 935-940.

Heymans, C. and Neil, E. (1958) Reflexogenic Areas of the Cardiovascular System. J & A Churchill, Ltd., London.

Ito, C.S. and Scher, A.M. (1974) Reflexes from the aortic baroreceptor fibers in the cervical vagus of the cat and the dog. Circulat. Res. 34, 51-60.

Ito, C.S. and Scher, A.M. (1981) Hypertension following arterial baroreceptor denervation in the unanesthetized dog. Circulat. Res. 48, 576-586, 1981.

Kalia, M. and Welles, R.V. (1980) Brain stem projections of the aortic nerve in the cat: a study using tetramethyl benzidine as the substrate for horseradish peroxidase. Brain Res. 188, 23-32.

Krieger, E.M. (1964) Neurogenic hypertension in the rat. Circulat. Res. 15, 511-521.

Laubie, M. and Schmitt, H. (1979) Destruction of the nucleus tractus solitarii in the dog: comparison with sinoaortic denervation. Amer. J. Physiol. 236, H736-H743.

McRitchie, R.J., Vatner, S.F., Heyndrickx, G.R. and Braunwald, E. (1976) The role of arterial baroreceptors in the regulation of arterial pressure in conscious dogs. Circulat. Res. 39, 666-670.

Nathan, M.A. and Reis, D.J. (1977) Chronic labile hypertension produced by lesion of the nucleus tractus·solitarii in the cat. Circulat. Res. 40, 72-81.

Nathan, M.A. and Reis, D.J. (1980) Baroreflex sensitivity--a new method of assessment; in Arterial Baroreceptors and Hypertension, P. Sleight, ed. Oxford University Press, Oxford, pp. 462-469.

Nathan, M.A., Tucker, L.W., Severini, W.P. and Reis, D.J. (1978) Enhancement of conditioned arterial pressure responses in cats after brainstem lesions. Science 201, 71-73.

Norman, R.A., Coleman, T.G. and Dent, A.C. (1981) Continuous monitoring of arterial pressure indicates sinoaortic denervated rats are not hypertensive. Hypertension 3, 119-125.

Panneton, W.M. and Loewy, A.D. (1980) Projections of the carotid sinus nerve to the nucleus of the solitary tract in the cat. Brain Res. 191, 239-244.

Sivertsson, R. and Olander, R. (1968) Aspects of the nature of increased vascular resistance and increased "reactivity" to noradrenaline in hypertensive subjects. Life Sci. 7, 1291-1297.

Copyright 1982 by Elsevier Science Publishing Co.,Inc.
Smith, Galosy, and Weiss, editors
CIRCULATION, NEUROBIOLOGY, AND BEHAVIOR

Behavioral Modulation of the Baroreceptor Reflex

ROBERT B. STEPHENSON
Department of Physiology, Michigan State University, East Lansing, Michigan

INTRODUCTION

The central nervous system (CNS) can facilitate or inhibit the arterial baroreceptor reflex. Specific supramedullary structures that are known to be important in organizing cardiovascular (CV) responses to behavioral states such as exercise or emotion are also capable of modulating baroreflex responses. Hypothalamic stimulation, for example, can facilitate or inhibit (depending on the site stimulated) the parasympathetic component of the baroreflex (Gebber and Snyder, 1970; Klevans and Gebber, 1970; Coote et al., 1979). Hypothalamic modulation of the sympathetic component of the baroreflex was first denied (Gebber and Snyder, 1970), but has since been demonstrated (Kumada et al., 1975; Coote et al., 1979; Hilton, 1980). The key question is: are there behavioral situations in which the CNS manifests its ability to modulate the baroreflex?

Despite all that is known about the baroreflex, there is persistent uncertainty about how behavioral state affects its function. As a negative feedback (homeostatic) control system, the baroreflex clearly has the potential to regulate blood pressure. Nevertheless, it does not prevent the changes in blood pressure that accompany normal changes in behavior. For example, blood pressure is higher during exercise and lower during sleep than during awake rest (Smith et al., 1980). Across a range of behavioral states blood pressure is positively correlated with heart rate, rather than negatively correlated as one would expect if the baroreflex were effectively buffering behaviorally induced changes in blood pressure (Smith et al., 1980; Anderson et al., 1979). This does not necessarily mean that the baroreflex is inhibited when behavioral state changes. It may simply be offset or reset by the many other mechanisms that affect blood pressure. These include psychogenic effects ("central command") which can alter the prevailing levels of sympathetic and parasympathetic tone, reflex influences that arise from numerous peripheral and central sensory receptors (in addition to the baroreceptors), and local factors that influence heart rate, stroke volume, and vascular resistance. Because complex mechanisms are involved in behavioral modulation of the baroreflex, demonstration of central facilitation or inhibition of the reflex in a behaving subject is difficult.

The role of the baroreflex in CV adjustments to various behavioral states has frequently been studied by surgically denervating the carotid and aortic baroreceptor afferents (Ferrario et al., 1969; McRitchie et al., 1976; Baccelli et al., 1981). The primary deficit that accompanies chronic denervation of baroreceptors is increased lability of blood pressure during any given behavioral state. These results imply that the primary role of the baroreflex is to stabilize blood pressure at levels determined for each behavioral state by non-baroreflex mechanisms. However, because of the potential for adaptation, it may be invalid to assume that the role of the baroreflex in the regulation of blood pressure is equal to the deficit in that regulation in the chronic absence of the baroreceptors. In order directly to measure the ability of the baroreflex to stabilize blood pressure in a particular behavioral state (i.e., to measure reflex gain or sensitivity), one must determine the effect on blood pressure of a standardized stimulus to the baro-receptors. The focus of this paper is therefore on specific methods for bringing the stimulus to the baroreceptors under experimental control. Data from several methods will be summarized and compared in the Results section. The Discussion will focus on whether or not central elements of the baroreflex are altered by behavior.

METHODS

In conscious experimental animals, electrical stimulation of the carotid sinus nerves has been used to simulate activation of the carotid baroreceptors (Vatner et al., 1970) and bilateral carotid artery occlusion has been used to deactivate the baroreceptors (Combs, this volume). By contrast, the classical method for study of the baroreflex in anesthetized animals has been to isolate the carotid sinus regions from the systemic circulation by the technique of Moissejeff (1926) and then to apply various static pressures to the isolated sinuses in order to determine the stimulus-response relation between carotid sinus pressure and arterial blood pressure (Fig. 1). If the isolation is reversible, then it is possible to compare the stimulus-response relation with the natural or control level of blood pressure. The stimulus-response curve shows, for a given experimental situation, the degree to which the carotid baroreflex can increase and decrease blood pressure relative to its control value. The slope of the curve defines the gain or sensitivity of the reflex. Threshold and saturation define the range of carotid sinus pressure over which the reflex responds. In the absence of baroreceptor activation (i.e., at carotid sinus pressures below threshold), blood pressure rises to the level that reflects the net effect of all the other factors that control blood presure. Graded increases in baroreceptor stimulation cause progressive decreases in blood pressure until the maximal ability of the baroreflex to depress blood pressure is reached. The control pressure is not necessarily in the middle of the response range, nor is the curve necessarily steepest at control pressure. Only if the control pressure lies away from the extremes of the curve can the baroreflex act to buffer both increases and decreases in blood pressure.

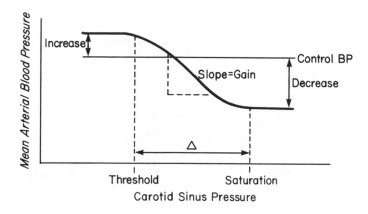

Fig. 1. Idealized stimulus-response curve for effect of pressure in isolated carotid sinuses on arterial blood pressure. Slope measured at steepest part of curve. Control BP: level of arterial pressure when the carotid sinuses are not isolated from the systemic circulation.

Stephenson and Donald (1980a,b) have developed surgical techniques that allow reversible isolation of the carotid sinus regions of dogs (Fig. 2) so that complete stimulus-response curves for the baroreflex can be derived in the conscious state (Fig. 3). Stimulus-response curves are derived using static carotid sinus pressures. Static pressures are easily controlled and repeated, and they allow systematic comparison of reflex responses to identical stimuli in different experimental situations, whereas pulsatile pressure would be much more difficult to standardize. A disadvantage of this technique is that aortic baroreceptors continue to be exposed to arterial blood pressure, so they would buffer changes in arterial pressure that are initiated by the carotid baroreceptors. Complete analysis would therefore require comparison of reflex responses with and without surgical denervation of aortic baroreceptors.

In an attempt to control carotid sinus distending pressure in human subjects, several investigators have applied an air-tight chamber around the neck (Bevegard and Shepherd, 1966; Ludbrook et al., 1978; Mancia et al., 1978). The chamber can be pressurized to decrease baroreceptor stimulation or partially evacuated to increase it. Although it has yielded useful data, the neck chamber technique has several limitations: (1) pressure at the aortic baroreceptors is not controlled, (2) pressure at the carotid baroreceptors is still pulsatile and therefore subject to uncontrolled influences, (3) corrections have to be made for incomplete transmission of the externally applied pressure through the tissue of the neck, and (4) only a limited portion of the entire baroreceptor response range can be studied.

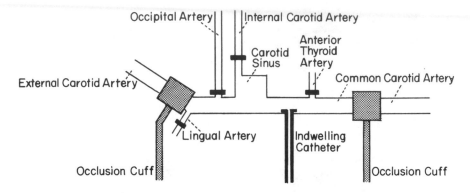

External Carotid Artery

Occipital Artery | | | Internal Carotid Artery

Carotid Sinus | Anterior Thyroid Artery

Common Carotid Artery

Lingual Artery

Indwelling Catheter

Occlusion Cuff

Occlusion Cuff

Fig. 2. Schematic of surgical preparation of carotid sinus region for subsequent, reversible isolation in conscious dogs. Heavy bars indicate points of ligation. When occluders are open, carotid sinus is exposed to arterial blood pressure. Inflation of the occluders isolates the sinus from the remainder of the circulation. Isolated sinus is pressurized to static levels between 50 and 250 mm Hg via the indwelling catheter. Preparation is bilateral. (From Stephenson and Donald, 1980, with permission.)

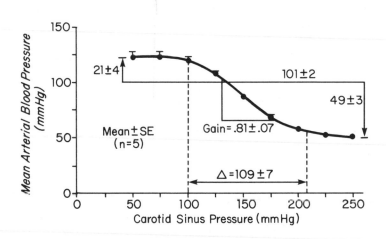

Fig. 3. Characteristics of carotid baroreflex in conscious, quiescent dogs; steady state responses.

The most common method used to study the baroreflex in humans and animals involves injection of vasoactive drugs to raise or lower arterial pressure; the magnitudes of the reflex changes in heart rate (or its reciprocal, heart interval) are taken to indicate baroreflex sensitivity (Robinson et al., 1966; Smyth et al., 1969). A definite advantage of this method is that both aortic and carotid baroreceptors are exposed to the same pressure stimulus. However, despite its simplicity and popularity, this method is limited to study of baroreflex control of heart rate (or heart interval). A change in the sensitivity of the cardiac component of the baroreflex does not necessarily imply a change in the ability of the reflex to control blood pressure. Also, it is difficult to control the timing and magnitude of blood pressure changes by injection of vasoactive drugs. The timing of the blood pressure stimulus has been brought under direct control in trained baboons by use of inflatable cuffs on the descending aorta or vena cava to increase and decrease arterial pressure transiently (Stephenson et al., 1981).

RESULTS

The effect of exercise is the most frequently studied behavioral influence on the baroreceptor reflex. The technique of reversible isolation of the carotid sinuses has been used to compare stimulus-response curves for the baroreflex in conscious dogs standing at rest and running on a treadmill (Melcher and Donald, 1981). Figure 4 (left) indicates that during exercise the control blood pressure and the curve relating blood pressure to carotid sinus pressure are shifted upward in a graded fashion, but the slope of the curve is not significantly altered. These data imply that blood pressure is elevated during exercise by pressor mechanisms that are independent of the baroreflex in the sense that even maximal stimulation of the baroreceptors cannot lower pressure to the levels reached during rest. Nevertheless, during exercise, the baroreflex retains the ability to increase and decrease blood pressure relative to control, and the potential for regulation of blood pressure by the baroreflex (i.e., reflex gain as indicated by the slope of the curves) is unaltered. These data corroborate the earlier findings in dogs that exercise did not change the magnitude of the depressor response that resulted from electrical stimulation of the carotid sinus nerves (Vatner et al., 1970). Also, data from human subjects, based on baroreflex manipulation using the neck chamber, have indicated that the baroreflex retains its ability to raise and lower blood pressure relative to control during dynamic treadmill exercise and during isometric handgrip exercise (Bevegard and Shepherd, 1966; Ludbrook et al., 1978).

Figure 4 (right) indicates that the responses of heart rate, like those of blood pressure, are shifted upward during exercise without a change in slope. Similar shifts were also found by Robinson et al. (1966), who administered infusions of phenylephrine and nitroglycerine to human subjects to obtain sustained increases or decreases in blood pressure during rest and during treadmill exercise (Fig. 5). Finally, Bevegard and Shepherd (1966) found that neck suction reflexly decreased heart rate by equivalent amounts during rest and exercise in human subjects.

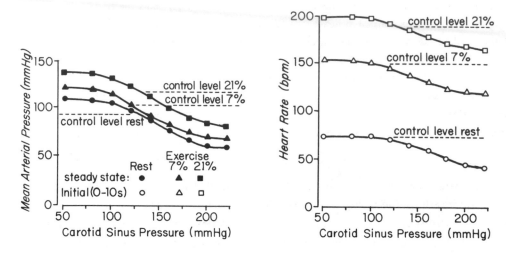

Fig. 4. Characteristics of carotid baroreflex in dogs standing at rest and during mild (5.5 km/hr, 7% grade) and moderately severe (5.5 km/hr, 21% grade) treadmill exercise. (From Melcher and Donald, 1981, with permission.

At least two major research groups have challenged the idea that the cardiac component of the baroreflex has equal sensitivity in rest and exercise. Mancia et al. (1978) found that the magnitude of cardiac slowing in response to neck suction in human subjects was smaller during hand-grip exercise than during rest, and Bristow et al. (1971) found less cardiac slowing in response to a transient, phenylephrine-induced rise in blood pressure in human subjects during supine bicycle exercise than during rest (Fig. 6). The major difference between these studies and those mentioned earlier is an analytical one. In the latter studies, heart interval (R-R interval) was used to measure the cardiac responses, whereas heart rate was used in the former studies. Heart rate and heart interval are reciprocals, each of the other, so the relation between them is hyperbolic (Fig. 7). Reflexly induced changes in heart rate might be equivalent during rest and exercise; but, since control heart rate is elevated during exercise, the corresponding reflex changes in heart interval would be smaller during exercise than during rest. There are no compelling theoretical grounds for asserting that heart rate or heart interval is the "proper" measure; therefore, the interpretation of such data remains arbitrary.

Since the heart rate/heart interval controversy derives from the unequal control rates in rest and exercise, some of the discrepancy can be reconciled by expressing reflex responses in terms of fractional or percent changes in interval or rate (Stephenson et al., 1981). No analysis, however, can overcome the inherent limitation that heart rate (or

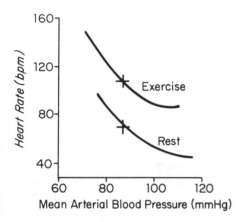

Fig. 5. Effect of treadmill exercise on baroreflex control of heart rate in human subject. **Cross:** control point. **Line:** regression of heart rate on mean arterial pressure during elevation of pressure with phenylephrine or reduction of pressure with nitroglycerine. (Adapted from Robinson et al., 1966.)

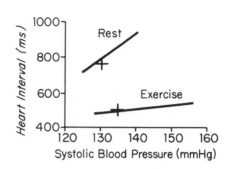

Fig. 6. Effect of bicycling in supine position on baroreflex regulation of pulse interval in human subject. **Cross:** control point. **Line:** regression of heart interval on systolic pressure during rising phase of pressor response to bolus injection of phenylephrine. (Adapted from Bristow et al., 1971).

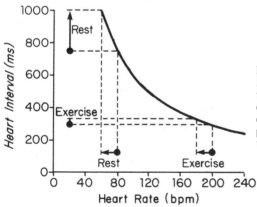

Fig. 7. Arithmetic relation between heart interval and heart rate. **Points:** hypothetical control values. **Arrows:** hypothetical reflex responses to standardized elevation of blood pressure. **Dashed lines:** projections of changes in heart rate onto the heart interval axis.

interval) is but one determinant of blood pressure. Therefore, it may be invalid to extrapolate from baroreflex control of the heart to baroreflex control of blood pressure. For example, in the transition from rest to exercise, an enhanced vascular contribution to the baroreflex could conceivably offset a diminished sensitivity of the cardiac component and account for the finding that the overall baroreflex gain (in terms of control of blood pressure) is equal in exercise and rest.

Cardiac, but not blood pressure, responses to baroreceptor stimulation have been studied during behavioral states other than exercise. The pressor effect of a bolus injection of phenylephrine elicits a reflex·prolongation of heart interval that is more pronounced during REM sleep and less pronounced during mental arithmetic than during awake rest in human subjects (Bristow et al., 1969; Smyth et al., 1969; Brooks et al., 1978). Of course, interpretation of heart interval data is equivocal here for the same reasons cited above in connection with the exercise studies. Another potential limitation on these studies is that only the first 1-15 sec of the rising phase of the pressor response is analyzed, and the systolic pressure on each beat is plotted against the duration of the very next heart interval. Parasympathetically mediated changes in heart rate are rapid enough to be expressed within these time restrictions, but sympathetic responses develop more slowly and may be undetected (Scher and Young, 1970). Indeed, atropine reduced reflex sensitivity essentially to zero (Pickering et al., 1972), indicating that only parasympathetically mediated responses were revealed by the transient analysis.

To clarify the interpretation of these experiments, we undertook studies in behaviorally trained baboons that were equipped with cuffs on the descending aorta (Stephenson et al., 1981). Cyclical inflation of aortic cuffs allowed blood pressure to be driven in sinusoidal patterns of controlled amplitude and frequency. Figure 8 shows typical responses to cyclic inflation of a cuff during four behavioral states. Despite nearly equal amplitudes of perturbation of blood pressure during each behavior, the amplitudes of the reflex responses of heart rate were larger during sleep and smaller during wheel turn than for the intermediate behavioral states of lever press (for food reinforcement) or eating. "Wheel turn" was a mild, dynamic leg exercise reinforced by shock avoidance. The mean levels of blood pressure and heart rate during wheel turn were inappropriately high for the degree of exercise involved, which suggests that the wheel turn involved strong emotion as well as mild exercise. Frequencies of sinusoidal forcing of blood pressure ranging from 0.032 Hz (low enough for expression of sympathetically mediated responses of heart rate) to 0.18 Hz (heart rate responses would be predominantly parasympathetic) were imposed during each behavior. Figure 9 shows that the reflex cardiac responses were affected both by behavioral state and by frequency of sinusoidal forcing. Differences in reflex sensitivity among behaviors were apparently greater when the cardiac responses were measured in terms of heart interval rather than heart rate; however, behavior significantly affected reflex sensitivity no matter which measure was used. In addition, when baroreflex sensitivities were calculated from fractional rather than absolute changes in rate and interval, the measures based on rate and interval became virtually identical; by either measure, baroreflex sensitivity was significantly depressed during wheel turn and enhanced during sleep.

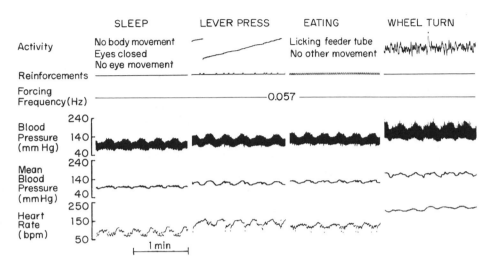

Fig. 8. Effect of cyclical inflation of cuff on descending aorta of baboon during four behavioral states. Degree of aortic constriction adjusted to achieve approximately ±12 mm Hg alterations in systolic blood pressure. Forcing frequency of 0.057 Hz (17 sec cycle). "Activity" shows cumulative lever presses during lever press and damped record of wheel velocity during wheel turn. "Reinforcements" shows delivery of applesauce. (From Stephenson et al., 1981, with permission.)

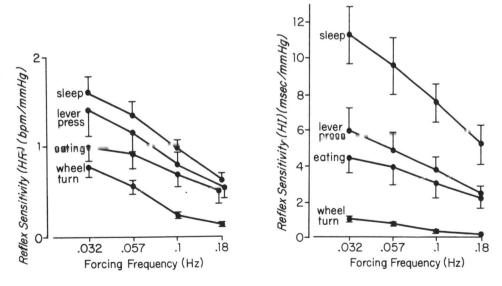

Fig. 9. Baroreflex sensitivity (mean ± SEM for 5 baboons) as function of behavioral state and frequency of alteration of blood pressure. Calculations based on heart rate (left) and heart interval (right). (From Stephenson et al., 1981, with permission.)

The analysis of sinusoidal patterns, such as those in Figure 8, also allows computation of the average time lag between a change in blood pressure and the ensuing reflex change in heart rate. Time lags were found to be short (less than 3 sec) during sleep and significantly longer during wheel turn, denoting parasympathetic dominance in the reflex responses during sleep and a relative increase in sympathetic participation in the reflex responses during wheel turn. However, the small magnitude of the reflex responses during wheel turn indicates that sympathetic participation in the reflex responses was relatively larger during wheel turn because of withdrawal of the parasympathetic contribution to the reflex responses rather than enlargement of the sympathetic contribution. This interpretation was corroborated through study of the effects of atropine and propranolol on the magnitudes and time lags of the reflex cardiac responses. The influence of behavior on reflex sensitivity was equivalent before and after beta sympathetic blockade with propranolol. By contrast, parasympathetic blockade with atropine reduced reflex sensitivity to low and nearly equal values in all four behavioral states.

DISCUSSION

The studies on behaviorally trained baboons (Stephenson et al., 1981) indicate that the sensitivity of the cardiac component of the baroreflex is increased during sleep and decreased during wheel turn (a behavior involving exercise and emotion). The differences in sensitivity are neither artifacts of the particular units used to measure the cardiac responses nor of the timing of transient stimuli to the baroreceptors. These results are consistent with the finding that reflex changes in heart interval following phenylephrine injection are enhanced during REM sleep and suppressed during mental arithmetic in human subjects (Bristow et al., 1969; Smyth et al., 1969; Brooks et al., 1978). The ability of the baroreflex to control blood pressure, not just heart rate, has yet to be fully studied during sleep or emotional behavior.

Dynamic exercise and hand-grip exercise apparently do not affect the sensitivity or gain with which the baroreflex controls blood pressure. Whether or not the cardiac component of the baroreflex is inhibited during exercise remains moot, due in large part to the heart rate/heart interval dilemma.

We come now to the question of whether or not central neural modulation is involved when behavior affects reflex sensitivity. The differences in sensitivity of the cardiac component of the baroreflex during the four different behavioral states in the baboon (Fig. 9) were primarily due to changes in the parasympathetic contribution to the reflex response. Alterations in blood pressure during sleep elicited substantial reflex changes in parasympathetic tone; similar alterations during wheel turn did not elicit substantial changes in either parasympathetic or sympathetic tone. A possible alternative explanation is that the baroreceptors themselves became less responsive to pressure stimuli when these stimuli were superimposed on already elevated pressure (as during wheel turn). Depressed reflex sensitivity persisted during wheel turn, however, when the elevated pressure was offset by propranolol or by partial, sustained constriction of the vena cava. Therefore, altered reflex sensitivity was attributable to central modulation of parasympathetic responsiveness rather than to unequal stimulation of the baroreceptors in the different behavioral states. Admittedly, this argument would be considerably strengthened had these experiments made use of reversibly isolated carotid sinuses, to which completely controlled and standardized stimuli could be delivered in each behavioral state.

To date, behavioral experiments with the isolated sinus preparation have been limited to study of rest and treadmill exercise in dogs. The finding (Fig. 4) that both the blood pressure and the heart rate curves are shifted upward in exercise with no change in slope would suggest that central modulation of reflex sensitivity does not occur in exercise. It could be, however, that the contribution of one neural component of the baroreflex (e.g., parasympathetic control of heart rate) is decreased during exercise (as suggested by Bristow et al., 1971), whereas the sympathetic cardiac and/or vasomotor components are enhanced (as suggested by Robinson et al., 1966). Alternatively, central inhibition of the baroreflex could be offset by increased responsiveness of the reflex effectors (e.g., vascular smooth muscle). Thus, the maintenance of overall reflex gain during exercise may reflect a complex balance among central and peripheral factors tending to increase gain and those tending to decrease gain. Central inhibition or facilitation of particular components of the baroreflex during exercise could be studied by (1) monitoring autonomic nerve activity in behaving animals or (2) the more usual pharmacologic techniques of selective autonomic blockade. To date, neither approach has been coupled with the isolated sinus preparation in the study of behavioral states other than awake rest. Thus, although it is clear that the CNS alters the prevailing levels of sympathetic and parasympathetic tone when behavioral state changes, much still needs to be learned about the extent to which the CNS may also modulate the responsiveness of sympathetic and parasympathetic neurons to baroreceptor input.

ACKNOWLEDGMENT

This work was supported in part by grant HL26628 from the National Institutes of Health.

REFERENCES

Anderson, D.E., Yingling, J.E. and Sagawa, K. (1979) Minute-to-minute covariations in cardiovascular activity of conscious dogs. Amer. J. Physiol. 236, H434-H439.

182

Baccelli, G., Albertini, R., Del Bo, A., Mancia, G. and Zanchetti, A. (1981) Role of sinoaortic reflexes in hemodynamic patterns of natural defense behaviors in the cat. Amer. J. Physiol. 240, H421-H429.

Bevegard, B.S. and Shepherd, J.T. (1966) Circulatory effects of stimulating the carotid arterial stretch receptors in man at rest and during exercise. J. Clin. Invest. 45, 132-142.

Bristow, J.D., Brown, E.B. Jr., Cunningham, D.J.C., Howson, M.G., Petersen, E.S., Pickering, T.G. and Sleight, P. (1971) Effect of bicycling on the baroreflex regulation of pulse interval. Circulat. Res. 28, 582-592.

Bristow, J.D., Honour, A.J., Pickering, T.G. and Sleight, P. (1969) Cardiovascular and respiratory changes during sleep in normal and hypertensive subjects. Cardiovasc. Res. 3, 476-485.

Brooks, D., Fox, P., Lopez, R. and Sleight, P. (1978) The effect of mental arithmetic on blood pressure variability and baroreflex sensitivity in man. J. Physiol. (Lond.) 280, 75P-76P.

Coote, J.H., Hilton, S.M. and Perez-Gonzalez, J.F. (1979) Inhibition of the baroreceptor reflex on stimulation in the brain stem defense centre. J. Physiol. (London) 288, 549-560.

Ferrario, C.M., McCubbin, J.W. and Page, I.H. (1969) Hemodynamic characteristics of chronic experimental neurogenic hypertension in unanesthetized dogs. Circulat. Res. 24, 911-922.

Gebber, G.L. and Snyder, D.W. (1970) Hypothalamic control of baroreceptor reflexes. Amer. J. Physiol. 218, 124-131.

Hilton, S.M. (1980) Inhibition of the baroreceptor reflex by the brainstem defense centre; in Arterial Baroreceptors and Hypertension, P. Sleight, ed. Oxford University Press, Oxford, pp. 318-323.

Klevans, L.R. and Gebber, G.L. (1970) Facilitatory forebrain influence on cardiac component of baroreceptor reflexes. Amer. J. Physiol. 219, 1235-1241.

Kumada, M., Schramm, L.P., Altmansberger, R.A. and Sagawa, K. (1975) Modulation of carotid sinus baroreceptor reflex by hypothalamic defense response. Amer. J. Physiol. 228, 34-45.

Ludbrook, J., Faris, I.B., Iannos, J., Jamieson, G.G. and Russell, W.J. (1978) Lack of effect of isometric handgrip exercise on the responses of the carotid sinus baroreceptor reflex in man. Clin. Sci. Mol. Med. 55, 189-194.

Mancia, G., Iannos, J., Jamieson, G.G., Lawrence, R.H., Sharman, P.R. and Ludbrook, J. (1978) Effect of isometric hand-grip exercise on the carotid sinus baroreceptor reflex in man. Clin. Sci. Mol. Med. 54, 33-37.

McRitchie, R.H., Vatner, S.F., Boettcher, D., Heyndrickx, G.R., Patrick, T.A. and Braunwald, E. (1976) Role of arterial baroreceptors in mediating cardiovascular responses to exercise. Amer. J. Physiol. 230, 85-89.

Melcher, A. and Donald, D.E. (1981) Maintained ability of carotid baroreflex to regulate arterial pressure during exercise in dogs. Amer. J. Physiol. 241, H838-H849.

Moissejeff, E. (1926) Zur Kenntnis des Carotissinusreflexes. Z. Gesamte Exp. Med. 53, 696-704.

Pickering, T.G., Gribbin, B., Petersen, E.S., Cunningham, D.J.C. and Sleight, P. (1972) Effects of autonomic blockade on the baroreflex in man at rest and during exercise. Circulat. Res. 30, 177-185.

Robinson, B.F., Epstein, S.E., Beiser, G.D. and Braunwald, E. (1966) Control of heart rate by the autonomic nervous system: studies in man on the interrelation between baroreceptor mechanisms and exercise. Circulat. Res. 19, 400-411.

Scher, A.M. and Young, A.C. (1970) Reflex control of heart rate in the unanesthetized dog. Amer. J. Physiol. 218, 780-789.

Smith, O.A., Astley, C.A., Hohimer, A.R. and Stephenson, R.B. (1980) Behavior and cerebral control of cardiovascular function; in Research Topics in Physiology, Neural Control of Circulation, M.J. Hughes and C.D. Barnes, eds. Academic Press, New York, pp. 1-21.

Smyth, H.S., Sleight, P. and Pickering, G.W. (1969) Reflex regulation of arterial pressure during sleep in man: quantitative method of assessing baroreflex sensitivity. Circulat. Res. 24, 109-121.

Stephenson, R.B. and Donald, D.E. (1980a) Reversible vascular isolation of carotid sinuses in conscious dogs. Amer. J. Physiol. 238, H809-H814.

Stephenson, R.B. and Donald, D.E. (1980b) Reflexes from isolated carotid sinuses of intact and vagotomized conscious dogs. Amer. J. Physiol. 238, H815-H822.

Stephenson, R.B., Smith, O.A. and Scher, A.M. (1981) Baroreceptor regulation of heart rate in baboons during different behavioral states. Amer. J. Physiol. 241, R277-R285.

Vatner, S.F., Franklin, D., Van Citters, R.L. and Braunwald, E. (1970) Effects of carotid sinus nerve stimulation on blood-flow distribution in conscious dogs at rest and during exercise. Circulat. Res. 27, 495-503.

Behavioral Modulation
of Arterial Baroreflexes

C. ANDREW COMBS
Regional Primate Research Center, University of Washington, Seattle, Washington

INTRODUCTION

It has long been recognized that certain behaviors are accompanied by marked changes in blood pressure, cardiac output, and regional blood flow. A recurrent theme in this volume has been that the central nervous system (CNS) is involved in initiating and maintaining these changes. However, it has also been recognized that any alterations in arterial blood pressure ought to be opposed by the baroreceptor reflexes. The means by which central activity can produce changes in blood pressure despite this opposition by the baroreflexes might be explained in either of two ways. One explanation would be that changes in blood pressure can be accomplished by simply overpowering the baroreflexes, that is, by producing more descending autonomic activity than would be required to produce equivalent changes in blood pressure in the absence of such reflexes. The second, and by far more intriguing, explanation would be that, in addition to its relatively direct effects on the autonomic motoneurons, CNS activity might also actively inhibit the baroreflexes.

Bard (1960) was apparently the first to entertain this notion that changes in baroreflex sensitivity might play a role in behavioral situations. "There can be no doubt," he stated, "that in emotional excitement suprabulbar influences inhibit the cardiovascular response to baroreceptor stimulation, for this state is characterized, as is muscular exercise, by the combination of high arterial pressure and high heart rates." Embodied in this relatively straightforward statement, however, were three key assumptions which left considerable room for doubt, and, more important, for experimentation.

The first assumption was that one could infer changes in reflex sensitivity ("inhibition") from changes in the extant values of blood pressure and heart rate. This notion has by now been thoroughly discredited by Korner (1979), whose analysis is adapted in Figure 1. As shown, two distinct types of reflex "modulation" may occur, either alone or in combination. The first is a shift of the baroreflex characteristic curve, without a change in its slope (sensitivity). Such a shift indicates that some reflex-independent mechanism influences the output and sums algebraically with the reflex. The second possible type of modulation is a change in the sensitivity of the reflex, manifested as a change in the slope of the curve. Such a change indicates a nonlinear interaction between

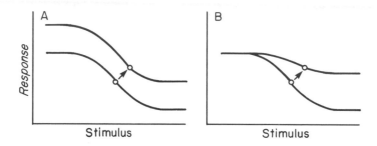

Fig. 1. Two possible types of baroreflex modulation. For both sets of curves, the stimulus is the blood pressure sensed by the baroreceptors. The response may be heart rate, regional resistance, or, in isolated-receptor experiments, systemic arterial blood pressure. Open circles represent conceivable "operating points," or extant values of pressure and response in the unperturbed system. **A**: curve shift, caused by algebraic summation of reflex and reflex-independent influences on the output. **B**: change in reflex sensitivity, caused by nonlinear interaction of reflex and nonreflex effects. Note that both types of modulation may cause indentical changes in the operating point. The two types of modulation may occur separately or in combination. (Adapted from Korner, 1979.)

reflex and nonreflex effects, an interaction that implies that the reflex and nonreflex pathways converge at some point.[1] As the arrows in Figure 1 show, the two types of modulation can conceivably be accompanied by identical shifts in the "operating point" values. Thus, while Bard was correct that simultaneous elevations of blood pressure and heart rate cannot be attributed to a single baroreflex curve, he was premature in concluding that a change in sensitivity, rather than a simple curve shift, occurs in emotional situations or exercise. To resolve this issue, one needs to measure reflex sensitivity by actually perturbing the baroreceptors. Indeed, several investigators who have measured reflex sensitivity by a variety of methods have reported a decreased sensitivity of the baroreflex influence on the heart during emotional situations (Brooks et al., 1978) and during exercise (Bristow et al., 1971; Pickering et al., 1971; Vatner et al., 1970; Geis and Wurster, 1980; Stephenson et al., 1981). Increases in sensitivity have been found during sleep (Smyth et al., 1969; Vatner et al., 1971; Stephenson et al., 1981). However, Stephenson (this volume) points out that there are conflicting results with regard to the changes during exercise (Robinson et al., 1966; Bevegard and Shepherd,

---

[1] The nomenclature of reflex modulation has become somewhat confusing. Shifts of the characteristic curves have been called "reflex resetting," a term which brings perhaps too much surplus meaning from engineering control theory; in this chapter, such shifts are simply called curve shifts. Some authors have referred to changes in reflex sensitivity as "inhibition" or "facilitation," terms which seem to imply that the neural mechanisms of reflex modulation are understood in somewhat more detail than they actually are; in this chapter, such changes are simply be called decreases or increases in sensitivity.

1966; Melcher and Donald, 1981) and that the interpretation of many of these results is hindered by methodological considerations.

Bard's second assumption was that suprabulbar mechanisms were needed to account for differences in reflex sensitivity that might occur between behaviors. Given that almost any interaction between reflex and nonreflex effects may manifest itself as a change in reflex sensitivity, and given that such interactions may occur at virtually any level of the neuraxis, or even at the receptor organ or effector organ level, this second assumption seems somewhat tenuous. Nonetheless, Bard was at least partly vindicated by several experiments showing that electrical stimulation of numerous suprabulbar loci could greatly attenuate baroreflex responses. Moruzzi (1940) had previously demonstrated that stimulation of the cerebellar cortex nearly abolished the reflex pressor response to carotid occlusion. More recently, attenuation of the baroreflex influence on heart rate has been observed to accompany stimulation of the cerebellar fastigial nucleus (Achari and Downman, 1970; Lisander and Martner, 1971), the inferior olivary nucleus (Smith and Nathan, 1967), the hypothalamic "defence area" (Hilton, 1963; Djojosugito et al., 1970; Humphreys et al., 1971; Coote et al., 1979), and the cerebral motor cortex (Achari and Downman, 1978). Evidence that true neural inhibition may be involved in some of these phenomena was obtained by Weiss and Crill (1969), who reported that stimulation in the fields of Forel caused presynaptic inhibition of carotid sinus nerve primary afferents. Similarly, McAllen (1976) found that "defence area" stimulation could inhibit the activity of baroreceptor-related units in or near the nucleus tractus solitarius (NTS), which contains the second-order neurons in the baroreflex arc. Increases in the baroreflex sensitivity have been obtained by stimulating other sites in the hypothalamus (Reis and Cuenod, 1965; Klevans and Gebber, 1970), the medullary reticular formation (Reis and Cuenod, 1965), the septal nuclei (Gebber and Klevans, 1972) and the amygdala (Gebber and Klevans, 1972). Although all these observations suggest that suprabulbar mechanisms can modulate the baroreflexes, it is not entirely clear which, if any, of these mechanisms or loci are actually used to produce the changes in reflex sensitivity accompanying various behaviors.

The third, and most tacit, assumption in Bard's hypothesis was that "the cardiovascular resonse to baroreceptor stimulation" could be adequately characterized by the heart rate response, ignoring the vasomotor responses. It is entirely conceivable that certain behaviors might attenuate the baroreflex effects on the heart while enhancing or leaving unaltered the effects on the systemic vasculature. For example, Vatner et al. (1970) found that exercise attenuated the heart rate response to carotid sinus nerve stimulation but did not change the regional flow responses. Conversely, the data of Bevegard and Shepherd (1966) show no exercise-induced changes in the heart rate response to neck suction, but a slightly larger forearm vasodilation than that observed at rest.

Geis and Wurster (1980) found that exercise decreased the sensitivity of both the heart rate and blood pressure responses to graded changes of carotid sinus pressure, but the heart rate response appeared to be attenuated to a greater extent.

These behavioral observations, as well as results from electrical stimulation experiments (Djojosugito et al., 1970; Humphreys et al., 1971; Humphreys and Joels, 1972; Lisander and Martner, 1971; Kumada et al., 1975) suggest the possibility of **differential modulation** of the various efferent components of the baroreflex. The importance of such a phenomenon is that it may provide a clue as to the level at which reflex modulation occurs. As illustrated schematically in Figure 2, the baroreceptor information diverges at some point in the nervous system to exert separate effects on the heart and on the systemic vasculature. If modulation were mediated by descending activity converging with reflex activity at some point **before** the pathway diverges (arrows 1 in Figure 2), one would expect equal effects on the sensitivity of cardiac and vasomotor limbs. This type of result would be predicted, for example, if modulation occurred by presynaptic inhibition (Weiss and Crill, 1969), by inhibition within the NTS, or even by changes in the sensitivity of the baroreceptors themselves (McCubbin et al., 1956). Alternatively, if

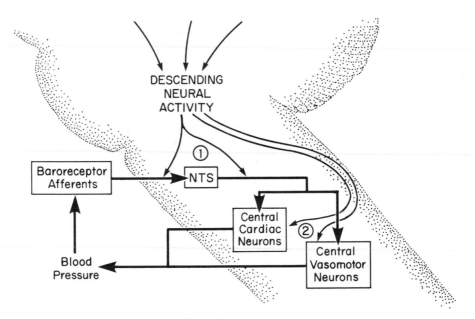

Fig. 2. Two possible models of baroreflex modulation by descending neural activity. Arrows 1 indicate modulation occurring by central activity impinging on reflex pathway before the latter diverges. Arrows 2 indicate central activity impinging on the reflex pathway after the divergence. Only model 2 allows differential modulation of cardiac and vasomotor limbs.

modulation were mediated by descending activity converging with reflex activity at some point **after** the pathway diverges (arrows 2 in Figure 2), then differential modulation would be possible. Such modulatory interactions could occur at the interneurons of the medulla or spinal cord, at the preganglionic neurons, in the autonomic ganglia, or even at the peripheral effector organs. These two types of possible interactions are not, of course, mutually exclusive, for certain behaviors may be accompanied by differential modulation while others may be accompanied by an equal modulation of the cardiac and vasomotor limbs.

The present experiments address Bard's hypothesis with particular attention to the possibility that changes in behavior may differentially modulate the different efferent limbs of the carotid sinus reflex. The effects of various behaviors on the cardiac responses and the hindlimb and renal responses to bilateral carotid occlusion (BCO) were tested in intact, unanesthetized baboons.

METHODS

Subjects and training. Four juvenile male baboons (*Papio cynocephalus*) were studied. During daily sessions in a sound-attenuating booth, each was trained to perform a 4-min dynamic leg exercise task, on cue, for applesauce reinforcement (for details see Hohimer and Smith, 1979). External sounds were masked by 45 dB of white noise. The animals were continuously observed via two closed-circuit video monitors.

Instrumentation and data collection. Following training, each subject was instrumented, under halothane anesthesia, for the measurment of arterial blood pressure, heart rate, renal blood flow, and terminal aortic blood flow. Cuff occluders were placed around the vessels distal to each electromagnetic flow probe for the determination of flow zero. In addition, cuff occluders were placed around the common carotid arteries bilaterally. The vagi were left intact. Three weeks recovery were allowed between the implantation of flow probes and the collection of data. During experimental sessions, each cardiovascular variable was recorded on an eight-channel stripchart recorder and simultaneously digitized, sampled at 100 Hz, averaged in 3-sec time bins, and stored on floppy disks. Renal vascular conductance and terminal aortic conductance were computed offline as the ratio of the respective flow to blood pressure for each time bin.

Experimental protocol. During each of several daily experimental sessions, each baboon performed the exercise task two or three times at random intervals. Quiet rest was observed during the intervals between or after exercises, after allowing several minutes for recovery to a stable baseline. Quiet, non-REM, nocturnal sleep was observed during separate overnight sessions in the sound-attenuating booth.

Each subject served as its own control. The experimental condition consisted of BCO performed during the middle 2 min of the 4-min exercise task or 2 min during rest or sleep. The control condition consisted of the same behaviors without BCO. The data collection format for experimental and control trials followed identical time-courses. Occasional trials during which the subject became visibly aroused by BCO or ceased performing the exercise task were excluded from analysis. At least five experimental trials and five control trials were obtained from each subject in each of the three behaviors.

Data analysis. Within each behavior, the bin-by-bin averages of all control and all experimental trials were computed for each subject. These 24 averages (4 animals X 3 behaviors X 2 conditions) constituted the data base for subsequent statistical analyses.

The effects of behavior alone (no BCO) on a given variable were determined from the control averages by taking the mean value during the 30-sec period that corresponded in time-course to the last 30 sec of BCO in the experimental trials. Significance of differences between behaviors was tested by a repeated measures analysis of variance and the Newman-Kuels multiple range test.

The steady-state response of a given variable to BCO was computed as follows. First, for the 12 experimental averages, the mean value during the 30 sec immediately preceding BCO was subtracted from the mean value during the last 30 sec of BCO. The corresponding difference was then computed for the control averages. The response to BCO was taken as the difference between these differences. This procedure controlled for the fact that BCO was performed before the steady state of exercise was fully reached, and also controlled for any systematic drift of a variable during rest or sleep. Within a behavior, significance of the response to BCO was tested with the Student t-statistic for paired data. Between behaviors, significance of differences in responses was tested with a repeated measures analysis of variance and the F-statistic for the interaction between behavior and BCO.

RESULTS

Each behavior resulted in a unique pattern of blood pressure, heart rate, and blood flow distribution. Table 1 summarizes the control values of each variable, obtained during the trials in which BCO was not performed.

BCO during the three behaviors resulted in the patterns of cardiovascular changes shown in Figure 3. Qualitatively, the responses to BCO were similar in all behaviors, with significant increases in heart rate and blood pressure and decreases in terminal aortic and renal conductance. Quantitatively, however, there were some differences in the responses across behaviors.

During all three behaviors, carotid occlusion caused a slight tachycardia, and there was a tendency, though not statistically significant, for this response to be smallest during leg exercise (4.3 ± 1.7 bpm), larger during rest (7.6 ± 2.4 bpm), and largest during sleep

TABLE 1

CARDIOVASCULAR RESPONSES TO THREE BEHAVIORS IN BABOONS

Variable	Behavior		
	Leg Exercise	Rest	Sleep
Heart rate (beats/min)	$190 \pm 7^{a,b}$	142 ± 8^{a}	113 ± 15^{b}
Terminal aortic flow (ml/min)	$1244 \pm 123^{a,b}$	501 ± 74	348 ± 104
Terminal aortic conductance (ml/min/mm Hg)	$11.4 \pm 1.3^{a,b}$	5.4 ± 0.7^{a}	4.1 ± 0.7^{b}
Renal flow (ml/min)	166 ± 17	184 ± 17	208 ± 64
Renal conductance (ml/min/mm Hg)	1.55 ± 0.23^{a}	2.02 ± 0.36	2.49 ± 0.55
Blood pressure (mm Hg)	110 ± 5^{a}	93 ± 2	81 ± 8

Means $\pm$ SE from four baboons
[a]Different from sleep (p<0.05, Newman-Kuels multiple range test)
[b]Different from rest (p<0.05, Newman-Kuels multiple range test)

(9.6 ± 3.7 bpm) (Fig. 4). The same trend was apparent whether the results were computed as heart rate or heart interval changes.

Terminal aortic flow was essentially unchanged by BCO during exercise or rest, and slightly elevated by BCO during sleep. Since these responses were undoubtedly influenced by the significant increases in perfusion pressure that accompanied BCO, conductance, rather than flow, is undoubtedly a better indicator of the vasomotor response of the terminal aortic bed. BCO caused decreases in terminal aortic conductance during all three behaviors, and this decrease was significantly greater during exercise (2.89 ± 0.89 ml/min/mm Hg) than during either rest (1.11 ± 0.25 ml/min/mm Hg) or sleep (0.35 ± 0.33 ml/min/mm Hg) (Fig. 4).

Both renal flow and renal conductance were decreased by BCO (Fig. 3), but neither response was significantly affected by behavior. Kirchheim (1976) has pointed out that the renal conductance changes accompanying BCO do not necessarily reflect true reflexogenic vasoconstriction, since the kidney has powerful autoregulatory mechanisms that tend to maintain constant flow in the face of changes in perfusion pressure. For this reason, renal flow, rather than conductance, is a more conservative indicator of the vasomotor response of the renal bed to BCO. There was no consistent effect of behavior on the renal flow responses (Fig. 4).

Finally, BCO elicited substantial increases in blood pressure during all three behaviors (Fig. 3), but this pressor response did not differ significantly across behaviors (Fig. 4).

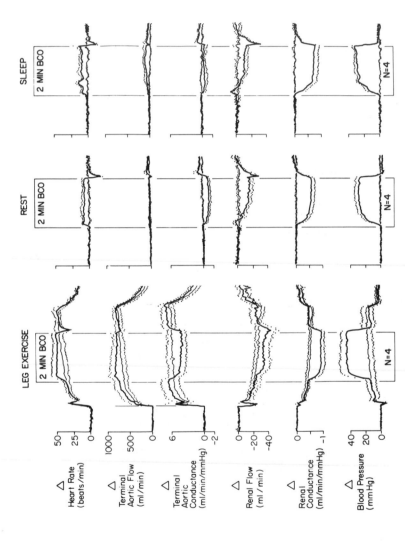

Fig. 3. Responses to BCO during three behaviors. Averages from four baboons. Each variable is plotted as change from the mean value during the first full minute. **Heavy lines:** trials in which BCO was performed during the time indicated. **Light lines:** control trials (no BCO). **Dots:** standard errors of the mean for each 3-sec time bin.

193

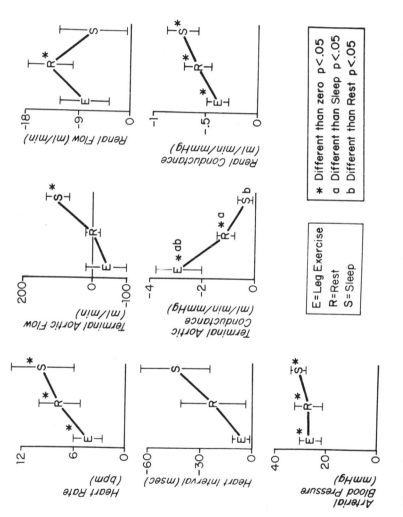

Fig. 4. Steady-state responses to BCO during three behaviors. Averages from four baboons. Values are the mean differences (±S.E.) between experimental and control trials over the last 30 sec of BCO. *Significant effect of BCO (p<0.05, Student's t-test, paired data). a, significant difference from sleep; b, significant difference from rest (p<0.05, F-test).

DISCUSSION

The heart rate response, hindlimb and renal vasomotor responses, and blood pressure response to BCO were employed in this study to indicate the ability of distinct efferent limbs of the carotid baroreflex to compensate for decreases in arterial pressure. While not statistically significant in this small number of subjects, the heart rate response to BCO was, on the average, somewhat depressed during leg exercise and somewhat exaggerated during sleep. The terminal aortic response, on the other hand, showed the opposite pattern, being largest during exercise and smallest during sleep. The renal and blood pressure responses were not significantly affected by the changes in behavior. The observation that the changes in behavior had opposite effects on the cardiac and terminal aortic responses, and no effect on the renal or pressor responses, is suggestive evidence for differential modulation of the various reflex components. Such modulation cannot be explained solely on the basis of differences in the magnitudes of the stimulus (BCO) or differences in the sensitivity of the receptors between behaviors. Further, these results are not compatible with a presynaptic inhibition model of baroreflex modulation. Any of these mechanisms would be expected to cause similar changes in all the reflex responses. This experiment does not, however, demonstrate whether the observed reflex modulation occurs as a result of central neural influences acting directly on the baroreflex pathways or whether it is a consequence of changes in the characteristics of the effector organs.

The apparent depression of the cardiac responses to baroreflex stimuli during exercise has been a matter of some controversy. Several investigators have reported that exercise causes a decrease in the sensitivity of this reflex limb (Pickering et al., 1970; Vatner et al., 1970; Bristow et al., 1971; Geis and Wurster, 1980; Stephenson et al., 1981) but others have reported negative results (Robinson et al., 1966; Melcher and Donald, 1981). Stephenson (this volume) has shown that some of the discrepancy is due to the reciprocal relation between heart rate and heart interval, since results expressed as heart intervals may show large apparent changes in reflex sensitivity across behaviors, whereas the same results expressed as heart rates may show no changes. The present data show evidence, on the average, of decreased cardiac responses to BCO during exercise, expressed as either heart rate or heart interval changes (Fig. 4). Stephenson et al. (1981) found a similar and highly significant effect of exercise in baboons. The failure of the present results to reach statistical significance may be due, in part, to the small number of subjects tested and, in part, to the relatively mild degree of exercise obtained (Table 1). Another potentially confounding influence was the competing effect of the intact aortic baroreceptors, which may have accounted for the small magnitude of all the responses.

The time-course of the heart rate changes (Fig. 3) suggests, however, that the depressed responses during exercise may have been due simply to a saturation effect, rather than a neurally mediated change in reflex sensitivity, since heart rate was already greatly elevated during exercise and may have been limited in the extent to which it could increase further in response to carotid occlusion. Although the heart may thus have been less responsive to decreases in carotid pressure, the same result would not necessarily have been found in an experiment involving increases in carotid pressure. This is an inherent limitation of experiments that perturb the baroreceptors in only one direction. To overcome this limitation, it is necessary to derive the full baroreflex characteristic curves during different behaviors. Two groups have done such an analysis in dogs and have, unfortunately, obtained different results. Melcher and Donald (1981) found that exercise, compared with rest, caused an upward shift in the curve relating heart rate and carotid sinus pressure, with no significant change in sensitivity. In contrast, Geis and Wurster (1980), using a similar preparation, reported both an upward shift and a decrease in sensitivity during exercise. Thus, the issue of a change in the sensitivity of the cardiac limb of the baroreflex during exercise seems to be nearly as unsettled today as when Bard proposed it two decades ago. It is clear, however, that any changes that may occur are quantitative rather than qualitative: the reflex continues to operate during exercise.

The terminal aortic response to carotid occlusion was greatly enhanced during leg exercise and depressed during sleep. The data of Bevegard and Shepherd (1966) similarly indicate that the forearm vasodilation caused by neck suction was larger during leg exercise than during rest, but their study was not designed to allow statistical comparisons between the two states. The large response during leg exercise in the present study was surprising, since it is usually difficult to elicit sympathetically mediated vasoconstriction in beds supplying working muscle, a phenomenon that has been termed "functional sympatholysis" (Remensnyder et al., 1962; Kjellmer, 1965; Strandell and Shepherd, 1967). However, the large carotid occlusion response observed here does not necessarily reflect neurogenic vasoconstriction, since local metabolic effects become important in controlling blood flow to working muscle. Thus, the large conductance change may be a kind of autoregulatory response to the large increase in perfusion pressure, a mechanism that would not be expected to be important during sleep or rest.

Another factor that confounds the interpretation of these changes is that they are dependent on whether one chooses to measure conductance or resistance. Since these two measures, like heart rate and heart interval, are reciprocally related, it is possible to bias the results by choosing one over the other. Figure 5 shows, for example, that although the terminal aortic conductance response to BCO was larger during leg exercise than during rest, the same results measured as resistances would have led us to the opposite conclusion. Since there are no compelling theoretical reasons to select one measure over the other, the interpretation of these data remains arbitrary.

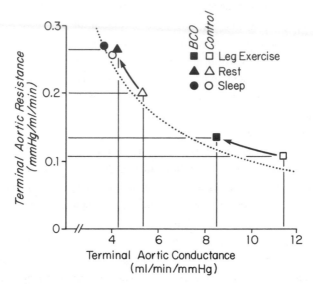

Fig. 5. Terminal aortic responses to carotid occlusion during three behaviors. Mean responses from four baboons. **Open symbols** show values of conductance and resistance during control trials (no BCO). **Solid symbols** show values during last 30 sec of BCO during experimental trials. **Dotted curve** shows expected reciprocal relation between conductance and resistance. Note that the response is much larger during exercise than during rest when expressed as a change in conductance, but smaller when expressed as a change in resistance. The response is quite small during sleep, regardless of which measure is used.

During sleep, on the other hand, the terminal aortic response to BCO was smaller than at rest, independent of whether conductance or resistance was measured. Again, however, the small responses during sleep can conceivably be due to a saturation effect, rather than central neural modulation of the reflex, since terminal aortic conductance was quite low during sleep and may have been limited in the extent to which it could decrease further in response to carotid occlusion (Myers and Honig, 1969). This is an example of a recurrent difficulty in studies of reflex modulation. Measurement of hemodynamic responses alone does not yield unequivocal information about the potential neural substrates, while measurement of central or peripheral neural activity alone cannot yield unequivocal information about the potential hemodynamic significance of any observed modulation. This difficulty will undoubtedly continue to challenge investigators for many years.

The renal responses to carotid occlusion, while not significantly affected by the changes in behavior, were noteworthy in one respect. Kirchheim (1969) and collaborators (Gross et al., 1979, 1981) have found that carotid occlusion in conscious dogs does not result in any renal vasoconstriction other than that attributable to autoregulation. The decrease in renal blood flow in the face of an increased perfusion pressure, as observed in all behaviors in the present study, cannot be attributed to autoregulation. To our knowledge, this is the first report of decreased renal blood flow in response to carotid occlusion in an unanesthetized preparation. This may reflect a species difference between baboons and dogs.

Finally, it is interesting that the pressor responses to carotid occlusion were virtually identical in all three behaviors. Similar results have been obtained for exercise in humans (Ludbrook et al., 1978) and in conscious dogs (Melcher and Donald, 1981). These findings suggest that although changes in behavior may be associated with changes in the responsiveness of particular effector organs to baroreflex stimuli, the overall ability of the reflex to compensate for changes in blood pressure may be relatively unaffected by behavior.

In conclusion, we may note that it is still uncertain whether Bard was correct in asserting that changes in behavior can alter the sensitivity of the baroreflexes. For those studies that seem to demonstrate changes in reflex sensitivity, it is unclear to what extent central neural mechanisms are involved or to what extent the changes may be attributable to altered responsiveness of the effector organs. The present data support the notion that changes in sensitivity of one efferent limb of the reflex need not be accompanied by parallel changes in sensitivity of the other limbs. However, we still have little understanding of the relative importance of reflex modulation, as opposed to more direct central neural influences on the heart and vasculature, in producing the patterns of cardiovascular changes that accompany various behaviors. It is hoped that this chapter has raised some general issues worthy of consideration in future investigations of reflex modulation, not only in behaviors such as exercise, rest, and sleep, but also in other classes of behavioral situations.

ACKNOWLEDGMENTS

I am indebted to Drs. Orville A. Smith and Eric O. Feigl for helpful discussions, to Dr. Gene P. Sackett for statistical advice, and to Clifford, Astley, David Taylor, and Deborah Baldwin for invaluable technical assistance. Dr. Robert B. Stephenson suggested the conductance-vs.-resistance analysis. Some of the statistical analyses were aided by Prophet, a computing resource of the National Institutes of Health. Supported by NIH grants HL16910, RR00166, and GM07266.

198

REFERENCES

Achari, N.K. and Downman, C.B.B. (1970) Autonomic effector responses to stimulation of nucleus fastigius. J. Physiol. (Lond.) 210, 637-650.

Achari, N.K. and Downman, C.B.B. (1978) Inhibition of reflex bradycardia by stimulation of cerebral motor cortex. Brain Res. 150, 198-200.

Bard, P. (1960) Anatomical organization of the central nervous system in relation to control of the heart and blood vessels. Physiol. Rev. 40 (Suppl. 4), 3-26.

Bevegard, B.S. and Shepherd, J.T. (1966) Circulatory effects of stimulating the carotid arterial stretch receptors in man at rest and during exercise. J. Clin. Invest. 45, 132-142.

Bristow, J.D., Brown, E.B., Cunningham, D.J.C., Howson, M.G., Peterson, E.S., Pickering, T.G. and Sleight, P. (1971) Effect of bicycling on the baroreflex regulation of pulse interval. Circulat. Res. 28, 582-592.

Brooks, D., Fox, P., Lopez, R. and Sleight, P. (1978) The effect of mental arithmetic on blood pressure variability and baroreflex sensitivity in man. J. Physiol. (Lond.) 280, 75P-76P.

Coote, J.H., Hilton, S.M. and Perez-Gonzales, J.F. (1979) Inhibition of the baroreceptor reflex on stimulation in the brain stem defence centre. J. Physiol. (Lond.) 288, 549-560.

Djojosugito, A.M., Folkow, B., Kylstra, P.H., Lisander, B. and Tuttle, R.S. (1970) Differentiated interaction between the hypothalamic defence reaction and baroreceptor reflexes: I. Effects on heart rate and regional flow resistance. Acta Physiol. Scand. 78, 376-385.

Gebber, G.L. and Klevans, L.R. (1972) Central nervous modulation of cardiovascular reflexes. Fed. Proc. 31, 1245-1252.

Geis, G.S. and Wurster, R.D. (1980) Baroreceptor reflexes during exercise; in Arterial Baroreceptors and Hypertension, P. Sleight, ed. Oxford University Press, Oxford.

Gross, R., Kirchheim, H. and Ruffman, K. (1981) Effect of carotid occlusion and of perfusion pressure on renal function in conscious dogs. Circulat. Res. 48, 777-784.

Gross, R., Ruffman, K. and Kirchheim, H. (1979) The separate and combined influences of common carotid occlusion and non-hypotensive hemorrhage on kidney blood flow. Pflügers Arch. 379, 81-88.

Hilton, S.M. (1963) Inhibition of baroreceptor reflexes on hypothalamic stimulation. J. Physiol. (Lond.) 165, 56P-57P.

Hohimer, A.R. and Smith, O.A. (1979) Decreased renal blood flow in the baboon during mild, dynamic leg exercise. Amer. J. Physiol. 236, R198-R205.

Humphreys, P.W. and Joels, N. (1972) The vasomotor component of the carotid sinus baroreceptor reflex in the cat during stimulation of the hypothalamic defence area. J. Physiol. (Lond.) 226, 57-78.

Humphreys, P.W., Joels, N. and McAllen, R.M. (1971) Modification of the reflex response to stimulation of carotid sinus baroreceptors during and following stimulation of the hypothalamic defence area in the cat. J. Physiol. (Lond.) 216, 461-482.

Kirchheim, H. (1969) Effect of common carotid occlusion on arterial blood pressure and on kidney blood flow in unanesthetized dogs. Pflügers Arch. 306, 119-134.

Kirchheim, H.R. (1976) Systemic arterial baroreceptor reflexes. Physiol. Rev. 56, 100-176.

Kjellmer, I. (1965) On the competition between metabolic vasodilatation and neurogenic vasoconstriction in skeletal muscle. Acta Physiol. Scand. 63, 450-459.

Klevans, L.R. and Gebber, G.L. (1970) Facilitatory forebrain influence on cardiac component of baroreceptor reflexes. Amer. J. Physiol. 219, 1235-1241.

Korner, P.I. (1979) Central nervous control of autonomic cardiovascular function; in Handbook of Physiology, Section 2, The Cardiovascular System, Volume I, The Heart. American Physiological Society, Washington, D.C.

Kumada, M., Schramm, L.P., Altmansberger, R.A., and Sagawa, K. (1975) Modulation of carotid sinus baroreceptor reflex by hypothalamic defence response. Amer. J. Physiol. 228, 34-35.

Lisander, B. and Martner, J. (1971) Interaction between the fastigial pressor response and the baroreceptor reflex. Acta Physiol. Scand. 83, 505-514.

Ludbrook, J., Faris, I.B., Iannos, J., Jamieson, G.G. and Russell, W.J. (1978) Lack of effect of isometric handgrip exercise on the responses of the carotid sinus baroreceptor reflex in man. Clin. Sci. Mol. Med. 55, 189-194.

McAllen, R.M. (1976) Inhibition of the baroreceptor input to the medulla by stimulation of the hypothalamic defence area. J. Physiol. (Lond.) 257, 45P-46P.

McCubbin, J.W., Green, J.H. and Page, I.H. (1956) Baroreceptor function in chronic renal hypertension. Circulat. Res. 4, 205-210.

Melcher, A. and Donald, D.E. (1981) Maintained ability of carotid baroreflex to regulate arterial pressure during exercise. Amer. J. Physiol. 241, H838-H849.

Moruzzi, G. (1940) Paleocerebellar inhibition of vasomotor and respiratory carotid sinus reflexes. J. Neurophysiol. 3, 20-32.

Myers, H.A. and Honig, C.R. (1969) Influence of initial resistance on magnitude of response to vasomotor stimuli. Amer. J. Physiol. 216, 1429-1436.

Pickering, T.G., Peterson, E.S., Gribbin, B., Cunningham, D.J.C. and Sleight, P. (1971) Comparison of the effects of exercise and posture on the baroreflex in man. Cardiovasc. Res. 5, 582-586.

Reis, D.J. and Cuenod, M. (1965) Central neural regulation of carotid baroreceptor reflexes in the cat. Amer. J. Physiol. 209, 1267-1277.

Remensnyder, J.P., Mitchell, J.H. and Sarnoff, S.J. (1962) Functional sympatholysis during muscular activity. Observations on influence of carotid sinus on oxygen uptake. Circulat. Res. 11, 370-380.

Robinson, B.F., Epstein, S.E., Beiser, G.D. and Braunwald, E. (1966) Control of heart rate by the autonomic nervous system. Studies in man on the interrelation between baroreceptor mechanisms and exercise. Circulat. Res. 19, 400-411.

Smith, O.A. and Nathan, M.A. (1967) Inhibition of the carotid sinus reflex by stimulation of the inferior olive. Science 154, 674-675.

Smyth, H.S., Sleight, P. and Pickering, G.W. (1969) Reflex regulation of arterial pressure during sleep in man: quantitative method of assessing baroreflex sensitivity. Circulat. Res. 24, 109-121.

Stephenson, R.B., Smith, O.A. and Scher, A.M. (1981) Baroreceptor regulation of heart rate in baboons during different behavioral states. Amer. J. Physiol. 241, R277-R285.

Strandell, T. and Shepherd, J.T. (1967) The effect in humans of increased sympathetic activity on the blood flow to active muscles. Acta Med. Scand. (Suppl. 472), 146-167.

Vatner, S.F., Franklin, D. and Braunwald, E. (1971) Effects of anesthesia and sleep on circulatory response to carotid sinus nerve stimulation. Amer. J. Physiol. 220, 1249-1255.

Vatner, S.F., Franklin, D., Van Citters, R.L. and Braunwald, E. (1970) Effects of carotid sinus nerve stimulation on blood flow distribution in conscious dogs at rest and during exercise. Circulat. Res. 27, 495-503.

Weiss, G.K. and Crill, W.E. (1969) Carotid sinus nerve: primary afferent depolarization evoked by hypothalamic stimulation. Brain Res. 16, 269-272.

Fastigial Nucleus and Its Possible Role in the Cardiovascular Response to Exercise

KENNETH J. DORMER AND H. LOWELL STONE
Department of Physiology & Biophysics, University of Oklahoma,
Oklahoma City, Oklahoma

INTRODUCTION

It has been approximately 15 years since it was proposed that the central nervous system (CNS) initiates and supports an integrated cardiovascular (CV) response under specific physiological conditions (Hilton, 1966). Since the initial description of the so-called "defense reaction," the nature of central CV control has remained a difficult issue. According to some (McC. Brooks, 1981), there are at least five fundamental CNS processes involved in autonomic function: (1) feedback to one of the afferent pathways; (2) interaction between "centers" in the spinal cord and brain; (3) central interaction between central representations of the two autonomic subdivisions; (4) reactions organizing and initiating patterns of efferent discharge; and (5) continuing actions that modify the activities started on the basis of feedback triggered by the effector activity.

The integrative autonomic response during exercise remains unresolved from the perspective of how these five processes relate to the response. Since the idea was first introduced by Paterson (1928), particular attention has been given to the role of afferents from skeletal muscle, which may function as ergoreceptors (see Mitchell et al., 1981). Furthermore, most studies relating muscle afferents to CV changes have been performed during isometric (static) exercise with attention given to fine muscle afferents. A greater increase in the heart rate (HR) and arterial blood pressure (AP) is observed during static than isotonic (dynamic) exercise. Surprisingly, no CNS component of the autonomic response to exercise has been described except for the central components of the arterial baroreflex and chemoreflex. ·Even the simplest paradigm, an "efference copy" of descending cortical motor projections to autonomic pathways, has not been demonstrated (Kotchabhakdi and Walberg, 1977).

If central control exists for the heart and circulation during exercise, we may expect it to respond to modulation from both higher CNS areas and peripheral afferents. Furthermore, because of the graded responses to different work loads, efferent autonomic activity should not only be initiated by, but also quantitatively related to, muscle activity. An ideal CNS location that may function in the control of the autonomic exercise response is the cerebellum. Anatomical relations between afferent information from numerous muscle and cutaneous receptor types and efferent projections to medullary nuclei involved in CV control exist through the fastigial nucleus (FN). Widespread but differentiated sympathoexcitation has been described following electrical stimulation of FN in the rat, cat, rabbit, dog and monkey, but the physiological role of FN remains unknown (Reis et al., in press).

In this paper, we shall discuss the results of studies on dogs that have been acutely and chronically implanted with cardiac and cerebellar instrumentation. We will describe the response to submaximal exercise before and after lesions in the FN region, and we will also discuss electrical stimulation of the FN in anesthetized and conscious dogs in relation to neural control of the circulation and its possible role in the exercise response. By relating the fastigial afferent and efferent projections, we hypothesize an FN role in exercise that incorporates two central command concepts: descending medullary projections (Krogh and Lindhard, 1913) and afferent neural activity from receptors in skeletal muscle (Paterson, 1928). Finally, based on all known FN physiological-behavioral responses, an hypothesis for the integrated somatovisceral role of the FN will be presented.

METHODS

Anesthetized Dogs

FN Stimulation. Mongrel dogs (13-15 kg) were anesthetized with alpha-chloralose (115 mg/kg) and placed in a stereotaxic head-holder. The FN was implanted with concentric electrodes using techniques previously described (Dormer and Stone, 1976). The area in rostromedial FN that elicited the greatest changes in HR and AP was located by stimulation using constant current, biphasic rectangular waveforms of 150 μsec duration, 80 pulses/sec, 30-500 μA. The AP was obtained through a saline-filled femoral artery cannula connected to a pressure transducer (Gould P23Id). Left ventricular pressure (LVP) was obtained by passing a miniature catheter-tip pressure transducer (Millar TCB100) retrogradely from a femoral artery into the left ventricle, and was differentiated to assess myocardial contractility (dLVP/dt). The HR was calculated from ECG or AP signals by a cardiotachometer. Either respiration was assisted by positive pressure ventilation, or its spontaneous rate was recorded by temperature excursions in an endotracheal thermistor.

Diving Response. The diving response was elicited in chloralose-urethane-anesthetized, tracheotomized dogs by perfusing the nasopharynx with tap water or saline (see Dormer and Stone, 1980). This response was elicited alone and during collision with FN stimulation so that the net effects on HR, AP, respiration and dLVP/dt could be observed.

FN-Medullary Projections. The FN efferent projections to medullary nuclei were identified by injecting a mixture of ^{3}H-labeled amino acids into rostral FN of beagle dogs. A 3:1 mixture of leucine and proline (60-120 μCi/μl) was injected during a sterile surgical procedure in which the FN response was first located by electrical stimulation. The electrode was then withdrawn and replaced with a micropipette containing the ^{3}H-leucine/proline (see Andrezik et al., 1982). Brain sections were processed using standard autoradiographic techniques and examined using dark-field microscopy.

Conscious Dogs

Exercise Response. Mongrel dogs (13-16 kg) were selected on the basis of their willingness to run on a motorized treadmill. In aseptic surgery, FN electrodes and CV instrumentation were implanted. Special 5-point, tubular array electrodes (0.1 mm diameter; 0.25 mm tip exposure, 1 mm separation) were implanted unilaterally or bilaterally in FN and fixed in place.

With a left thoracotomy, solid-state pressure transducers were implanted in either the apex of the left ventricle or the descending aorta (Dormer, 1980). Directional Doppler blood flow meters (L&M Electronics 1012) were placed on the left circumflex coronary artery (LCA) or left renal artery. All wires exited in the neck region except for the pressure transducer, which contained a percutaneous connector plug (Konigsberg P5CK).

The dogs recovered for 2 weeks before resuming the treadmill exercise. They were conditioned to run for 3-min intervals at increasing work loads which approached submaximal exercise. After one to five control exercise tests had been done, lesions were placed through the indwelling electrodes using either DC current (10-50 volts) or radio-frequency current (Radionics RG). If a motor deficit resulted from the lesion, the dog was rehabilitated so that it could readily perform the treadmill exercise again. One to five exercise tests were repeated and compared with controls. The extent of each lesion was histologically verified.

Chronic Stimulation. Mongrel dogs were instrumented with solid-state pressure transducers in the aorta and FN electrodes for observation of behavioral and autonomic changes during intermittent, low-level stimulation. Once each dog had recovered and adjusted to the laboratory environment, HR and AP were recorded (1-5 hr) over 1 week, then the FN was stimulated by a programmable stimulator carried in a vest worn by the dog. This stimulation was continued for 2 weeks while AP, HR and behavior were observed. Stimulus parameters consisted of a charge-balanced, biphasic, rectangular waveform, 20 pulses/sec, 50-150 μA with a 10-sec duty cycle, delivered to the pair of electrodes evoking the greatest CV response.

RESULTS

Anesthetized Dogs

The response to FN stimulation in dogs is similar to that observed in other species (Del Bo et al., 1981; Koyama et al., 1980; McKee et al., 1976) except for HR and respiration. The sympathoexcitation that results causes a sustained, stimulus-locked increase in AP, LVP, dLVP/dt and LCA blood flow, but the rapid-onset tachycardia is buffered by the baroreceptor reflex, resulting in bradycardia. Tachypnea is frequently observed during FN stimulation. Threshold for the CV response was near 20 μA and the greatest changes were observed at 70-100 pulses/sec (Fig. 1).

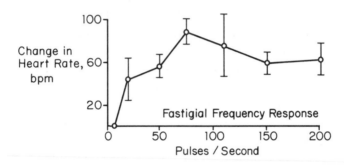

Fig. 1.   Increase in heart rate for various frequencies of FN stimulation; optimal frequency response was 70-90 square wave pulses/sec.

The AP, LVP and dLVP/dt increased approximately 40% when stimulation was 5 times threshold (Fig. 2), primarily because of direct neural influences on the heart and vasculature. Beta-adrenergic blockade (propranolol, 1 mg/kg i.v.) eliminated about 80-90% of the increases in HR and dLVP/dt, while alpha-adrenergic blockade (phenoxybenzamine, 1 mg/kg i.v.) substantially reduced the AP increase. Left stellate ganglionectomy substantially reduced the increase in dLVP/dt, while right stellate ganglionectomy severely reduced the tachycardia. Bilateral lesions placed in descending sympathetic pathways located in the cervical dorsolateral funiculus of the spinal cord completely abolished the response (Dormer et al., in press).

Two other contributors to FN sympathoexcitation are adrenal catecholamines and renal renin-angiotensin. The increase in HR, LVP and dLVP/dt 10-15 sec after stimulus onset (Fig. 2) is most likely due to catecholamines. This supports recent observations on the FN release of catecholamines in other species (Del Bo et al., 1981). The renin-angiotensin contribution is less clear, but neural release of renin has been shown to occur in dogs that were stimulated at rates below the threshold for HR and AP increases (Ohata

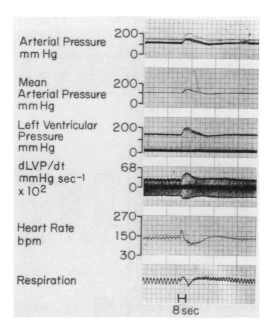

Fig. 2. Fastigial cardiopulmonary response produced by 8 sec of stimulation (0.4-0.7 mA) in anesthetized dogs. (From Dormer and Stone, 1980, with permission).

et al., 1978). More recently, Koyama et al. (1981) demonstrated a relation between the FN and baroreceptors influencing plasma renin activity in cats.

The rapid-onset tachycardia that occurs during the first 3 sec of FN stimulation can exceed 300 beats/min with maximal stimulation. This, however, is immediately buffered by baroreceptor reflexes and prolonged stimulation will result in bradycardia which is maintained as long as the AP is elevated (Fig. 2). Vagotomy results in sustained tachycardia during FN stimulation, while bilateral vascular isolation of the carotid sinuses at normotensive pressures will augment both the rate of rise in HR and the peak tachycardia during FN stimulation (Dormer and Stone, 1976). Baroreceptor buffering of the hypertension, though not noticeable in the organ response, has also been demonstrated by recording preganglionic activity during FN stimulation (Dormer et al., in press).

Tachypnea (60-70 breaths/min) is often observed along with the CV changes, but never alone. This "gasping," shallow breathing, evident in Fig. 2, is too rapid for endotracheal thermistor rate detection. Interestingly, the respiratory changes are less frequently observed in the conscious dog during FN stimulation, but always occur in conjunction with sympathoexcitation.

To examine the physiological relation of FN to particular medullary nuclei, we simultaneously evoked an opposing CV response that was expressed through medullary nuclei known to influence CV control (Dormer and Stone, 1980). The nasal-perfusion diving response that produced bradycardia, decreased contractility and hypotension was also evoked during FN stimulation (Fig. 3). All of the CV increases, especially HR, were significantly reduced by superimposition of the two responses, although precise algebraic cancellation of the FN response was not demonstrable.

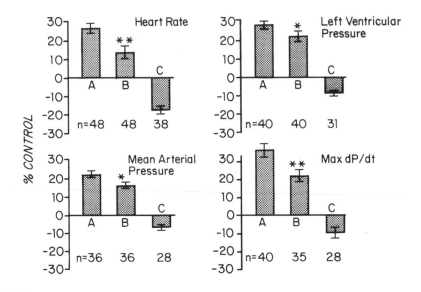

Fig. 3. Fastigial stimulation and nasal-perfusion. A, electrical stimulation of FN; B, stimulation during nasal perfusion; C, nasal perfusion alone. The significantly reduced FN sympathoexcitation in B suggested NTS was involved in the expression of both the nasal perfusion (diving) and FN responses. "n," number of trials in 14 dogs. (From Dormer and Stone, 1980, with permission.)

Previous anatomical studies indicate that FN projects to medullary regions implicated in CV control, including locus ceruleus, parabrachial region, lateral reticular nucleus, nucleus of the solitary tract (NTS), and paramedian reticular nucleus. Of these, the latter two are involved in baroreceptor function. Since the dive response apparently is initiated by trigeminal-NTS afferents, and since the FN has reciprocal connections with NTS and is subject to baroreceptor intervention, we concluded that the diving and FN responses were modulated by a common site, the NTS. The apnea during nasal perfusion was also more powerful than the FN tachypnea.

Conscious Dogs

The dogs receiving partial unilateral (n=6) or bilateral (n=2) FN lesions performed submaximal treadmill exercise up to 6.45 km/hr and 16% grade. Comparisons of the pre- and postlesion changes in HR, LVP, dLVP/dt and LCA flow are shown in Fig. 4. Although some deficits were observed in all of the parameters measured, the most remarkable was a significantly lower HR throughout exercise. The lack of significant changes at all work loads may be attributed to the small number of dogs, or to the nature of the lesions; i.e., the discrete lesions did not encompass the rostral 20% of FN, and the unilateral lesions

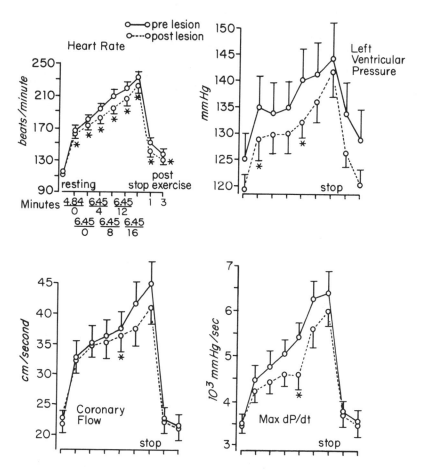

Fig. 4. CV response to submaximal exercise before and after partial FN lesions. Increases in HR, LVP, dP/dt max and coronary flow are shown as treadmill exercise was increased from rest to 6.45 km/hr and 16% grade, then discontinued for 1 and 3 min. The deficit in CV performance was most demonstrable in HR, less so in LVP, dP/dt and LCA flow. Asterisks indicate p<0.05.

permitted full function of the remaining FN, which has bilateral medullary projections. In the animals with bilateral lesions, CV deficits were greater. More experiments are needed on animals with bilateral lesions, but early evidence suggests the total response will be modified but not obliterated (Foreman et al., 1980). Lesions were confined near the rostral FN to minimize vestibular and motor deficits. In cases where the lesions were extensive or produced irreparable motor-vestibular deficits, exercise produced increases in HR and AP compared with those levels in controls.

Although some steady-state CV changes were recorded during exercise in dogs with FN lesions, the FN may function more importantly during transient changes in activity. A trend toward decreased CV responses during exercise was evident at the immediate onset (first 10 sec) of exercise. A group of dogs with incomplete rostral FN lesions had a nonsignificant but consistent decrease in HR and AP compared with those in prelesion exercise (Fig. 5). These are preliminary observations and only serve as potential clues of a role for FN during exercise.

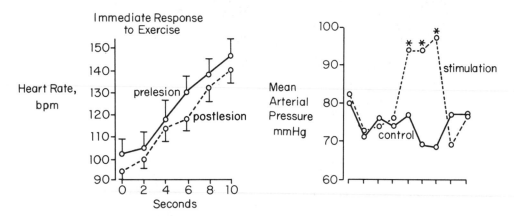

Fig. 5. Initial 10 sec of treadmill exercise in dogs before and after partial FN lesions (n=6).

Fig. 6. Mean AP changes during treadmill exercise and FN stimulation. This dog received a 7-10 x threshold stimulus for 10 sec following 3 min of exercise at 6.45 km/hr and 8, 12 and 16% grade (same abscissa as in Fig. 4).

The relative magnitude of the sympathoexcitation from FN is demonstrated in representative AP data from a dog that received FN stimulation (200-400 μA) during treadmill exercise at work loads of 6.45/8, 6.45/12 and 6.45/16 (Fig. 6). HR and AP increased significantly, while renal blood flow decreased, suggesting that the level of sympathoexcitation is less than optimal during submaximal treadmill exercise.

Distribution of Cardiac Output. Distribution of the cardiac output during FN stimulation is not well understood, but three local circulations have been studied: cerebral, coronary and renal. Neurogenic cerebrovasodilatation in the anesthetized monkey (McKee et al., 1976) and rat (Reis et al., in press) is reported to be unrelated to metabolism and possibly evoked by an intrinsic neural pathway in the brain. As might be expected, the LCA blood flow in conscious dogs increases in parallel with the increase in cardiac metabolism from increased HR and contractility (Fig. 7). Profound vaso-constriction in the renal artery observed in eight conscious dogs (Fig. 8) supports a second FN mechanism for the release of renin, underperfusion of the kidney. Renal flow actually was reduced to zero for several seconds with FN stimuli of 200-500 μA. Thus, from the studies available, it appears that blood flow during FN-induced sympathoexcitation is reduced in the periphery, but that coronary and cerebral perfusion match or exceed the metabolic requirements of that organ.

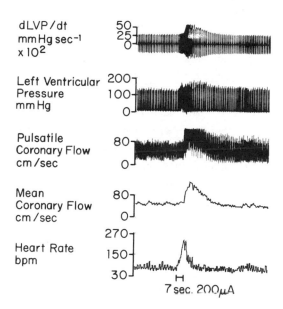

Fig. 7. FN stimulation and coronary flow in a conscious dog. The increase in LCA blood flow accompanies increases in HR and dLVP/dt during 7 sec of 200-μA stimulation. This flow increase is due primarily to an increase in cardiac metabolism.

Behavioral Response. Another approach toward elucidation of the physiological role of FN has been behavioral analysis during intermittant stimulation in unrestrained, conscious cats and dogs. No autonomic or behavioral role for FN has been identified in

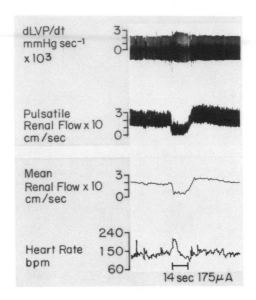

Fig. 8. FN stimulation and renal blood flow in a conscious dog. Renal blood flow may reach zero in the absence of any muscle contraction during FN stimulation (4 x threshold, 175 μA).

the quiet, resting state, but others have described a graded behavioral response to electrical stimulation of FN that began with grooming, alerting and orienting at low level stimulation and culminated with agression, attack and eating behaviors at maximal stimulation (Berntson and Paulucci, 1979; Reis et al., 1973). Similar behavior patterns were found during stimulation in unrestrained dogs. When stimulated at 20 pps and 25–150 μA, the dogs displayed alerting, licking, grooming, biting, eating, and "anxious" whining behaviors. These behaviors ceased immediately when the stimulation was stopped. Concomitant with the behaviors were episodic increases in AP and tachycardia (Fig. 9). Thus, the FN also seems to have a higher behavioral function, which may be an integral part of the overall autonomic response observed during natural stimulation.

DISCUSSION

The understanding of neural CV control during exercise has eluded man for nearly 100 years. From studies of FN in anesthetized or conscious exercising dogs, and earlier observations from cat and rat on the sympathoexcitation resulting from electrical stimulation in FN, it appears that a selective redistribution of the cardiac output can be achieved and may be related to an autonomic role during exercise. Both medullary nuclei and higher CNS levels may be influenced by FN. If it is true that the cerebellum is a

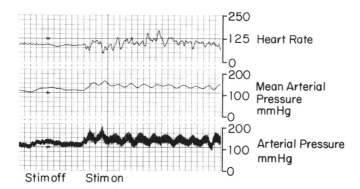

Fig. 9. Effects of intermittant FN stimulation on HR and AP changes in conscious dogs. Total stimulation time represents 230 sec (10 sec on, 10 sec off) during which HR and AP oscillated above normal.

somato-visceral integrator or, as the evidence suggests, a fine tuner of CV parameters during exercise, then we may speculate about the overall FN role in mammals.

If the FN is a contributor to the central control of CV function during exercise it must have appropriate anatomical connections. Thus, consideration should be given to muscle (mechanoreceptor or chemoreceptor) and joint afferents postulated to support HR and AP during exercise and their relative input to the cerebellum and brain stem.

Rowell (1980) suggested that CV control during exercise may operate in the absence of feedback (central command), while others have suggested that CV control is related to the recruitment activity of muscles (Crayton et al., 1981). Since the CV requirements of the working muscle are, in fact, directly proportional to the number of active motor units, the CV response could be a direct function of somatic afferent activity. The cerebellum receives substantial group III and IV afferent information from joint receptors, which is believed to support cardiopulmonary reflexes (increased HR, AP and ventilation) during exercise (Coote, 1975). Thus the cerebellum, in addition to receiving both afferent information from muscles or joints and the "efference copy" of descending cortical motor programs, could provide its own proportional "autonomic efference copy" to medullary regions subserving the CV system.

Identification of the muscle afferents influencing the CV system, along with their origin and destination, is an active area of research. The high-threshold group III and IV fibers from muscle have been implicated in HR and AP changes during exercise, as a result of their activation by stretching, contraction or chemical means (Mitchell et al., 1981). In a review, Sato and Schmidt (1973) emphasized the role of both medullary and supramedullary regions for reflexes involving myelinated (groups I-III) afferents, but only supramedullary regions for reflexes with unmyelinated (group IV) afferents. The ultimate question remains: where do the exercise-related afferents project in order to initiate autonomic efferent traffic--to medullary or to supramedullary regions?

The cerebellum and FN receive a rich supply of afferents from both dynamically and statically exercising muscles. This information is proprioceptive from muscle spindles and Golgi tendon organs, and exteroceptive from joint and cutaneous receptors. For example, the dorsal spinocerebellar tract relays proprioceptive and exteroceptive, as well as slowly conducting, flexor reflex afferents (group III) from dorsal column nuclei to the FN and lateral reticular nucleus (Gilman et al., 1981). These FN projections are from spinal laminae IV and V, which are believed to relay the muscle afferents involved in cardiopulmonary reflexes (Mitchell et al., 1981). The cuneocerebellar tract, forelimb equivalent of the dorsal spinocerebellar tract, relays information to FN through the external cuneate nucleus, also recently implicated in HR control (Galosy et al., 1981). The spino-reticulo-cerebellar tract from laminae VI and VII also conveys cutaneous and flexor reflex afferent information to the FN via the lateral reticular nucleus.

Another population of muscle afferents arises from dorsal column nuclei and projects to FN via direct or polysynaptic spino-olivo-cerebellar pathways. These group III afferents enter the cerebellum exclusively as olivary climbing fibers. Specific projections exist from the medial accessory olive to the rostral FN (Gilman et al., 1981) which are potentially important for autonomic control during exercise. These projections have been confirmed using autoradiography in the dog (Andrezik et al., in press). Recent studies using pharmacological excitation of portions of the inferior olive with harmaline revealed CV changes resembling those in exercise (Dormer, 1981). Harmaline also produces rhythmic bursts of neuronal spike activity that are identical to spike trains occurring in FN.

The lateral reticular nucleus, which receives FN efferents and integrates somatic and visceral afferent information, not only has been shown to elicit sympathetic excitation (Galosy et al., 1981), but may produce a deficit in the CV response to static exercise after lesions (Iwamoto et al., 1981).

In summary, group III and IV afferents predominantly affect CV changes during exercise but some contribution to cardiopulmonary reflexes ultimately may be made by all afferents. The cerebellum receives all group I-IV afferents and is physiologically associated with medullary nuclei affecting HR and AP. Several spino-cerebello-medullary anatomical relations that may be important in CV control during exercise are summarized in Figure 10.

What can we conclude regarding the neurobiological and behavioral functions of the fastigial nucleus? If we consolidate all the animal observations, a physiological role begins to emerge that depicts the archi- and paleocerebellar regions as a somatovisceral

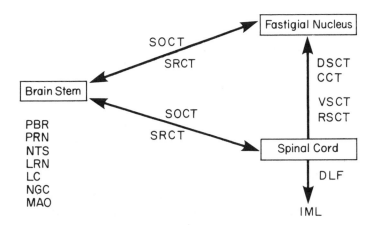

Fig. 10. Summary of major nuclei receiving FN projections and spinal afferent pathways potentially important in CV control during exercise. Although this summary is anatomically incomplete, most brain stem regions indicated have reciprocal FN or cerebellar connections. **Abbreviations:** PBR, parabrachial regions; PRN, paramedian reticular nucleus; NTS, nucleus of the solitary tract; LRN, lateral reticular nucleus; LC, locus ceruleus; NGC, nucleus gigantocellularis; MAO, medial accessory olive; SOCT, spino-olivo-cerebellar tract; SRCT, spino-reticulo-cerebellar tract; DSCT, dorsal spino-cerebellar tract; CCT, cuneocerebellar tract; VSCT, ventral spinocerebellar tract; RSCT, rostral spinocerebellar tract; DLF, dorsolateral funiculus; IML, intermediolateral cell column.

integrator during movement. No physiological parameters are yet known to be affected by FN in the resting state. We see a substantial involvement of the caudal FN and flocculonodular lobe in vestibulo-oculomotor activity (precision control of the head and neck, even on a moving body platform). Neural, behavioral and CV data indicate that alertness and mental acuity would be enhanced by increased cerebrovascular blood flow and circulating catecholamines, as a result of rostral FN excitation. Redistribution of the cardiac output during rostral FN-induced sympathoexcitation and a decrement in the CV response to exercise after partial FN lesions support the hypothesis that the cerebellum contributes fine tuning to exercise heterostasis since, under these conditions, FN is maximally excited by afferent input. Postural reflexes (orthostatic tolerance) are also active during exercise (Johnson et al., 1974). Finally, aggressive capture, attack and eating behavior would also come under the aegis of both the visceral and somatic nervous systems and, potentially, the cerebellum, as demonstrated in two species thus far.

Speculatively, these observations may be compiled to describe the very primitive physiological and behavioral response of "food-getting." A paradigm for this response could be any mammalian carnivore whose survival depends on skillful detection, capture, killing and eating of its prey. Visual and mental acuity and visual tracking during pursuit would be supported by FN vestibulo-oculomotor mechanisms and cerebrovasodilatation. The muscular coordination, work, and increased cardiac output involved in the capture would all be supported by natural FN sympathoexcitation in proportion to the amount of muscle activity. Finally, behavior supporting the kill itself, aggressive defense against intruders and devouring of the prey are remarkably similar to the responses observed during FN stimulation. Thus, the relatively primitive regions of the cerebellum, to the exclusion of the neocerebellum, may be supportive of the somatic and visceral activity involved in "food-getting," a primitive integrated behavioral response.

ACKNOWLEDGMENTS

The portable stimulator used in these studies was designed by Drs. J. Zehr and A. Livnat, Department of Physiology, University of Illinois, and graciously offered for our use. We gratefully acknowledge the technical assistance of Dan Smith, Mel Gower and Vicki Parrish. This work was supported by NIH grants HL 22747 (Young Investigators Award) and HL 24082.

REFERENCES

Andrezik, J.A., Dormer, K.J., Foreman, R.D. and Gower, M.D., Jr. (in press) Fastigial nucleus projections to the brain stem in beagles. Fed. Proc.

Berntson, G.G., Paulucci, T.S. (1979) Fastigial modulation of brainstem behavioral mechanisms. Brit. Res. Bull. 4, 549-552.

Coote, J. (1975) Physiological significance of somatic afferent pathways from skeletal muscle and joints with reflex effects on the heart and circulation. Brain. Res. 87, 139-144.

Crayton, S.C., Mitchell, J.H. and Payne, F.C., III (1981) Reflex cardiovascular response during injection of capsaicin into skeletal muscle. Amer. J. Physiol. 240, H315-H319.

Del Bo, A., Ross, C., Pardal, J., Saavedra, J. and Reis, D. J. (1981) Neural and humoral components of the pressor response elicited by electrical stimulation of fastigial nucleus (FN) in rats before and after sympathectomy. Soc. Neurosci. Abst. 7, 632.

Dempsey, J.A., Vidruk, E.H. and Mastenbrook, S.M. (1980) Pulmonary control systems in exercise. Fed. Proc. 39, 1498-1505.

Dormer, K.J. (1980) Technique for the surgical implantation of solid-state pressure transducers. Med. Electron. (Oct.) pp. 69 75.

Dormer, K.J. (1981) Reduction of the harmaline cardiovascular response by diazepam administered in the cerebellum. Soc. Neurosci. Abstr. 7, 821.

Dormer, K.J., Foreman, R.D. and Ohata, C.A. (in press) Fastigial nucleus stimulation and excitatory spinal sympathetic activity in the dog. Amer. J. Physiol.

Dormer, K.J. and Stone, H.L. (1976) Cerebellar pressor response in the dog. J. Appl. Physiol. 41, 574-580.

Dormer, K.J. and Stone, H.L. (1980) Interaction of the fastigial pressor response and depressor response to nasal perfusion. J. Autonom. Nerv. Syst. 2, 269-280.

Foreman, R.D., Dormer, K.J., Ohata, C.A. and Stone, H.L. (1980) Neural control of the heart during arrhythmias and exercise. Fed. Proc. 39, 2519-2525.

Galosy, R.A., Clark, L.K., Vasko, M.R. and Crawford, I.L. (1981) Neurophysiology and neuropharmacology of cardiovascular regulation and stress. Neurosci. Behav. Rev. 5, 137-175.

Gilman, S., Bloedel, J.R. and Lechtenberg, R. (1981) Disorders of the Cerebellum. F.A. Davis Co., Philadelphia.

Hilton, S.M. (1966) Hypothalamic regulation of the cardiovascular system. Brit. Med. Bull. 22, 243-248.

Iwamoto, G.A., Kaufman, M.P., Botterman, B.R. and Mitchell, J.H. (1981) Effect of lesions in lateral reticular nucleus on the exercise pressor reflex. Physiologist 24, 80.

Johnson, J.M., Rowell, L.B., Niederberger, M. and Eisman, M. (1974) Human splanchnic and forearm vasoconstrictor responses to reductions of right atrial pressure. Circulat. Res. 34, 515-524.

Kotchabhakdi, N. and Walberg, F. (1977) Cerebellar afferents from neurons in motor nuclei of cranial nerves demonstrated by retrograde axonal transport of horseradish peroxidase. Brain Res. 137, 158-163.

Koyama, S., Ammons, W.S. and Manning, J.W. (1981) Visceral afferents and the fastigial nucleus in vascular and plasma renin adjustments to head up tilt. J. Autonom. Nerv. Syst. 4, 381-392.

Krogh, A. and Lindhard, J. (1913) The regulation of respiration and circulation during the initial stages of muscular work. J. Physiol. (Lond.) 51, 59-90.

McC. Brooks, C. (1981) Introduction: Control of the autonomic nervous system and the multiple integrative roles it plays in regulating cardiovascular functions. J. Amer. Neurol. Soc. 4, 115-120.

McKee, J.C., Dunn, M.J. and Stone, H.L. (1976) Neurogenic cerebral vasodilatation from electrical stimulation of the cerebellum in monkey. Stroke 7, 179-186.

Mitchell, J.H., Blomqvist, C.G., Lind. A.R., Saltin, B. and Shepard, J.T., eds. (1981) Static (isometric) exercise: cardiovascular responses and neural control mechanisms. Circulat. Res. 48, I1-I179.

Ohata, C.A., Dormer, K.J., Foreman, R.D. and Kem, D.C. (1978) Effect of fastigial nucleus stimulation on plasma renin activity. Physiologist 21, 86.

Paterson, W.D. (1928) Circulatory and respiratory changes in response to muscular exercise in man. J. Physiol. (Lond.) 66, 323-345.

Reis, D.J., Doba, N. and Nathan, M.A. (1973) Predatory attack: grooming and consummatory behavior evoked by electrical stimulation of cerebellar nuclei in cat. Science 182, 845-847.

Reis, D.J., Iadecola, C., MacKenzie, E., Mori, M., Nakai, M. and Tucker, L.W. (in press) Primary and metabolically coupled cerebrovascular dilation elicited by stimulation of two intrinsic systems of brain; in Symposium on Cerebral Blood Flow: Effects of Nerves and Neurotransmitters, D. Heistad and M. Marcus, eds.

Rowell, L. B. (1980) What signals govern the cardiovascular response to exercise? Med. Sci. Sports Exercise 12, 307-315.

Sato, A. and Schmidt, R. F. (1973) Somatosympathetic reflexes: afferent fibers, central pathways, discharge characteristics. Physiol. Rev. 53, 916-947.

Central Command During Exercise: Parallel Activation of the Cardiovascular and Motor Systems by Descending Command Signals

STUART F. HOBBS

Department of Physiology and Biophysics, and Regional Primate Research Center, University of Washington, Seattle, Washington

INTRODUCTION

This chapter deals with how the central nervous system (CNS) might produce a tightly coupled interaction between cardiovascular (CV) and motor systems during exercise. One idea expressed nearly 100 years ago was that the motor outflow from the cerebral cortex might interact with the centers that elicit CV responses to exercise (Johansson, 1895). This motor outflow was called central command and was described as "irradiation of descending motor impulses onto cardiovascular control centers" (Krogh and Lindhard, 1913). Descending motor signals were thought to activate CV control centers via collaterals from the descending motor pathways. The first objective of this chapter is to express the central command concept as an experimentally testable hypothesis. The second objective is to report the results of two experiments that tested our central command hypothesis.

What is Central Command?

The concept of central command has never been explicitly defined in terms of measurable variables. Several studies provide indirect evidence that descending motor signals activate motor and CV systems in parallel during exercise (Krogh and Lindhard, 1913; Asmussen et al., 1965; Freyschuss, 1970; Goodwin et al., 1972; Schibye et al., 1981; McCloskey, 1981). However, quantification of any relation between motor and CV commands must be expressed in terms of direct measures of some responses within the CV and motor systems. Measures of muscle function such as EMG and force production, and factors that control motor unit recruitment must be examined. The motor unit, defined as a motoneuron and the muscle fibers that it innervates, is the basic building block of muscle. Based on twitch contraction times and fatigability, motor units have been segregated into three main types: slow-twitch, nonfatiguing units (S); fast-twitch, fatigue-resistant units (FR); and fast-twitch, fatiguing units (FF) (Burke et al., 1973). As type S units seem to depend on aerobic metabolism to meet their energy needs, the force produced by these units depends on the blood flow to them. Type FF units seem to use primarily glycolysis to meet their metabolic demands, and to fatigue regardless of the blood flow to them. Type FR units probably use a mixture of aerobic and glycolytic metabolism and exhibit fatigue characteristics that are partially dependent on blood flow (Burke et al., 1973; Barclay et al., 1979). During a voluntary contraction of progressively increasing force, recruitment follows the order of S to FR and finally to FF units (Milner-Brown et al., 1973; Grimby and Hannerz, 1977). During brief static contractions, each motor unit seems to have a rather specific force threshold below which the unit is not active and above which the unit is always active. At relatively low forces, only S and some FR units may be active, but at higher forces all three types are active. One hypothesis that follows from this is that the magnitude of the command signals may be estimated from the number of motor units activated during contractions.

Under certain circumstances, force production could provide a reasonable estimate of motor unit recruitment. An example of the relations among descending motor signals, motor unit activation and force production is illustrated in Figure 1. If only six muscle fibers were required to hold a light load, motor command would have to increase only until the three lowest threshold motor units, or 60% of the motor unit pool, were activated. To lift the heavier load, which requires activation of all ten muscle fibers, the descending motor command must activate not only the motor units used for the light-load contraction, but also the two higher threshold motor units, or 100% of the motor unit pool. Thus, the greater the number of motor units that are needed, the greater the magnitude of the descending motor command required to activate them. Consequently, the magnitude of the descending motor command should also be directly related to the force production or load as well as to the number of motor units recruited. However, such a unique relation between descending motor command and force production during static contractions occurs only if muscle fatigue is not present.

When muscles fatigue, the magnitude of descending motor command could be estimated if there were some reproducible end point for motor unit recruitment. A subject's endurance limit (i.e. the time at which the muscles can no longer generate the required tension) may provide such an end point. Regardless of how fatigue occurs, additional motor units must be recruited if a constant force production is to be maintained (Schibye et al., 1981; Grimby et al., 1981). Because of the order in which types of motor units are recruited (S, then FR, then FF) as fatigue progresses, the additional motor units that are recruited fatigue at faster rates as more and more FF motor units are needed to maintain force (Grimby and Hannerz, 1977). Once a certain number of motor units are recruited, a progressive cycle of motor unit fatigue and recruitment occurs. During fatiguing tests that require a constant output of muscle

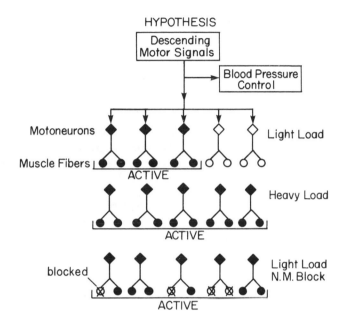

Fig. 1. Schematic diagram of our central command hypothesis, showing the relation of descending command signals to both motor unit recruitment and arterial pressure. Note that motor units are recruited sequentially from left to right. N.M., neuromuscular.

tension or work, this cycle continues until a point is reached at which force can no longer be maintained. If voluntary performance of the task always ends after the same number of motor units has been recruited, regardless of the endurance time and force production, then at the endurance limit the descending motor command should always be the same. Therefore, the motor unit recruitment shown for the heavy load in Figure 1 could indicate the recruitment at the endurance limit for both heavy- and light-load contractions; the former could be held for only a few seconds and the latter could be held for several minutes.

From the foregoing, one hypothesis for central command can be stated as follows: The magnitudes of CV and motor command signals are directly related to the number of motor units activated during a normal voluntary muscle contraction. This chapter focuses now on two questions: (1) Are the magnitudes of CV response and motor unit recruitment actually directly related? (2) Do the motor and CV commands descend from supra-medullary centers along separate pathways?

Relation between CV Responses and Motor Unit Recruitment

To test our central command hypothesis, we need some measure of the CV command. We chose arterial blood pressure because it is crucial for adequate muscle perfusion, and is one of the key regulated variables under the control of the autonomic nervous system during exercise. Under well-controlled conditions such as static exercise, the increases in blood pressure and motor outflow are highly reproducible and seem to be directly related (Stenberg et al., 1967; Funderburk et al., 1974). The common practice in human subjects has been to relate pressor responses to the percent of maximum voluntary contraction force developed during a static contraction (Funderburk et al., 1974). One problem with this approach is that factors other than central command might explain the rise in blood pressure so that any relation to centrally generated signals might be fortuitous.

An alternative hypothesis is that reflexes originating from within the contracting muscle might cause the blood pressure and other circulatory responses to exercise. For example, a muscle chemoreflex (see Rowell and Kaufman et al., this volume) can elicit marked pressor responses that are directly related to the muscle mass rendered ischemic (Freund et al., 1978) and to the degree of oxygen deficiency within the muscle (Rowell et al., 1976). The afferent arm of the reflex seems to be those Group III and IV fibers that are sensitive to mechanical, chemical and thermal stimuli (McCloskey and Mitchell, 1972; Kumazawa and Mizumura, 1977; Kniffki et al., 1978). The role (if any) of this reflex during normal exercise is not yet known.

We have attempted to separate the effects of a central CV command signal from those that might arise from a muscle reflex by employing partial neuromuscular blockade (NMB) of contracting muscle. The basic idea is that for a given motor task, we can force the use of more and more motor units as the degree of NMB increases, while the force of muscle contraction remains constant; that is, as a first approximation any contribution from a mechano- or chemoreflex should be constant (some qualifications are given later). This idea is depicted at the bottom of Figure 1. If the activation of some of the muscle fibers that were used to hold a light load are pharmacologically blocked, a greater number or fraction of the motor units would have to be recruited in order to hold the same load. Also, NMB might be expected to decrease the endurance time for holding a light load because of an increased recruitment of FF motor units.

Our central command hypothesis predicts for a given motor task that: (1) the pressor response during a heavy-load contraction with short endurance time is greater than that during a light-load contraction with a relatively long endurance time; (2) the pressor response to a light-load contraction will be increased by NMB if the endurance time is reduced; and (3) the pressor response at any given time during muscle contraction should be the same for contractions with similar endurance times regardless of the load.

The last point is true only if the assumption about reproducibility of motor unit recruitment at the endurance limit is also true.

METHODS

The experimental setup used to test our central command hypothesis is shown in Figure 2. Five baboons were trained by operant techniques to respond to a light by using their left arms to pull a handle that was attached to weights. The animals were given food rewards for holding the handle within a preset range of displacement distances. Static exercise was chosen because the motor unit recruitment patterns are better understood for this form of exercise and the task could be defined in terms of an all-or-nothing response; i.e., the baboon either does or does not hold the load. The animals were trained to hold the loads to their voluntary endurance limit or until 3 min had elapsed. A 3-min limit was chosen because it allowed a wide range of endurance times but did not permit too many food rewards during a single contraction. Loads selected for each baboon produced endurance times ranging from a minimum of 30 sec to well over 3 min. The minimum endurance time was set at 30 sec because it exceeded the duration of

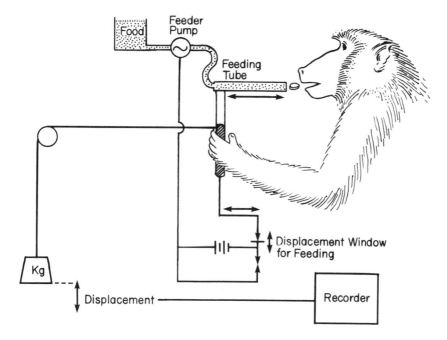

Fig. 2. Diagram showing the experimental setup used to test our central command hypothesis.

transient responses attending the transition from rest to exercise (Fig. 3). This range of endurance times corresponds to those for humans producing contraction forces within the range of near maximal to relatively light or nonfatiguing (Humphreys and Lind, 1963).

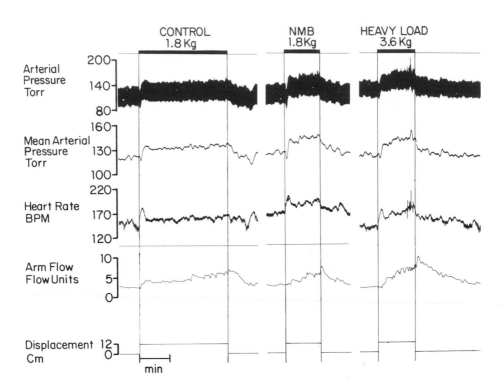

Fig. 3. CV responses in one animal to contraction with a light load (control), a light load during NMB, and a heavy load. BPM, beats per minute. Flow units are arbitrary. The displacement trace has been retouched.

Once a baboon's behavior was reproducible at different loads, the animal was anesthetized with Halothane, and pressure- and flow-measuring devices were implanted during aseptic surgery. A catheter was placed in a femoral artery for the measurement of blood pressure. An electromagnetic flow probe and an occluder for checking zero flow were placed around the left subclavian artery for measurement of blood flow to the working arm. Another catheter was placed in the left axillary artery for infusion of neuromuscular blocking agents. Heart rate and mean arterial pressure were derived electronically from the pulsatile pressure signal. The animal was allowed to recover for 3 weeks after surgery so that tissue growth could stabilize the implants.

The experimental procedure was as follows. The animal was placed in a sound-attenuating booth. The measurement devices were connected for recording purposes and the animal was allowed to rest until it appeared calm and relaxed. A light in the booth was then activated and the animal responded by pulling the handle. Food rewards were provided throughout the contraction until the handle could no longer be kept in the prescribed position, at which time the task was terminated. The animal was allowed to rest for about 3 min before another contraction was initiated. Three or four different loads were used and the animals performed two or three contractions at each. Exercise began at the heaviest load and proceeded to progressively lighter loads until one was reached that could be held easily for 3 min; these light-load contractions served as controls. The animal then began to receive bolus injections of neuromuscular blocking agent (gallamine, d-tubocurarene, succinylcholine, or decamethonium) into the left axillary artery. After each injection, the animal was signaled to perform a contraction at the preselected light load. The cycle of injection of a neuromuscular blocking agent followed by contraction continued until the baboon could hold the load for only 90 sec or less. After a period of recovery, the baboon continued to perform contractions until normal strength and endurance had returned.

RESULTS

Typical responses from one baboon holding a light load and one twice as heavy are shown in Figure 3. Endurance time was shorter and the pressor response greater when the heavier load was held. The heavy load could be held for only 75 sec and generated a 22-Torr increase in pressure at the endurance limit. In contrast, the light load could be held for the full 3 min and generated an increase in pressure of only 14 Torr. Heart rate and blood flow to the working arm rose in proportion to the contraction load. More importantly, the postcontraction hyperemia was considerably larger after the heavy-load contraction.

The middle panel of Figure 3 shows the augmented pressor response to a light-load contraction during NMB. NMB also reduced endurance time from 3 min to 70 sec. In fact, the responses during light-load contractions with NMB seem quite similar to those during heavy-load contractions; the endurance times and the pressor responses are almost identical. However, an important difference is that postcontraction hyperemia was not augmented along with the pressor response after a light-load contraction during NMB. This suggests that the metabolic demand was not augmented along with the rise in blood pressure.

The average blood pressure responses to contractions at heavy loads and light loads with and without NMB are shown for five animals in Figure 4. This figure reveals that the pressor responses were greater for heavy-load than for light-load contractions. In

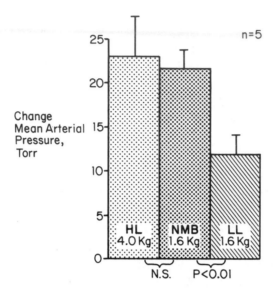

Fig. 4. Average change in arterial pressure in five animals in response to holding a heavy load (HL), light load during NMB (NMB), and a control light load (LL). The pressor responses during NMB were significantly greater ($p < 0.01$) than those during the control light-load contractions. There was no significant difference (N.S.) between the pressor responses during heavy-load contractions and during light-load contractions with NMB when their endurance times were the same.

contrast, there was no significant difference between the pressor responses to contractions at heavy loads and light loads with NMB at similar endurance times. The pressor response was always measured at the 30th sec of each contraction. Comparisons at this time permitted the inclusion of all contractions meeting the prescribed minimum endurance limit. Results from contractions at the heavy and light loads with NMB were paired for analysis based on three criteria: first, contractions were performed on the same day; second, the heavy load weighed at least twice as much as the light load; and third, endurance times for the two loads did not differ by more than 20% (the means were 42 and 45 sec for heavy- and light-load contractions, respectively).

DISCUSSION

The results are consistent with our central command hypothesis. Based on our present knowledge, they cannot be explained by reflexes originating from within the muscle, e.g., muscle mechano- or chemoreflexes. A muscle mechanoreflex cannot explain why NMB increased the blood pressure response to light-load contractions even though force or muscle tension was the same during all of these contractions. Also, were the augmented pressor response to contraction during NMB to result from an increase in muscle metabolism, then the postcontraction hyperemia of the contraction during NMB should be greater than that of the light-load contraction and should approach that of the heavy-load contraction (Donald et al., 1967). Yet, NMB did not result in an increase in the postcontraction hyperemia following a light-load contraction. However, the rise in blood pressure paralleling the need to recruit more and more motor units during contraction supports the hypothesis that the central CV command is somehow related to the number of motor units used to perform a static contraction.

To determine the role of a central CV command during different types of muscle contraction, we must integrate other factors in addition to fatigue into our scheme of analysis. Local factors affect the relations of the command signals to their measured output. The relation between motor command and force production depends not only on fatigue processes but also on muscle mechanics. Both the muscle length and the rate of shortening of the muscle affect the maximum force a muscle can produce (Joyce et al., 1969). The shorter the muscle length at the onset of contraction and the faster the muscles shorten, the more motor units are required to produce a given force. Consequently, the fraction of motor units used during a given task can be estimated only if the force at which a task is performed can be described in terms of a fraction of the maximum force that can be generated during the task. Thus, if the magnitude of both motor unit recruitment and motor command are to be estimated, the motor output for all tasks must be quantified as a fraction of the maximum muscle force that can be generated during a given task, and for tasks performed at relatively high intensities, the endurance time should also be determined.

Arterial pressure may also be influenced by local factors. The decrease in systemic vascular resistance due to muscle vasodilation opposes the effects of central CV command on arterial pressure. The powerful effect of muscle vasodilation on the arterial pressure is indicated by the fact that arterial pressure increases less than half as much during maximum dynamic exercise with both legs as during maximum static exercise with the forearm muscles (Stenberg et al., 1967; Funderburk et al., 1974). However, arterial pressure increases linearly with motor unit activation during both static and dynamic exercise (Stenberg et al., 1967; Funderburk et al., 1974). Therefore, arterial pressure does not seem to provide a unique measure of central CV command during different tasks, but within a given task pressure seems to provide an adequate measure.

Changes in the reflex control of either the motor or CV systems might also be expected to affect the relation of a command signal to its respective output variable. Both the motor and CV systems seem to be at least partially under reflex control during both rest and exercise, and manipulation of these reflexes during exercise has been shown to alter the CV responses to exercise. For example, to decrease the motor and central CV command during a constant force contraction, Goodwin et al. (1972) used vibration of muscle spindles to facilitate the motoneurons that were eliciting the contraction. During this increase in afferent input, the CV response to the contraction was decreased and this decrease was attributed to a reduction in the central CV command. Nevertheless, the relation between force production and the CV response was altered by manipulation of muscle afferent activity. Likewise, manipulation of the carotid baroreceptors alters arterial pressure during exercise while both the motor and central CV commands should be constant (Ludbrook et al., 1978; Melcher and Donald, 1981). Therefore, any manipulation of the normal reflex control of either the motor or CV system may alter the relation between motor unit recruitment and arterial pressure.

Another factor to consider is the effect of muscle blood flow on both motor unit fatigue and the command signals. Force production by both type S and FR motor units is dependent on aerobic metabolism (Barclay et al., 1979). With inadequate blood flow these units fatigue, which would require an increase in the motor command to recruit additional motor units to maintain force production (Armstrong and Peterson, 1981). The increase in the command signals would result in an increase in arterial pressure and blood flow to the active muscle. Fatigue related to blood flow would continue to result in progressively greater command signals until they generated a muscle blood flow that was adequate to support a constant force production by each motor unit. Blood-flow-dependent fatigue is an important factor primarily during dynamic and static exercise that can be performed for prolonged periods.

A final factor to be considered is the possibility that the motor command may modulate the CV reflexes originating from within contracting muscle. Muscle Group III and IV afferent input onto ascending pathways can be powerfully inhibited by descending motor activity (Arshavskii et al., 1977). Although it is not known if the descending motor activity inhibits the afferent pathways of the muscle pressor reflexes, it cannot be assumed that the input-output function of a reflex such as the muscle chemoreflex will be the same during the resting or anesthetized state and during exercise.

Because of the complex interactions of all of these factors, determination of many of the actions of the central CV command may require the ability to directly manipulate the central CV signal directly. Direct manipulation might be possible if the pathway used by the command for the CV response were separate from that for the motor response. If such a pathway exists, its destruction should eliminate the CV responses to exercise. We adopted this traditional neurophysiological approach in the following experiments.

An Experiment to Isolate the CV Command Pathway

There are several general patterns of neural organization that a central CV command might use. Pathways 1 and 2 in Figure 5 can be considered equivalent to what has classically been called central command or "irradiation of cortical motor impulses onto brainstem CV control centers" (Krogh and Lindhard, 1913). Collaterals from the descending motor tracts that transmit the motor command impinge on these two pathways. However, pathway 1 has a direct input onto CV centers, whereas pathway 2 activates other nuclei such as the hypothalamic nuclei (see Smith et al., this volume) or fastigial nuclei which can then affect CV control centers. Pathway 3 in Figure 5 differs from pathways 1 and 2 in that the CV command does not depend on the motor command, but the commands may be related by having a common origin. Thus, as the motor cortex, thalamus, cerebellum, basal ganglia and other integrative nuclei develop the integrated behavioral response to an external cue, they may develop separate command signals for the motor and CV systems.

Pathway 4 in Figure 5 introduces another degree of complexity: a spinal loop may be involved with synthesis or effectiveness of the command signal. Such a loop is suggested by the failure of subjects who attempt to contract paralyzed leg muscles to generate a pressor response (Gasser and Meek, 1914; Freund et al., 1979). The lack of response in subjects with spinal block could not be attributed to a lack of autonomic function because their heart rates and blood pressures during rest were not markedly changed by spinal blockade. On the other hand, subjects with intact spinal cords do generate a pressor response when they attempt to contract forearm muscles that are blocked by a neuromuscular blocking agent (Freyschuss, 1970). Presence or absence of a pressor response in these cases could be explained if spinal cord feedback generated by descending motor command activity were important for the normal manifestation of command signals.

We wanted to determine whether the CV command descended from supramedullary centers. To prove the existence of a supramedullary command signal, one would like to be able to abolish the CV response to exercise without affecting the motor response and without disrupting normal CV control during rest. We attempted to do this by placing bilateral subthalamic lesions in five behaviorally trained baboons. The subthalamus was chosen because previous studies on the CV and respiratory systems indicated that this area may be involved with integrating motor, CV and respiratory functions (Smith et al., 1960; Eldridge et al., 1981). The site chosen for lesions in each animal was identified during sterile surgery by the stereotaxic and electrical stimulation techniques mentioned by Smith et al. (this volume).

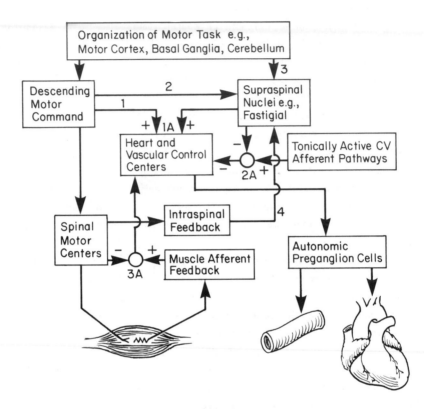

Fig. 5. Schematic diagram of possible pathways and actions of a central CV command. Pathways are labeled 1-4; actions are labeled 1A-3A. 1A indicates direct action on both brain stem centers and autonomic preganglionic cells that control both the heart and the vasculature. 2A indicates modulation of tonically active CV afferent pathways, e.g., baroreceptors. 3A indicates modulation of the afferent limb of the muscle pressor reflex pathways.

After recovery from the surgery, all animals displayed normal motor functions; however, the pressor response to exercise was abolished in one and reduced by 50% in another. The most impressive effect is shown in Figure 6. After the lesion the pressor response to exercise was abolished during both heavy- and light-load contractions, whereas the motor performance at the two loads was essentially unchanged. Note also that the resting blood pressure was normal after the lesion. We do not yet know whether the lesion destroyed cells or axons of cells involved with the transmission of the CV command, but we do know that the lesion did not destroy the animal's ability to increase its blood pressure: the baboon showed a marked increase in blood pressure when startled (Fig. 6, bottom).

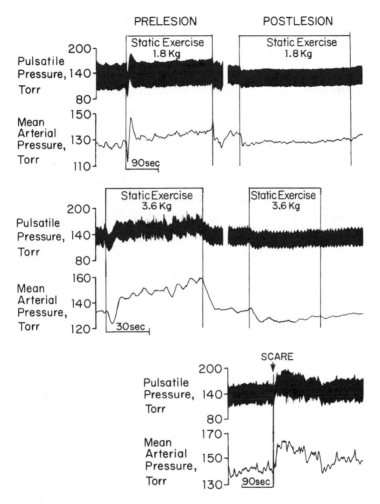

Fig. 6. Effect of lesions in the subthalamus on the arterial pressure response to contractions with light and heavy loads. The bottom right panel shows the postlesion pressure response to a scare. Note the difference in the time scales.

These results indicate that the CV response to exercise is elicited by a central signal that can be separated from the motor command signal, but they do not indicate whether the CV command is dependent on the motor command. The results also suggest that the muscle chemoreflex does not by itself elicit the pressor responses to these levels of static contraction force. This muscle reflex is still present even in midcollicular decerebrate animals, so we assume it must still be intact in our baboons. Since the pressor response was abolished with relatively small lesions above the midcollicular level in our baboon, we assume this result could not be associated with any peripheral defect. These results indicate that a command signal is probably important in eliciting the CV responses during all intensities of exercise.

CONCLUSION

Although command signals cannot be measured, measurement of motor unit recruitment and arterial pressure provides a crude method for expressing the magnitude of command signals. Our experimental results show that the change in arterial pressure is directly related to the magnitude of motor unit recruitment and cannot be explained by muscle reflexes. These results indicate that a CV command may elicit much of the CV response to static exercise. However, the application of this type of analysis to other motor tasks involves many complicating factors that must be considered before the relative importance of a central CV command during various motor tasks can be determined. Finally, lesions placed in the subthalamus can abolish the pressor response to static exercise. Although this result needs further confirmation, it does tend to indicate that the central CV command utilizes a separate pathway from that of the motor command. Future identification and isolation of this pathway may allow direct manipulation of the central CV command for more quantitative and detailed studies of its actions.

ACKNOWLEDGMENTS

I wish to thank Drs. L. B. Rowell and O. A. Smith for the support and advice they provided for these experiments and their critical review of this manuscript. I would also like to thank Cliff Astley, Dave Taylor, Sue King, and Debbie Baldwin for technical assistance, and Pam Stevens and Phyllis Wood for art work.

This research was supported by NIH grants RR00166, HL16910 and HL07090.

REFERENCES

Armstrong, R.B. and Peterson, D.F. (1981) Patterns of glycogen loss in muscle fibers: response to arterial occlusion during exercise. J. Appl. Physiol. 51, 552-556.

Arshavskii, Y.I., Gelfand, I.M., Orlovskii, G.N. and Pavlova, G.A. (1977) Activity of the neurones of the lateral reticular nucleus on scratching. Biophysics 22, 184-186.

Asmussen, E., Johansen, S.H., Jorgensen, M. and Nielsen, M. (1965) On the nervous factors controlling respiration and circulation during exercise. Experiments with curarization. Acta Physiol. Scand. 63, 343-350.

Barclay, J.K., Boulianne, C.M., Wilson, B.A. and Tiffin, S.J. (1979) Interaction of hyperoxia and blood flow during fatigue of canine skeletal muscle in situ. J. Appl. Physiol. 47, 1018-1024.

Burke, R.E., Levine, D.N., Tsairis, P. and Zajac, F.E. (1973) Physiological types and histochemical profiles in motor units of the cat gastrocnemius. J. Physiol. (Lond.) 234, 723-748.

Donald, K.W., Lind, A.R., McNicol, G.W., Humphreys, P.W., Taylor, S.H. and Staunton, H.P. (1967) Cardiovascular responses to sustained (static) contractions. Circulat. Res. (Suppl. 1) 20, 115-132.

Eldridge, F.L., Millhorn, D.E. and Woldrop, T.G. (1981) Exercise hyperpnea and locomotion: parallel activation from the hypothalamus. Science 211, 844-846.

Freund, P.R., Hobbs, S.H. and Rowell, L.B. (1978) Cardiovascular responses to muscle ischemia in man--dependency on muscle mass. J. Appl. Physiol. 45, 762-767.

Freund, P.R., Rowell, L.B., Murphy, T.M., Hobbs, S.F. and Butler, S.H. (1979) Blockade of the pressor response to muscle ischemia by sensory nerve block in man. Amer. J. Physiol. 237, H433-H439.

Freyschuss, U. (1970) Cardiovascular adjustments to somatomotor activation. The elicitation of increments in heart rate, aortic pressure and venomotor tone with the initiation of muscle contraction. Acta Physiol. Scand. Suppl. 342, 1-63.

Funderburk, C.F., Hipskind, S.G., Welton, C. and Lind, A.R. (1974) Development of and recovery from fatigue induced by static effort at various tensions. J. Appl. Physiol. 37, 392-396.

Gasser, H.S. and Meek, W.J. (1914) A study of the mechanisms by which muscular exercise produces acceleration of the heart. Amer. J. Physiol. 34, 48-71. See Ref. 2.

Goodwin, G.M., McCloskey, D.I. and Mitchell, J.H. (1972) Cardiovascular and respiratory responses to changes in central command during isometric exercise at constant muscle tension. J. Physiol. (Lond.) 226, 173-190.

Grimby, L. and Hannerz, J. (1977) Firing rate and recruitment order of toe extensor motor units in different modes of voluntary contraction. J. Physiol. (Lond.) 264, 865-879.

Grimby, L., Hannerz, J. and Hedman, B. (1981) The fatigue and voluntary discharge properties of single motor units in man. J. Physiol. (Lond.) 316, 545-554.

Humphreys, P.W. and Lind, A.R. (1963) The blood flow through active and inactive muscles of the forearm during sustained hand-grip contractions. J. Physiol. (Lond.) 166, 120-135.

Johansson, J.E. (1895) Ueber die Einwirkung der Muskelthätigkeit auf die Athmung und die Herzthätigkeit. Skand. Arch. Physiol. 5, 20-66.

Joyce, G.C., Rack, P.M.H. and Westbury, D.R. (1969) The mechanical properties of cat soleus muscle during controlled lengthening and shortening movements. J. Physiol. (Lond.) 204, 461-474.

Kniffki, K-D., Mense, S. and Schmidt, R.F. (1978) Responses of Group IV afferent units from skeletal muscle to stretch, contraction and chemical stimulation. Exp. Brain Res. 31, 511-522.

Krogh, A. and Lindhard, J. (1913) The regulation of respiration and circulation during the initial stages of muscular work. J. Physiol. (Lond.) 47, 112-136.

Kumazawa, T. and Mizumura, K. (1977) Thin-fibre receptors responding to mechanical, chemical and thermal stimulation in the skeletal muscle of the dog. J. Physiol. (Lond.) 273, 179-194.

Ludbrook, J., Faris, J.B., Iannos, J., Jamieson, G.G. and Russel, W.J. (1978) Lack of effect of isometric handgrip exercise on the responses of the carotid sinus baroreceptor reflex in man. Clin. Sci. Mol. Med. 55, 189-194.

McCloskey, D.I. (1981) Centrally-generated commands and cardiovascular control in man. Clin. Exp. Hypertension 3, 369-378.

McCloskey, D.I. and Mitchell, J.H. (1972) Reflex cardiovascular and respiratory responses originating in exercising muscle. J. Physiol. (Lond.) 224, 431-441.

Melcher, A. and Donald, D.E. (1981) Maintained ability of carotid baroreflex to regulate arterial pressure during exercise. Amer. J. Physiol. 241, H838-H849.

Milner-Brown, H., Stein, R. and Yemm, R. (1973) The orderly recruitment of human motor units during voluntary isometric contractions. J. Physiol. (Lond.) 230, 359-370.

Rowell, L.B., Hermansen, L. and Blackmon, J.R. (1976) Human cardiovascular and respiratory responses to graded muscle ischemia. J. Appl. Physiol. 41, 693-701.

Schibye, B., Mitchell, J.H., Payne, F.C. and Saltin, B. (1981) Blood pressure and heart rate response to static exercise in relation to electromyographic activity and force development. Acta Physiol. Scand. 113, 61-66.

Smith, O.A., Rushmer, R.F. and Lasher, E.P. (1960) Similarity of cardiovascular responses to exercise and to diencephalic stimulation. Amer. J. Physiol. 198, 1139-1142.

Stenberg, J., Astrand, P-O., Ekblom, B., Royce, J. and Saltin, B. (1967) Hemodynamic response to work with different muscle groups, sitting and supine. J. Appl. Physiol. 22, 61-70.

Cardiovascular Control Centers in the Brain: One More Look

O. A. SMITH, J. L. DE VITO AND C. ASTLEY

Regional Primate Research Center at the University of Washington, Seattle, Washington

For those of us working in the overlapping areas of central nervous system (CNS), behavior, and cardiovascular (CV) control, the fundamental thesis is that when there is organized central nervous activity dedicated to producing integrated somatic behavior, there will also be organized central neural activity to provide the metabolic adjustments to support that ongoing behavior. Just how the nervous system is put together, anatomically and functionally, to produce this organized central neural activity which results in the pattern of CV adjustment to support that behavior is really one of the major foci of attention for this conference.

Given the complexity of the CNS, there are obviously myriads of ways that this organization could be achieved. However, wouldn't it be convenient if there were a circumscribed group of nerve cells located in proximity to one another that had the capability of organizing the complete pattern of CV responses required to support a particular behavior? If there were such a group of cells, we would probably refer to them collectively as a "center." The center concept has been applied to neural control of CV responses many times before, and it is one of the most primitive ideas that developed shortly after the recognition that the mind is located in the head. It is a concept that recurs periodically, but as our awareness of the complexity of the brain increases, the idea is rejected more rapidly each time it appears until now it is viewed as completely naive, passe and unworthy of serious consideration.

Despite this view, however, let us examine the concept one more time, establish some criteria for postulating such an anatomically delimited function, and determine whether recent experimental results contribute any validity to the idea. To do this, it will be necessary first to define the precise behavior to be dealt with, the environmental circumstances in which it is elicited, and the set of CV responses that accompany and support that behavior. Figure 1 illustrates the standard baboon preparation from which measurements of renal flow, terminal aortic flow, arterial pressure, heart rate and O_2 consumption are recorded during seven different behaviors including dynamic and static exercise, lever pressing, sleeping, eating, resting quietly, and the conditioned emotional response (CER). These recordings are made in an environmentally controlled booth, and all are under close stimulus control.

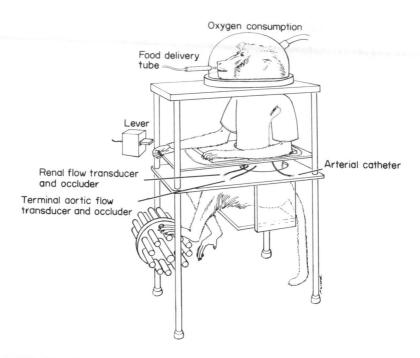

Oxygen consumption

Food delivery
tube

Lever

Renal flow transducer
and occluder

Terminal aortic flow
transducer and occluder

Arterial catheter

Fig. 1. Experimental setup for measurement of CV responses in the restrained baboon.

The CER, upon which we will focus, is an operationally defined measure of emotion. First, the animal is trained to press a lever to receive food reinforcement. Then at a specific time, a signal (visual or auditory) comes on for 1 min, and the termination of that signal coincides with a brief peripheral electric shock. After several combinations of signal and shock, suppression of the lever pressing occurs, i.e., the animal stops pressing the lever during the signal and sits quietly until the shock is delivered, then begins pressing the lever again. This suppression of the lever pressing provides an operational definition of emotion in the somatic system, but in addition there is a characteristic set of CV responses that accompany the suppression of lever pressing. Figure 2 shows the increased terminal aortic flow; a biphasic response in the renal flow that is first a rapid, neurally mediated flow decrease, then a return to normal followed by a delayed second decrease for the duration of the signal presentation. An increased blood pressure and a tachycardia invariably accompany the other CV responses. These CV changes provide an additional operational definition of emotion, this time in the visceral system.

Having defined the experimental situation, the specific behavior, and the well-characterized CV responses that accompany the behavior (CER), we can stipulate the

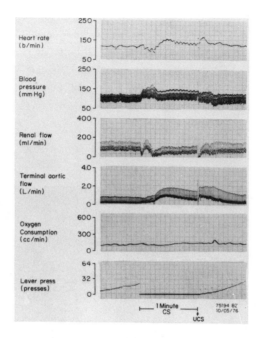

Fig. 2. CV response to a conditioned emotional response. (Reproduced, with permission, from Smith et al., Fed. Proc., 1980, 39, 2487.)

following set of criteria that must be satisfied if we are to postulate that there is an anatomically circumscribed set of neurons acting as an organizing, integrating center in the brain that controls these CV responses accompanying the CER:

1. The response pattern involving the adjustment in all of the neurally mediated CV variables appropriate to the behavior must be controlled by the center.

2. There must be multiple sources of relevant information providing input to the center.

3. The center must consist of neural elements capable of integrating a variety of inputs.

4. There must be multiple outputs from the center that affect the various autonomic motor nuclei that ultimately produce the changes in the effector organs.

5. The CV responses associated with other behaviors should not be affected by elimination of the center.

There are two corollaries of the first criterion. First, electrical stimulation of the center should reproduce the complete CV response normally associated with the CER. This has been done in the baboon by using a ventriculographic approach to electrode placement, as demonstrated in Figure 3. Metrizamide, a radio-opaque material, is introduced into the lateral ventricle via a stainless steel cannula. The material flows through the foramen of Munro into the third ventricle, outlining the anterior commissure, optic chiasm, mammillary body, massa intermedia, posterior commissure, etc. Once the complete third ventricle is outlined and the exact location of the cannula is known, stimulating electrodes may be placed accurately in any structures in the vicinity of the third ventricle.

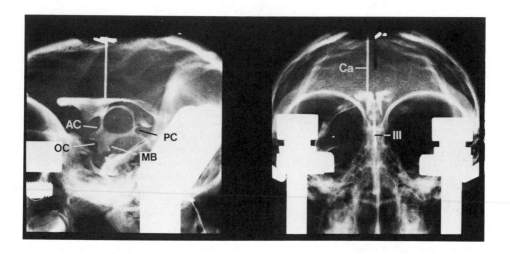

Fig. 3. Lateral (left) and frontal (right) X-rays showing ventricular system full of contrast medium (metrizamide). An 18-gauge stainless steel cannula (Ca) used to inject metrizamide into lateral ventricle is shown exiting top of skull. AC, anterior commissure; PC, posterior commissure; OC, optic chiasm; MB, mammillary body; III, third ventricle.

If one then explores the brain with a stimulating electrode, one can locate the precise hypothalamic site that, upon brief electrical stimulation, produces a tachycardia, increased arterial pressure, biphasic constriction in the kidney (i.e., a fast decrease, recovery, a slower maintained decrease), and increased terminal aortic flow (Fig. 4). This is the exact pattern that occurs during the CER. Therefore, the first corollary of the first criterion is fulfilled.

The second corollary is that if this center is destroyed, then the total CV response associated with the CER should be eliminated. It would not be adequate for just heart rate or just blood pressure or just renal flow to be eliminated; the whole response should

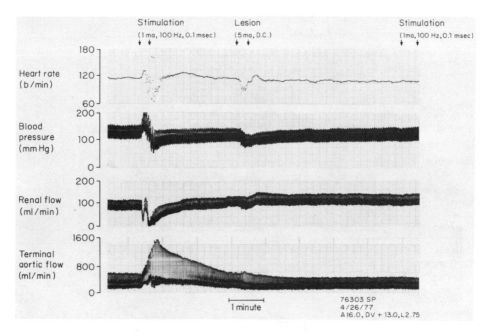

Fig. 4. CV responses to stimulation of hypothalamus before and after an electrolytic lesion. Animal was anesthetized with chloralose (65 mg/kg). (Reproduced, with permission, from Smith et al., Fed. Proc., 1980, 39, 2487.)

be gone. Figure 5 shows the results of bilateral ablation of this same hypothalamic area that, when stimulated, produces the CV response mimicking the CER response. On the left of the figure is shown the prelesion CER response. After a week's postsurgical recovery, the animal was returned to the testing situation. On the right is the postlesion CER response. When the signal comes on, the baboon stops pressing as usual and does not press the lever until after the shock is delivered. However, there is no increased TA flow, no decrease in renal flow, no change in pressure, no change in heart rate. The totality of the CV response normally associated with the CER has been eliminated, fulfilling the second corollary of the first criterion.

The second criterion is that there must be multiple inputs to the center. If the nerve cells that make up this center are really going to provide an integrative function, then they must receive relevant information from many sources and put it together in a fashion that produces the pattern of CV responses characterizing the CER. This anatomical area cannot be only a pass-through system, but must have inputs from places that are important for production of the response that is appropriate to the ongoing behavior. To determine the sources of inputs to this hypothalamic area, we have used the horseradish peroxidase (HRP) retrograde transport technology. To locate the appropriate

238

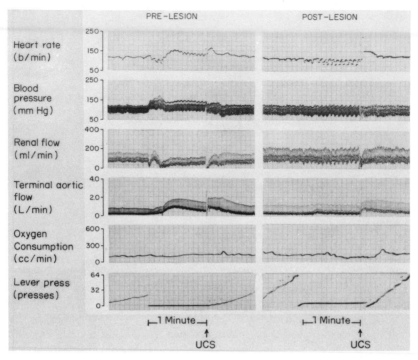

PRE-LESION   POST-LESION

Heart rate (b/min)

Blood pressure (mm Hg)

Renal flow (ml/min)

Terminal aortic flow (L/min)

Oxygen Consumption (cc/min)

Lever press (presses)

Fig. 5. The "pre-lesion" panel shows the complex CV pattern associated with emotion, including tachycardia, biphasic arterial blood pressure increase, a triphasic renal flow response (rapid decrease, recovery to normal and a second decrease with slow recovery) and a bimodal increase in terminal aortic flow. The "post-lesion" panel illustrates the disappearance of these CV changes in response to the CS (conditional stimulus) after destruction of a discrete area of the hypothalamus. (Reproduced, with permission, from Smith et al., in Morrison and Struck, Changing Concepts of the Nervous System, Academic Press, 1982, 569.)

site we introduce a stimulating electrode through a cannula and, when the CER response occurs, we withdraw the electrode, insert a small-gauge needle through the cannula to the identical location, and inject 4% HRP into the site. After a transport time of 48-72 hr the animal is euthanized and the tissues are prepared by the Mesulam technique.

Figures 6 and 7 illustrate the locations of cell bodies that provide axons to the area of the hypothalamus that controls the CV response to the CER. Some of these include the diagonal band of Broca (DBB), lateral septal area, an accumulation of cells in the organum vasculosum lamina terminalis (OVLT), the supraoptic nucleus, the amygdala, the sub-fornical organ (SFO), and the subiculum of the hippocampus. All these sources are relevant to the production of a CV response associated with emotion. The amygdala and the septal regions have been implicated repeatedly in the control of emotional behavior, the inputs from OVLT and SFO provide information about levels of circulating

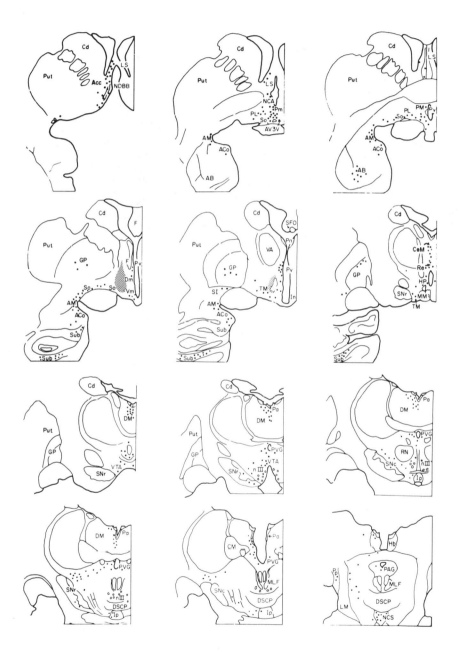

Fig. 6.   Sites of retrograde transport of horseradish peroxidase after injection into the hypothalamus (shaded area).   Abbreviations defined on following page.

ABBREVIATIONS

Ab	nucleus	PAG	periaqueductal grey
AB	basal amygdaloid nucleus	PbL	lateral parabrachial nucleus
ACo	cortical amygdaloid nucleus	PbM	medial parabrachial nucleus
AM	medial amygdaloid nucleus	PL	lateral preoptic area
CT	central tegmentum	PM	medial preoptic area
DR	dorsal raphe nucleus	PuM	medial pulvinar nucleus
GPi	internal segment of globus pallidus	Pv	paraventricular nucleus
Ip	interpeduncular nucleus		of hypothalamus
LC	locus ceruleus	RF	reticular formation
LM	medial lemniscus	PVG	periventricular grey
LS	lateral septal nucleus	MD	dorsomedial nucleus
MM	medial mamillary nucleus	SFO	subfornical organ
NCS	superior central nucleus	SN	substantia nigra
NTS	nucleus of the solitary tract	So	supraoptic nucleus
NX	dorsal motor nucleus of vagus nerve	Sub	subiculum
OT	optic tract	TM	tuberomamillary nucleus
OVLT	organum vasculosum lamina terminalis	VTA	ventral tegmental area
Pa	paraventricular nucleus of thalamus	ZI	zona incerta

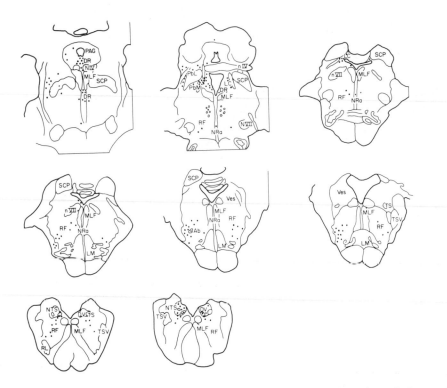

Fig. 7. Locations of cell bodies that provide axons to the area of the hypothalamus that controls the CV response to the CER.

angiotensin, and the supraoptic nucleus is involved in regulation of blood volume. Farther down the brain stem there are cells in the ventral tegmental area, periaqueductal gray, parabrachial nuclei, locus ceruleus, the dorsal raphe. Several of these midbrain and pontine regions are potentially important in CV regulation; for instance, the parabrachial nuclei have been implicated in the neural control of renal flow, the locus ceruleus is the major source of noradrenergic cells in the CNS, the dorsal raphe cells are involved in sleep--and therefore possibly alerting as well. In the medulla there are cells located in the vicinity of the nucleus ambiguus, the nucleus of the solitary tract, and the dorsal motor nucleus of the vagus. The medullary inputs are particularly relevant because these nuclei provide the source of cardiac efferents and primary afferent terminations for the baroreflexes. It makes sense for a CV regulatory center to receive information from those neurons controlling heart rate and those providing information about the status of the levels of systemic arterial pressure.

The third criterion for a "center" is that it has to be truly integrative. The responses derived from stimulation or destroyed by ablation cannot simply be due to a chance accumulation of fiber bundles passing through the area. For this center to have a true integrating function, there must be neuronal cell bodies present with dendritic fields upon which facilitatory and inhibitory inputs act to raise and lower the firing thresholds of those neurons. How can this be determined? It is difficult, because the cells have not yet been precisely identified, and so no one has recorded intracellular potentials from them. Therefore, we adapted the conditioning-testing procedure classically used in studying spinal reflexes. One electrode was placed in the hypothalamic area and another was placed in one of the sites that was proven by the HRP technique to project strongly to the hypothalamus. The nucleus of DBB showed a strong input to that hypothalamic area; therefore the conditioning electrode was placed there. The testing electrode was positioned in the hypothalamic site.

Figure 8 shows that low-current stimulation of the hypothalamus produces a small, fast renal response and a small pressure response; the slower renal response is more substantial. With this low current strength, not all the neural elements are being stimulated. A higher stimulating current would have produced a much larger response by recruiting more cells. However, the low current level excites a set of cells at a subthreshold level. Figure 8 also shows that stimulation of DBB by itself produces no CV response, but when stimulation of the DBB precedes and overlaps the hypothalamic stimulation there is a marked facilitation of the hypothalamic response. The amplitude of the fast renal response is now 350% of control and both blood pressure and heart rate are facilitated by approximately 50%. These data strongly suggest that the CV response controlled by this hypothalamic region depends on the presence of cell bodies and

242

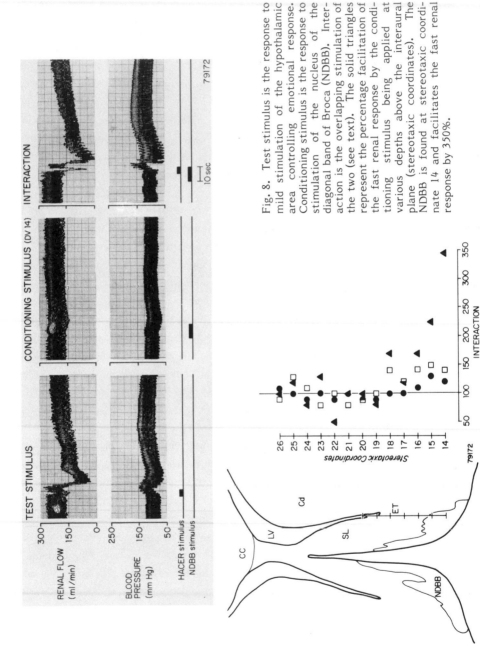

Fig. 8. Test stimulus is the response to mild stimulation of the hypothalamic area controlling emotional response. Conditioning stimulus is the response to stimulation of the nucleus of the diagonal band of Broca (NDBB). Interaction is the overlapping stimulation of the two (see text). The solid triangles represent the percentage facilitation of the fast renal response by the conditioning stimulus being applied at various depths above the interaural plane (stereotaxic coordinates). The NDBB is found at stereotaxic coordinate 14 and facilitates the fast renal response by 350%.

therefore has the potential of serving an integrative function in much the same fashion as the ventral horn cells do for simple motor reflexes. There is a facilitatory interaction between these two sites. Although we are not absolutely certain that the facilitation occurs at the hypothalamic site rather than at some other location, the strong anatomical connection between the two locations demonstrated by the HRP studies suggests that the hypothalamic site probably is the locus of interaction.

The fourth criterion demands that there be multiple outputs from the hypothalamic center, inasmuch as a variety of structures must be excited throughout the brain stem and spinal cord if the unique patterning of the CV response associated with the CER is to be produced. To study the efferents, we mixed tritiated proline and leucine, which are transported in an anterograde fashion, with some of the HRP injections, and processed them with autoradiography. Figure 9 shows plots of both the hypothalamic afferents determined with HRP technique and hypothalamic efferents determined with tritiated amino acids. This figure strikingly demonstrates the extent of reciprocal connections, with many nuclei providing afferents to the hypothalamic area and also receiving efferents from it. As one would expect, there are multiple outputs from the hypothalamic area. There is an output to the zona incerta, which has been implicated in baroreflex control, and outputs ascending the midline in the thalamus, going to the central gray and the reticular formation. We have not yet examined the spinal cord; however, one would expect from Loewy's and Swanson's work (this volume) that there will be inputs at the level of the intermediolateral cell column. The analysis is not yet complete, but apparently there will be little trouble showing multiple outputs to the important structures involved in autonomic control.

The final criterion for a "center" refers to the specificity issue, i.e., if this center is concerned with the CV responses accompanying only one kind of behavior, then the CV responses associated with other behaviors should not be affected by the lesions in this area. Figure 10 shows the average CV responses of six animals during exercise and eating before and after receiving lesions that eliminated the CER response. It is apparent that other than some random variability, there are no pre- and postlesion differences in the CV responses accompanying these behaviors. It is this result that establishes the unique function of this area of the hypothalamus. It seems to control the CV responses associated with emotional behavior alone, having no effects on other behaviors or their CV sequelae.

DISCUSSION

If one accepts that the criteria presented in this chapter are valid, then one would be hard pressed not to admit that the data provide strong support for the existence of an anatomically delimited set of nerve cells that subserve a unique integrative physiological

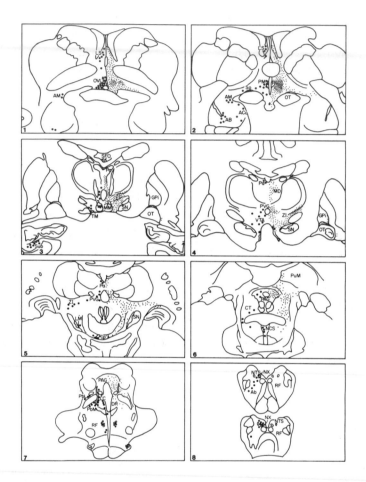

Fig. 9. Brain sections showing afferent sources of neurons projecting to the hypothalamic area controlling emotional response (large dots on left of each drawing) and efferent projection targets and pathways emanating from the same area (small stipple on right of each drawing). Abbreviations as previously listed. (Reproduced, with permission, from Smith et al., in Morrison and Struck, Changing Concepts of the Nervous System, Academic Press, 1982, 569.)

function. It would also be reasonable to designate such an area as a "center," as that term seems to embody the ideas inherent in the concept.

At one time, neurobiologists despaired of finding extensive functional localization in the CNS and settled for "equipotentiality" and more gestalt concepts. Just recently, however, using higher-level technology, we are discovering a great deal of functional specificity. The analysis of the visual system, the discovery of functionally specific

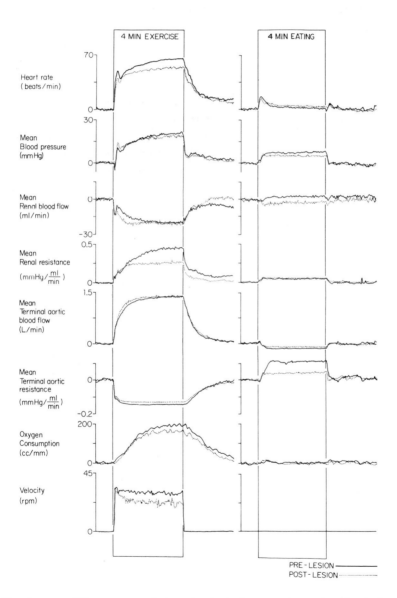

Fig. 10. Average CV responses of six animals during exercise and eating before and after receiving lesions that eliminated the CER response. (Reproduced, with permission, from Smith et al., Fed. Proc., 1980, 39, 2487.)

dominance columns in cerebral cortex, the extensive investigations of hemispheric lateralization of function--particularly those based on gender--and, in general, finding highly specific anatomical connections and systems of interrelations based on particular chemical transmitters, all contribute to a return toward the notion of a greater degree of specificity of function within the CNS. This does not imply that one "center" after another will be revealed, but it makes the idea of centers rest a bit more comfortably within our general understanding of the biology of the nervous system.

The task of analyzing the neural control of circulation would be simplified greatly if there were a series of "centers" that could be associated with various behaviors; but then again, it is entirely conceivable that it is **only** response to emotion-producing situations that requires the immediacy of a centrally organized CV response. It may well be, however, that more peripheral mechanisms and simple feedback to low-level reflexes are the way CV adjustments to other behaviors are produced. Elsewhere in this volume, Hobbs suggests that there may be a system for the control of the CV response to exercise that parallels this system described for the CER, and Simpson implies a similar integrative system related to drinking behavior. Clearly, the center concept cannot yet be interred.

ACKNOWLEDGMENTS

The studies described here were supported by NIH grants RR00166 and HL1690.

Behavioral Hypertension Mediated by Salt Intake

DAVID E. ANDERSON
Department of Psychiatry and Behavioral Sciences, University of South Florida College of
Medicine, Tampa, Florida

The search for the environmental determinants of essential hypertension has led epidemiologists to focus on two major research areas.   One encompasses the broad category of psychological stress and includes studies on the cultural prevalence of hypertension as a function of pervasive social changes (e.g., Henry and Cassell, 1969), the effects of occupational stress on blood pressure (e.g., Kasl and Cobb, 1967), and personality characteristics of patients with hypertension (e.g., Esler et al., 1977; Sullivan et al., 1981).   In general, this literature is consistent with the view that events in the individual's environment can exert long-term effects on the central nervous system that mediate the pathogenesis of chronic hypertensive adaptations.   The other major area of research concerns the cardiovascular (CV) effects of dietary sodium.   Numerous studies have shown that prevalence of hypertension among members of a culture is a function of dietary sodium intake levels (Costa et al., 1981).   These studies are consistent with the view that hypertension involves changes in renal regulation of fluid volume.

At first glance, it might appear that psychological stress and dietary sodium intake represent independent and alternative environmental influences in the development of chronic hypertension.   However, a growing body of research is revealing complex interactions between the sympathetic nervous system, on the one hand, and electrolyte metabolism, on the other, which suggest that a complete understanding of the role of either psychological stress or sodium intake in long-term control of blood pressure may not be possible without concomitant consideration of the other.

Over the past 20 years, experimental studies of long-term blood pressure regulation in laboratory animals have been facilitated by the combined application of behavioral science methodology and modern electronic monitoring technology.   These studies have shown that aversive behavioral conditioning can produce acute but sustained elevations in arterial pressure, which are accompanied by alterations in sympathetic nervous system activity (Kelleher et al., 1972), renal blood flow (Forsyth, 1971) and associated renal (Blair et al., 1976) and adrenal (Mason, 1968) hormones.   Grignolo (1980) reported that dogs on shock-avoidance procedures showed increased sodium and fluid retention compared with levels when they were performing exercise that produced comparable cardiac activation.

Their glomerular filtration rates were unchanged during avoidance, suggesting that the retention may have involved altered renal tubular activity.

A number of attempts have been made to develop chronic hypertension in laboratory animals by repeated exposure to aversive behavioral conditioning procedures. These efforts have not been without success (Forsyth, 1969; Herd et al., 1969), but many months usually are required to produce significant blood pressure elevations in individual animals, and several studies have not produced positive findings (Findley et al., 1971; Buchholz et al., 1981). In no study to date has there been a systematic attempt to determine the effects of the behavioral procedures as a function of the animal's level of salt intake. Similarly, hypertension was found to develop in rats exposed for periods of months to a high-salt diet with no specific stress conditioning (Meneeley et al., 1953), but is more difficult to obtain in larger animals without genetic or surgical bias of the preparation.

Both the acute and long-term CV effects of the sympathetic neurotransmitter norepinephrine (NE) are a function of the subject's recent level of salt intake. In one recent study (Cowley and Lohmeier, 1979), effects of intravenous (i.v.) and intrarenal infusion of NE on arterial pressure, plasma renin activity, and renal function of uninephrectomized dogs were investigated at four levels of sodium intake. After 3 days of continuous intrarenal infusion, mean arterial pressure had increased in proportion to the level of salt intake, while effective renal plasma flow and glomerular filtration rate were decreased and renal vascular resistance was increased. Smaller but similar effects were observed with i.v. infusions of NE. Extension of these results to human subjects was recently reported in studies of i.v. infusions of NE under four levels of dietary sodium intake (Rankin et al., 1981). This study also showed that basal levels of arterial pressure were higher in the high salt group, though sympathetic nervous system activity was decreased compared with the low salt group. Previously, it had been found that a high salt diet increased forearm vascular resistance and arterial pressure of borderline hypertensive humans and augmented reflexive vasoconstriction (Mark et al., 1975). Since aversive conditioning alters sympathetic influences on the heart and peripheral vasculature, the CV effects of emotional behavioral interactions might also be a function of the concurrent intake of sodium.

Conversely, changes in nervous system functions are observed in experimental hypertension produced by techniques which include salt loading. For example, hypertension induced by administrations of salt-retaining hormones (DOCA) and salt has been associated with increased levels of plasma catecholamines (deChamplain, 1972). Moreover, DOCA-salt hypertension can be prevented by pre-treatment of the brain with 6-hydroxydopamine, a neurotoxin that selectively destroys catecholaminergic neurons (Finch et al., 1972). Recently, Buckley et al. (1981) showed that intracerebroventricular administrations of angiotensin II to dogs produced a hypertensive response (28/14 mm Hg) over a 4-week period, but only if accompanied by substitution of saline for drinking water. This hypertension was associated with an increase in femoral and renal arterial resistance, increases in serum calcium, and decreases in serum sodium levels. It is well established that the hypertensive effects of clipping renal arteries, removing renal mass, or administering steroids are enhanced if the animal is provided with increased sodium in the diet.

In rodents, early experience can importantly determine blood pressure levels later in life (Henry et al., 1967), even in genetically susceptible subjects. For example, if spontaneously hypertensive rats are reared in a quiet, protected environment, the rate of rise in blood pressure with age is significantly attenuated (Lais et al., 1974). Conversely, if they are exposed to aversive stimulation or restraint, the hypertension is increased (Yamori et al., 1969). Operant conditioning studies of genetically susceptible rats have shown that experimentally programmed behavioral interactions can also be important in determining the magnitude of hypertension. Friedman and Dahl (1975) reported that a conflict situation (i.e., a behavioral response produced both food and electric shock) significantly elevated blood pressure levels over a 13-week period in the Dahl S-strain of hypertensive rats. This hypertension was reversible over 8 subsequent weeks without experimental conflict. In addition, Lawler et al. (1981) mated spontaneously hypertensive rats with Kyoto Wistar normotensive rats and found that the offspring developed borderline hypertension. Systolic pressure levels increased more than 30 mm Hg above this borderline hypertensive baseline if the rats were exposed 2 hr per day for 15 weeks to a conflict procedure in which either the occurrence or the omission of an operant response resulted in electric shock. The stress-mediated hypertension persisted for 10 weeks after termination of the conflict procedure, and resulted in degenerative CV changes.

Over the past several years, we have studied CV adaptations of dogs with no genetic predisposition to hypertension. Studies of avoidance conditioning of these chronically instrumented subjects have revealed two basic patterns of hemodynamic response, each associated with a specific aspect of the experimental conditions. Avoidance conditioning procedures require the subject to emit an operant response to reset a recycling 20-sec timer which, if permitted to complete its cycle, would present a brief electric shock. The shock intensity is the minimum required to sustain avoidance behavior. With training, subjects become very proficient at this task and will generate and maintain stable patterns of responding during prolonged intervals with a minimum of aversive stimulation. The performance of avoidance is associated with a sustained increase in blood pressure, mediated by an increase in heart rate and cardiac output, but not peripheral resistance (Anderson and Tosheff, 1973). The CV response during avoidance sessions can be modified by the administration of adrenergic blocking drugs (Anderson and Brady, 1976; Anderson et al., 1976), either alpha (which decreases blood pressure but not heart rate) or beta (which decreases heart rate but not blood pressure).

However, periods immediately **preceding** avoidance sessions are accompanied by progressive behavioral inhibition together with a gradual rise in arterial pressure, mediated by a concomitant rise in total peripheral resistance (Anderson and Tosheff, 1973; Lawler et al., 1975). Heart rate and cardiac output decrease over the same period. This divergent change in blood pressure and heart rate is accompanied by a decrease in respiratory rate, and can emerge gradually over prolonged intervals of up to at least 16 hr (Anderson and Brady, 1973). The rise in blood pressure and fall in heart rate occurring during pre-avoidance periods are not prevented by the administration of adrenergic blocking drugs (Anderson and Brady, 1976; Anderson et al., 1976).

The CV changes during pre-avoidance periods are apparently associated with the animal's motivation to respond quickly to an anticipated stimulus, since they are not observed until the subject has learned to make the first avoidance response immediately after the panel light signals the avoidance contingency, and before the occurrence of any electric shocks. Moreover, this CV response pattern was not observed when animals were required to wait in the experimental environment before the onset of an operant conditioning procedure in which panel-pressing behavior was maintained by food reinforcement (Anderson and Brady, 1972). Novel stimulus conditions can also evoke acute, divergent changes in vascular resistance and cardiac rate (i.e., orienting reflexes), but repeated elicitation of this hemodynamic response may require an experimental condition involving signal detection, such as the onset of an avoidance session or a reaction time paradigm.

It has long been known that total peripheral resistance increases markedly while heart rate and cardiac output decrease in animals during immersion of the head in water. The traditional view is that the hemodynamic changes in diving conserve oxygen for critical organs such as the brain and heart, but Kanwisher et al. (1981) recently demonstrated that there is apparently an emotional component as well. When animals were forced to submerge their heads in water, the magnitude of effects was much greater than when they were permitted to dive spontaneously. During diving there is a significant decrease in renal blood flow and an increase in plasma potassium levels, which could influence aldosterone metabolism (reviewed by Andersen, 1966). It will be of interest to determine whether renal and adrenal functions during extended pre-avoidance periods resemble those observed during brief intervals of diving and inhibit renal excretion of fluid volume in response to the observed increases in total peripheral resistance and arterial pressure.

Some years ago, Coleman and Guyton (1969) showed that hypertension developed in dogs under conditions of saline infusion (3-4 liters per day) or increases in dietary salt intake if renal functions were also impaired by surgical excision of renal mass. If, in fact, the behavioral procedures described here reduce the ability of the kidney to excrete fluid volume, an increase in sodium intake might have comparable effects upon blood pressure as observed in nephrectomized dogs. We are now testing this hypothesis by concurrently exposing dogs to recurrent avoidance sessions (which maintain elevated peripheral resistance but not cardiac ouput levels between sessions) and an increase in intake of salt and water. The dogs live in a kennel throughout the experimental period, and blood pressure and heart rate are monitored directly and continuously over periods of weeks (Kearns et al., 1981). These experiments require dogs to avoid electric shocks by panel-pressing at least once every 20 sec during each of three daily 30-min sessions. The first occurs at 12 a.m., the second at 8 a.m. and the third at 4 p.m. Each is signaled by turning off the chamber light and turning on the panel light. During experimental periods of 15 days or more, isotonic saline is infused into the arterial catheter at a rate of 50 ml/hr, resulting in 185 mEq sodium per 24 hr. This amount of saline provides 10.8 g of sodium chloride per day. The amount of salt infused into the circulation in these experiments, while more than that consumed daily by most Americans, is still in the physiological range. A comparable amount of salt is consumed by some individuals, for example in cultures that have a diet high in oceanic fish.

We have completed experiments with six dogs exposed to avoidance schedules and increased saline infusion for 14 or more days, and have analyzed data in terms of changes in arterial pressure (systolic and diastolic in mm Hg) and heart rate (bpm) over successive 24-hr intervals. Figure 1 shows the effects averaged for the group of six dogs for six days of baseline monitoring and 15 days of exposure to the experimental procedures. Systolic and diastolic pressure levels remained stable during the six days of baseline monitoring (group mean of 107/66 mm Hg) and then increased in response to the presentation of avoidance sessions and increased saline infusion. Typically, systolic and diastolic pressure increased about 10 mm Hg over the first 72 hr of the experimental period (range: 8-14 mm Hg) with smaller increases thereafter for some dogs. By the 15th day of exposure, systolic pressure levels were, on the average, 23.2 mm Hg higher and diastolic pressure levels averaged 11.2 mm Hg higher than during the last day of baseline monitoring. Heart rate levels did not change significantly, either during the baseline interval or in response to the experimental procedures.

It should be emphasized that the changes in blood pressure described in these experiments are based on continuous measurements made 24 hr per day, including during sleep, and do not reflect the peak pressure levels observed during avoidance sessions. Preliminary analyses of the data indicate that the magnitude of acute increase during avoidance sessions in hypertensive dogs was not significantly different from that observed when they were normotensive. While all 6 dogs showed an increase in 24-hr mean levels of blood pressure in response to the experimental procedure, substantial variability in magnitude of effect was observed between subjects, with one showing an increase of 49/25 mm Hg and another only 12/11 mm Hg. Linear regression analyses were performed on the 24-hr means of each CV measure over the 15-day experimental period. The slopes of systolic and diastolic pressure trends were significantly positive for each dog.

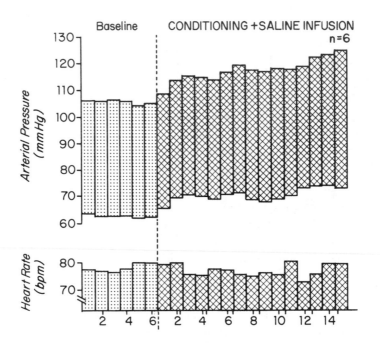

Fig. 1. Twenty-four-hour mean levels of arterial pressure and heart rate over six days of baseline monitoring followed by 15 days of exposure to avoidance conditioning and saline infusion, averaged for the group of six dogs.

In three dogs for which the avoidance sessions and high salt intake were terminated after 14 days, blood pressure fell towards the normotensive range, in some cases gradually but in others within 24 hr. (Hypertension of 4 months duration in rats produced by the Goldblatt procedure may also be totally reversed within 24 hr of removal of the renal artery clip (Russell et al., 1981)). This indicates that the increases in blood pressure were not accompanied by structural changes in the peripheral vasculature. Three other dogs experienced a cerebral hemorrhage during the third week on the procedure (Anderson, 1981). Of interest was the observation that in two of these dogs, the stroke occurred at a period of inordinately elevated presure associated with an unscheduled change in discriminative stimuli used in avoidance sessions. Two of these hemorrhages occurred in the basal ganglia and occipital cortex.

Exposure to avoidance conditioning alone or high salt intake alone did not produce a comparable hypertensive response in any of the three dogs exposed to each of these conditions. Figure 2 shows the group effects of 15 days of avoidance conditioning with sodium restriction immediately following 3 days of baseline monitoring (no avoidance sessions). The rise in pressure observed during day 1 of avoidance sessions seems to have been due to a transient physiological arousal associated with the onset of the contingency, since pressure levels drifted downwards on subsequent days. Figure 3 shows the group effects of 3 days of baseline monitoring followed by 15 days of saline infusion at a rate that produced hypertension in behaviorally conditioned dogs: this quantity of salt infusion alone did not produce significant change in blood pressure levels over these intervals.

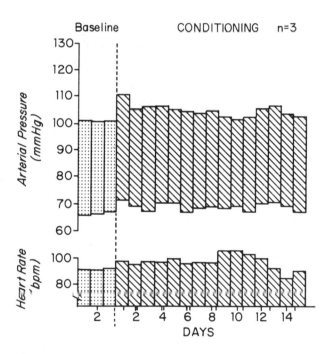

Fig. 2. Twenty-four-hour mean levels of arterial presure and heart rate over three days of baseline monitoring followed by 15 days of avoidance conditioning under conditions of sodium restriction, averaged for the group of three dogs.

Variable results have been reported in previous studies in which high salt intake or aversive stimulation was scheduled for laboratory animals over extended periods of time. This variability in results may have reflected nonsystematic control of one of these two

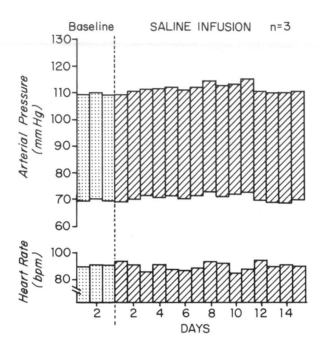

Fig. 3. Twenty-four-hour mean levels of arterial pressure and heart rate over 3 days of baseline monitoring followed by 15 days of saline infusion (1.2 1/24 hr), averged for the group of three dogs.

variables (psychophysiological state, salt intake) in the study of the other. For example, one previous study reported that salt loading alone produced hypertension in laboratory dogs (Vogel, 1965). This study reported that a first exposure to the high salt condition elevated arterial pressure significantly, but that an attempt to replicate this finding at a later date with the same subjects was unsuccessful. Our experience with laboratory animals has shown that even so-called "resting" hemodynamic states of individual animals normally change substantially over a period of weeks as the subject becomes accustomed to the laboratory environment, and that 24-hr means of arterial pressure levels may fall 10 mm Hg or more over this habituation period. Thus, initial attempts to produce sodium hypertension in this previous study may have been successful due to the physiological arousal associated with the novelty of the environment, experimenters, etc., and the lack of replication of this effect may have been due to extinction of the novelty-induced emotional state, with subsequent improvement in circulatory functions.

The results of these studies are consistent with the hypothesis that behavioral contingencies on individuals can exert sustained effects on physiological regulatory systems which alter the metabolism of ingested sodium. The interpretation of the results is based on the hypothesis that the CV state **between** avoidance sessions was as important as (or more important than) the acute CV changes observed **during** avoidance sessions, when blood pressure was typically at daily peaks. It is suggested that the elevation in vascular resistance occurring between avoidance sessions with a hypothesized reduction in renal functions provided sufficient conditions for maladapted sodium and fluid retention. Other stressful procedures that also elevate blood pressure acutely but via alternative hemodynamics (e.g., associated with increased beta adrenergic activity) may not result in comparable long-term CV adaptations. This concept of associated behavioral inhibition, vigilance and increased vascular resistance seems to fit with existing data on the incidence of CV disease in persons such as air traffic controllers, police and firemen, whose occupations require sustained vigilance and immediate response. Similarly, it also seems to be consistent with the traditional psychosomatic concept of suppressed emotionality as a personality characteristic of hypertensives (Weiner, 1977).

In summary, the results of the present research are consistent with the view that the effects of sodium intake on long-term blood pressure regulation depend on the emotionally induced physiological "state" of the subject, and conversely, that the effects of emotional stress on circulatory functions are dependent on intake of sodium. The manner in which these variables interact with genetic predisposition to engender chronic hypertension remains to be determined, but the present experiments provide a basis for investigation of pathophysiological processes involved in long-term blood pressure elevation in a large laboratory animal preparation. Such studies may ultimately provide a rational basis for preventive behavioral interventions.

ACKNOWLEDGMENTS

This research was supported by grant HL17970 from the National Heart, Lung and Blood Institute. I am grateful to William Kearns and Warren Better for their expert technical assistance.

REFERENCES

Andersen, H.T. (1966) Physiological adaptations in diving vertebrates. Physiol. Rev. 46, 212-243.
Anderson, D.E. (1981) Experimental behavioral hypertension in the dog. 3rd Joint U.S.-U.S.S.R. Symposium on Hypertension. National Institutes of Health, Bethesda, Maryland.
Anderson, D.E. and Brady, J.V. (1972) Differential preparatory cardiovascular responses to aversive and appetitive behavioral conditioning. Condit. Reflex 7, 82-96.
Anderson, D.E. and Brady, J.V. (1973) Prolonged preavoidance effects upon blood pressure and heart rate in the dog. Psychosom. Med. 35, 4-12.
Anderson, D.E. and Brady, J.V. (1976) Cardiovascular responses to avoidance conditioning: effects of beta adrenergic blockade. Psychosom. Med. 38, 181-189.

Anderson, D.E. and Tosheff, J.G. (1973) Cardiac output and total peripheral resistance changes during pre-avoidance periods in the dog. J. Appl. Physiol. 35, 650-654.

Anderson, D.E., Yingling, J.E. and Brady, J.V. (1976) Cardiovascular responses to avoidance conditioning: effects of alpha adrenergic blockade. Pavlov. J. Biol. Sci. 11, 150-161.

Blair, M.F., Feigl, E.O. and Smith, O.A. (1976) Elevations of plasma renin activity during avoidance performances in baboons. Amer. J. Physiol. 231, 772-776.

Buchholz, R.A., Lawler, J.E. and Barker, G.F. (1981) The effects of avoidance and conflict schedules on the blood pressure and heart rate of rats. Physiol. Behav. 26, 853-864.

Buckley, J.P., Lokhandwala, M.F., Steenberg, M., Francis, J.S. and Tadepalli, A.S. (1981) Cardiovascular effects of chronic administration of angiotensin II in dogs. Clin. Exp. Hypertension 3, 1001-1018.

deChamplain, J. (1972) Hypertension and the sympathetic nervous system; in Perspectives in Neuropharmacology, S. Snyder, ed. Oxford University Press, Oxford.

Coleman, T.G. and Guyton, A.C. (1969) Hypertension caused by salt loading in the dog. III. Onset transients of cardiac output and other variables. Circulat. Res. 25, 153-160.

Costa, F.V., Ambrosioni, E., Montebugnoli, L., Paccaloni, L., Vasconi, L. and Magnani, B. (1981) Effects of a low-salt diet and of acute salt loading on blood pressure and intralymphocytic sodium concentration in young subjects with borderline hypertension. Clin. Sci. 61, 21s-23s.

Cowley, A.W. Jr. and Lohmeier, T.E. (1979) Changes in renal vascular sensitivity and arterial pressure associated with sodium intake during long-term intrarenal norepine-phrine infusions in dogs. Hypertension 1, 549-558.

Dahl, L.K. (1977) Salt intake and hypertension; in Hypertension, J. Genest, E. Koiw and O. Kuchel, eds. McGraw-Hill, New York, pp. 548-558.

Esler, M., Julius, S., Zweifler, A., Randall, O., Harburg, E., Gardiner, H. and deQuattro, V. (1977) Mild high-renin essential hypertension: a neurogenic human hypertension. New Engl. J. Med. 296, 405-411.

Finch, L., Haeusler, G. and Thoenen, H. (1972) Failure to induce experimental hypertension in rats after intraventricular injection of 6-hydroxydopamine. Brit. J. Pharmacol. 44, 356-357.

Findley, J.D., Brady, J.V., Robinson, W.W. and Gilliam, W. (1971) Continuous cardiovascular monitoring in the baboon during long-term behavioral performances. Commun. Behav. Biol. 6, 49-58.

Forsyth, R.P. (1969) Blood pressure responses to long-term avoidance schedules in the restrained rhesus monkey. Psychosom. Med. 31, 300-309.

Forsyth, R.P. (1971) Regional blood flow changes during 72-hour avoidance schedules in the monkey. Science 173, 546-548.

Friedman, R. and Dahl, L.K. (1975) The effect of chronic conflict on the blood pressure of rats with a genetic susceptibility to experimental hypertension. Psychosom. Med. 37, 402-416.

Grignolo, A. (1980) Renal function and cardiovascular dynamics during treadmill exercise and shock avoidance in dogs. Unpublished doctoral dissertation. University of North Carolina at Chapel Hill.

Henry, J.P. and Cassel, J.C. (1969) Psychosocial factors in essential hypertension: recent epidemiologic and animal experimental evidence. Amer. J. Epidemiol. 90, 171-200.

Henry, J.P., Meehan, J.P. and Stephens, P.M. (1967) The use of psychosocial stimuli to induce prolonged systolic hypertension in mice. Psychosom. Med. 29, 408-432.

Herd, J.A., Morse, W.H., Kelleher, R.T. and Jones, L.G. (1969) Arterial hypertension in the squirrel monkey during behavioral experiments. Amer. J. Physiol. 217, 24-29.

Kanwisher, J.W., Gabrielson, G. and Kanwisher, N. (1981) Free and forced diving in birds. Science 211, 717-719.

Kasl, S.V. and Cobb, S. (1967) Blood pressure changes in men undergoing job loss: a preliminary report. Psychosom. Med. 32, 19-38.

Kearns, W.D., Better, W.E. and Anderson, D.E. (1981) A tether system for cardiovascular studies in the behaving dog. Behav. Res. Instr. Meth. 13, 323-327.

Kelleher, R., Morse, W. and Herd, J.A. (1972) Effects of propranolol, phentolamine, and methylatropine on cardiovascular function in the squirrel monkey during behavioral experiments. J. Pharmacol. Exp. Ther. 182, 204-207.

Lais, L.T., Bhatnagar, R.K. and Brody, M.J. (1974) Inhibition by dark adaptation of the progress of hypertension in the spontaneously hypertensive rat (SHR). Circulat. Res. 34 (Suppl. I), 155.

Lawler, J.E., Barker, B.A., Hubbard, B.S. and Schaub, R.G. (1981) Effects of stress on blood pressure and cardiac pathology in rats with borderline hypertension. Hypertension 3, 496-505.

Lawler, J.E., Obrist, P.A. and Lawler, K.A. (1975) Cardiovascular function during pre-avoidance, avoidance and post-avoidance in dogs. Psychophysiology 12, 4-11.

Mark, A.L., Lawton, W.J., Abboud, F.M., Fitz, A.E., Connor, W.E. and Heistad, D.D. (1975) Effects of high and low sodium intake on arterial pressure and forearm vascular resistance in borderline hypertension. Circulat. Res. 36 (Suppl I), 194-198.

Mason, J.W. (1968) Urinary aldosterone and urine volume responses to 72-hour avoidance sessions in the monkey. Psychosom. Med. 30, 733-745.

Meneeley, G.R., Tucker, R.G., Darby, W.J. and Auerbach, S.H. (1953) Chronic sodium chloride toxicity in the albino rat. II. Occurrence of hypertension and a syndrome of edema and renal failure. J. Exp. Med. 98, 71-80.

Rankin, L.I., Luft, F.C., Henry, D.P., Gibbs, P.S. and Weinberger, M.H. (1981) Sodium intake alters the effects of norepinephrine on blood pressure. Hypertension 3, 650-656.

Russell, G.I., Brice, J.M., Bing, R.F., Swales, J.D. and Thurston, H. (1981) Hemodynamic changes after surgical reversal of chronic two-kidney, one-clip hypertension in the rat. Clin. Sci. 61, 117s-119s.

Sullivan, P.A., Procci, W.R., DeQuattro, V., Schoentgen, S., Levine, D., Van Der Meulen, J. and Bornheimer, J.F. (1981) Anger, anxiety, guilt and increased basal and stress-induced neurogenic tone: causes or effects in primary hypertension. Clin. Sci. 61, 389s-392s.

Vogel, J.A. (1965) Salt-induced hypertension in the dog. Amer. J. Physiol. 210, 186-190.

Weiner, H. (1977) Psychobiology and Human Disease. Elsevier, New York.

Yamori, Y., Matsumoto, M., Yamabe, H. and Okamoto, K. (1969) Augmentation of spontaneous hypertension by chronic stress in rats. Jap. Circulat. J. 33, 399-409.

Published 1982 by Elsevier Science Publishing Co., Inc.
Smith, Galosy, and Weiss, editors
CIRCULATION, NEUROBIOLOGY, AND BEHAVIOR

Area-Specific Contingent Control of Pressor-Cardioacceleratory Responses to Electrical Stimulation of the Brain in the Rhesus Macaque

J. A. JOSEPH AND B. T. ENGEL

Gerontology Research Center, Baltimore, Maryland; National Institute on Aging, National Institutes of Health, U.S. Department of Health and Human Services, Bethesda, Maryland; and Baltimore City Hospital, Baltimore, Maryland

There is growing evidence that the central nervous system (CNS) provides a high degree of plasticity for peripheral cardiovascular (CV) and motor functions. Responses that ordinarily occur in one way under one set of conditions may occur in another way under other conditions. For example, Ainslie and Engel (1974) showed that a tachycardia classically conditioned to a warning click (conditioned stimulus) was changed through instrumental conditioning to a bradycardia in monkeys taught to slow heart rate. Thus, learning is an important process that can operate through the nervous system to modulate peripheral function. To investigate the role of learning in the modification of CV responses, we have used rhesus macaques (*Macaca mulatta*) to investigate (1) reflex modulation of CV function by examining baroreceptor sensitivity during sessions in which animals are operantly conditioned to slow or speed their heart rate (Engel and Joseph, 1981), (2) constraints on physical exercise produced by instrumental CV conditioning (Perski et al., in press), and (3) the effects of electrical stimulation of the brain (ESB), which produces changes in CV function under control conditions and during instrumental heart rate conditioning (Joseph and Engel, 1981).

In this chapter, we will consider the latter subject, the effects of instrumental conditioning of heart rate on the heart rate and blood pressure responses to ESB. An examination of the effects of instrumental conditioning on CV responses during ESB is important because, although numerous investigators have attempted to use ESB to assess the circuitry of central CV control in anesthetized nonprimates (e.g., Hilton, 1975; McAllen and Spyer, 1976) and baboons (Smith et al., 1974, 1979), few have attempted this assessment in the awake animal where a contingency was placed on CV control (e.g., Joseph and Engel, 1981). Therefore, there was no chance to observe the possible relations among ESB, CV changes, and behavior of the animal. If it is true that environmental and behavioral stimuli demand as careful control and consideration as the individual electrode placements within the animal (Korner, 1979), then CV responses to stimulation in certain brain areas in the anesthetized animal may show differences from those in the awake animal and also from those in the animal contingently trained to control heart rate.

Each of four animals was trained to slow or speed its heart rate, or had its heart rate monitored (control condition) in experimental sessions that were divided into a baseline (512 sec) and a conditioning or monitoring (control) phase (2048 sec) which, in turn, was divided into sixteen 128-sec segments (Engel, 1974, 1980; Engel and Gottlieb, 1970; Joseph and Engel, 1981). Each monkey had a polyethylene catheter surgically implanted into the abdominal aorta via the external iliac artery (Engel and Gottlieb, 1970). The catheter was kept patent by continuous infusion of heparinized saline (1 ml/hr). The blood pressure signal was detected by a P23 DB Statham pressure transducer. The signal was fed through devices interfaced with a Raytheon 704 computer, which operated on-line to control experiments and to record heart rate and blood pressure. (In this paper, blood pressure will be reported as derived mean pressure: systolic plus two times diastolic, divided by three.) Animals were signaled to slow heart rate by a red cue light or to speed it by a green cue light. If the training contingency was to speed the heart rate, the system was set so that the animal could successfully avoid shock as long as its heart rate was greater than baseline by 20 bpm--e.g., if its rate was 120 bpm, the avoidance criterion was 100 bpm. Correct performance was signaled by a yellow light and incorrect performance was punished by a 10-mA, 0.45-sec shock to the tail delivered on an 8-sec fixed interval schedule. The control condition was unsignaled and unreinforced. The monkeys were housed in Plexiglas^R restraining chairs, which were maintained in standard primate booths throughout the experiments.

Following training, an acrylic platform containing holes drilled to prespecified anterior-posterior and lateral coordinates (D. Bowden, personal communication) corresponding to one of four brain regions was stereotaxically mounted on the monkey's skull and cemented in place under aseptic conditions. The four brain regions selected were the striatum (AP +14-16, LAT 1.5-4.0), the anterior hypothalamus (AP +13.5, LAT 1.5-3.0), the posterior hypothalamus (AP +8.5-10.0, LAT 1.5-4.5), and the subthalamic nucleus (AP +7.0-8.5, LAT 3.0-4.5) (Snider and Lee, 1965). All coordinates were measured from ear bar zero; all lateral coordinates were measured from the midline of the skull. We selected the striatum because of its involvement with motor control, and because we were interested in somatomotor effects on heart rate during instrumental CV conditioning. We chose the hypothalamus because of its influence on autonomic function (Hilton, 1975), and the subthalamic nucleus because pilot work showed that stimulation in this area is associated with strong autonomic responsivity.

A week after the platform was in place, the monkey received an intramuscular injection of phencyclidine (0.1 mg/kg), and the skull was drilled at the prespecified points in the platform using a pin vise and a No. 79 drill. Since it was impossible under these

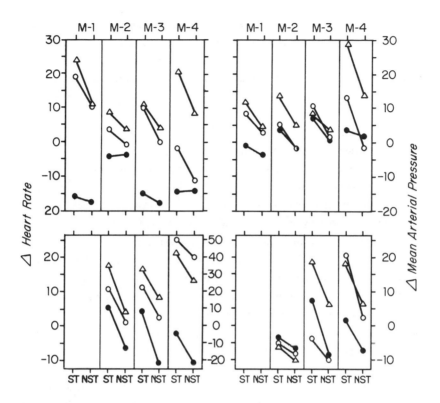

Fig. 1. Changes in heart rate (left panels) and mean blood pressure (right panels) responses during speeding (triangles), no feedback, or control (open circles), and slowing (closed circles) conditions following posterior hypothalamic (top panels) and anterior hypothalamic (bottom panels) stimulation (Hilton, 1975).

conditions to mount the animal's head in the stereotaxic instrument and lower the electrode with the aid of a standard electrode holder, the bipolar electrodes were lowered into the brain by holding them with the thumb and forefinger while pushing them down 1 mm at a time until a site was found that produced a tachycardia and pressor response when stimulated at an intensity between 50 and 1000 μA. The lowest current intensity was chosen that would produce reliable heart rate and blood pressure changes of about 10-20%. The electrode was cemented in place. CV changes were examined in the fully awake animal during slow, control and speed sessions in which ESB was delivered to one of the sites during alternate segments beginning with the second segment. The ESB sessions consisted of a 256-sec baseline period and a 1024-sec conditioning or monitoring period (sixteen 64-sec segment). The ESB was delivered for the entire 64-sec segment. The ESB sessions were carried out daily in sets of three, i.e., one control, one slow and one fast session per set on a particular brain area. Two brain areas were examined per day on alternate days. Sessions within a set were counterbalanced across days so that each type of session was given first, second, or third. Thus, over the course of the experiment each type of session was given equal representation at each position, and the chance of any bias due to a decrease in sensitivity to ESB as a result of repeated presentations was minimized.

At the completion of the sessions, lesions were made at the electrode sites with a radio-frequency lesion generator (50 mA/60 sec). The animals were given an overdose of sodium pentobarbitol and perfused intracardially with 20% formalin in saline. The brains were removed, embedded in paraffin, sectioned at 5 μm, stained with hematoxylin eosin, and examined under low-power magnification.

Data were analyzed by subtracting each stimulation (ST) and nonstimulation (NST) score on each segment from the baseline for the session to produce difference scores for heart rate (ΔHR) and mean blood pressure (ΔMBP). Two (ST, NST) by three (control, speed, slow) analyses of variance were carried out for each site in each monkey, followed by Duncan's (1975) post tests where significant statistical interactions were found. Baseline heart rate prior to each type of session for animals 2, 3 and 4 were not significantly different. Animal 1 showed a significantly different baseline heart rate ($p < 0.05$) owing to a higher baseline heart rate prior to slowing.

The results were consistent across the four animals: each was able to attenuate or even abolish the effects of the ESB on heart rate in the striatal and posterior hypothalamic areas during slowing, but not with stimulation in the anterior hypothalamic or subthalamic areas. Figure 1 (left side) illustrates these findings for ΔHR during ST and NST segments for the anterior and posterior hypothalamus. Heart rate differences were greater during ST and NST segments under speed and control conditions than under the slow condition when the posterior hypothalamus was stimulated. These findings contributed to significant interactions between stimulation condition and session type for each animal. To explore these differences further, Duncan's tests were done on the means computed by subtracting the control scores for the ST and NST segments from their respective segments under the speed and slow conditions, and also by subtracting the speed and slow scores under ST and NST conditions. Results of these tests showed that ESB did not have differential effects between speed and control conditions; however, both of these conditions differed from the slow condition ($p < 0.05$). Figure 2 further illustrates these results for the posterior hypothalamus: increases in heart rate occurred following ESB during the speed and control conditions but not during the slow condition. There was no selective attenuation of ESB effects on heart rate during the slow condition when ESB was delivered to the anterior hypothalamus (Fig. 1). Subsequent analyses of variance showed that there were no statistically significant interactions between stimulation condition and session type for animals 2 and 4. In monkey 3 this interaction was significant (F(2,89) = 4.09, p<0.025), although the difference in ΔHR between ST and NST was greater under the slow condition than under speed and control conditions (Fig.1). (Monkey 1 died before experiments were completed in the anterior hypothalamus or subthalamic areas.)

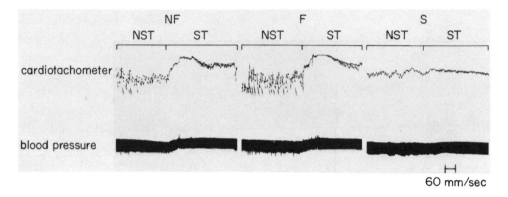

Fig. 2.   Change in heart rate and mean blood pressure responses during posterior hypothalamic stimulation and nonstimulation segments for speeding, no feedback, and slowing conditions. Note that the ESB was in effect for all portions labeled ST.

The right portions of Figure 1 show the results for Δ MP as a function of type of session and stimulation condition. The Δ MP following posterior hypothalamic ESB did not necessarily parallel those seen in Δ HR (left panel). Two animals showed significant interactions between session type and stimulation condition. Subsequent Duncan's tests showed the difference between ST and NST was less under the slow condition than under the fast and control conditions, indicating some attenuation of Δ MP under the slow condition. Anterior hypothalamic stimulation produced changes in blood pressure similar to those in heart rate, as can be seen by comparing the left and right lower portions of Figure 1: there was no tendency for any animal to attenuate the ESB effects on blood pressure during slowing. There were significant interactions between session type and stimulation condition for the three animals, but subsequent Duncan's post tests indicated that the ST-NST differences were greater under slow than under speed and control conditions for monkey 2, control for monkey 3, or speed condition for monkey 4.

The results of striatal stimulation were similar to those seen following posterior hypothalamic stimulation for both heart rate and blood pressure. For example, in monkey 2 the ST heart rate values (mean ± SD) were 3.6 ± 0.7 (control), -3.7 ± 1.2 (slow) and 8.8 ± 1.2 (speed), while the NST values were 0.9 ± 0.7 (control), -2.8 ± 0.6 (slow) and 3.3 ± 0.8 (speed). Note that ESB was attenuated under the slowing condition. This finding contributed to a significant interaction between stimulation condition and session type for this animal (p<0.01). Similar interactions were seen for the other animals as well, indicating attenuation during slowing. As with posterior hypothalamic stimulation, Δ MP did not parallel ΔHR following stimulation in the striatum. Subthalamic stimulation effects on heart rate were similar to those in the anterior hypothalamus. Strong effects were seen on heart rate and the animals were not able to attenuate these effects during slowing. ESB effects on ΔMP in the subthalamic nucleus were inconsistent and variable across animals and conditions. Subsequent analyses of electrode sites in two other animals within these four regions have yielded similar results. Table 1, which summarizes the results to date of all of the electrode penetrations into active "controllable" and "non-controllable" sites, shows that animals can significantly attenuate their heart rate responses to stimulation delivered to two regions of the brain (striatum and posterior hypothalamus) during conditions in which shock avoidance is contingent on heart rate slowing. Several regions, such as the subthalamus and amygdala, are not subject to this control and the animal cannot attenuate its heart rate during the slowing sessions. Moreover, attenuation seems to be selective to the parameter upon which the contingency is placed, i.e., heart rate but not blood pressure. For two reasons, the attenuation does not seem to be the result of threshold changes in the stimulation sites with repeated stimulation. First, care was taken to counterbalance all of the sessions so that control or a speed session did not always occur first and a slowing session last. Thus, any stimulus fading within a day's testing would be as likely to occur during control or speed sessions as it would during slowing. Second, analyses of variance carried out by comparing ΔHR during the first stimulus segment in the control sessions with the last stimulus segment (2 (segment) X 4 (brain area) for each brain area in each animal) showed neither segment differences nor segment differences as function of the brain area for ΔHR in any animal.

Other investigators have shown that stimulation in the anterior hypothalamus and subthalamic nucleus evokes affective as well as CV responses. For example, McBride and Larsen (1980) found that the subthalamic nucleus is a complex area that contains motor as well as CV functions and may receive selective input from the anterior hypothalamus and striatum, while Smith and colleagues (1980; this volume) have shown that lesions in the baboon in areas corresponding to our anterior hypothalamic sites create deficits in the animal's ability to generate a conditioned CV emotional response, i.e., ΔHR or ΔBP to a conditioned stimulus that was given prior to the administration of an electric shock. Lesions outside this zone did not have similar effects. It is possible in the present experiments that affective responses elicited by stimulation in these areas are stronger than the reinforcement strength of shock avoidance. However, the striatal or posterior hypothalamic stimulations can be overriden because they are associated primarily with CV effects. Posterior hypothalamic stimulation may involve only the outputs from the

TABLE 1

SUMMARY OF "CONTROLLABLE" AND "NONCONTROLLABLE SITES"
IN THE ANIMALS EXAMINED THUS FAR

"Controllable" sites	"Noncontrollable" sites
Striatum	Anterior amygdala
Caudate nucleus	
Lenticular nucleus	Thalamus
Lateral portion of the area tegmentum	Ventral posterior inferior nucleus
Globus pallidus	
	Subthalamus
Internal capsule lateral to the area tegmentum	Anterior hypothalamus
	Dorsomedial hypothalamus
Posterior hypothalamus	Supraoptic area of the hypothalamus
Mamillary nuclei	Paraventricular hypothalamus
Posterior dorsomedial hypothalamus	Parafascicular nucleus
Mamillothalamic fasciculus	

anterior hypothalamic area (Smith et al., 1979). It is interesting to note that Smith has defined a localizable area of the hypothalamus that is critical to the expression of a conditioned emotional response and extends caudally from the entry point of the postcommissural fornix to a point just rostral to the anterior tip of the mamillary bodies. Penetrations caudal to or in the mamillary bodies were not shown to be critical to this response. Our animals were always able to control stimulation delivered to these more caudal hypothalamic placements.

We are now examining the inputs and outputs to these areas, and one conclusion is clear: CNS-autonomic interactions in the unanesthetized animal are not invariant and can be modified by training. We believe that our findings provide strong evidence for Korner's (1979) speculation that environmental and behavioral stimuli demand as careful control and consideration as the individual electrode placements within the animal. Differences in response to ESB suggest that there are a variety of mechanisms operating within the brain that mediate plasticity such as that seen here. Heart rate responses, even in the face of ESB, can be different depending on the environmental contingencies and the demands made on the animals.

REFERENCES

Ainslie, G.W. and Engel, B.T. (1974) Alteration of classically conditioned heart rate by operant reinforcement in monkeys. J. Comp. Physiol. Psychol. 87, 373-382.
Duncan, J.B. (1975) T-tests and intervals for comparisons suggested by the data. Biometrics 31, 339-344.
Engel, B.T. (1974) Electroencephotographic and blood pressure correlates of operantly conditioned heart rate in the restrained monkey. Pavlov. J. Biol. Sci. 9, 222-232.

Engel, B.T. (1980) Somatic mediation of heart rate: a physiological analysis; in Biofeedback and Self-Regulation, N. Birbaumer and H.D. Kimmel, eds. Lawrence Erlbaum Associates, Hillsdale NJ, pp. 265-271.

Engel, B.T. and Gottlieb, S.H. (1970) Differential operant conditioning of heart rate in the restrained monkey. J. Comp. Physiol. Psychol. 73, 217-225.

Engel, B.T. and Joseph, J.A. (1981) Modulation of baroreceptor sensitivity during operant cardiac condition. Adv. Physiol. Sci. 17, 177-180.

Hilton, S.M. (1975) Ways of viewing the central nervous control of the circulation--old and new. Brain Res. 87, 213-219.

Joseph, J. and Engel, B.T. (1981) Instrumental control of cardio-acceleration induced by central electrical stimulation. Science 214, 341-343.

Korner, P.I. (1979) Central nervous control of autonomic cardiovascular function; in Handbook of Physiology: The Cardiovascular System (The Heart), R.M. Berne, ed. The American Physiology Society, Bethesda, Maryland.

McAllen, R.M. and Spyer, K.M. (1976) The location of cardiac vagal preganglionic motoneurons in the medulla of the cat. J. Physiol. (Lond.) 258, 187-204.

McBride, R.L. and Larsen, K.D. (1980) Projections of the feline globus pallidus. Brain Res. 189, 3-14.

Perski, A., Engel, B.T. and McCroskery, J.H. (in press) The modification of elicited cardiovascular responses by operant conditioning of heart rate; in Perspectives in Cardiovascular Psychophysiology, J.T. Cacioppo and R.T. Petty, eds.

Smith, O.A., Astley, C.A., DeVito, J.L., Stein, J.M. and Walsh, H.E. (1980) Functional analysis of hypothalamic control of the cardiovascular responses accompanying emotional behavior. Fed. Proc. 39, 2487-2494.

Smith, O.A., Hohimer, A.R., Astley, C.A. and Taylor, R.J. (1979) Renal and hindlimb vascular control during acute emotion in the baboon. Amer. J. Physiol. 236, R189-R205.

Smith, O.A., Stephenson, R.B. and Randall, D.C. (1974) Range of control of cardiovascular variables by the hypothalamus; in Recent Studies of Hypothalamus Function, K. Lederis and K.E. Cooper, eds. Karger, Basel, pp. 294-305.

Snider, R.S. and Lee, J.C. (1965) Stereotaxic Atlas of the Monkey. University of Chicago Press, Chicago.

Published 1982 by Elsevier Science Publishing Co., Inc.
Smith, Galosy, and Weiss, editors
CIRCULATION, NEUROBIOLOGY, AND BEHAVIOR

Psychosocial Stimulation of Mice in Complex Population Cages and the Mechanism of Cardiomyopathy

JAMES P. HENRY

Department of Physiology and Biophysics, University of Southern California, School of Medicine, Los Angeles, California

INTRODUCTION

Psychosocial stimulation as a result of emotionally arousing interactions between males in the presence of females in Henry-Stephens complex population cages leads to chronic high blood pressure and is accompanied by hypertrophy of the heart and myocardial fibrosis (Henry and Stephens, 1977a). The mice double their adrenal catecholamine synthetic enzymes (Henry and Stephens, 1977a), and the increased levels of plasma catecholamines are greatest in mice with the most social interaction (R. Campbell, unpublished observations). The renin-angiotensin system is chronically aroused (Vander et al., 1978); the adrenal gland is hypertrophied; and plasma corticosterone is increased, especially in older animals that have been exposed to social disorder for long periods (Henry and Stephens, 1977a).

Pathophysiological observations have been made of the hearts of these chronically aroused animals subjected to repeated episodes of dominance-subordination conflict. In one of our papers (Henry et al., 1971), Ratcliffe described the lesions as follows:

> The degeneration observed in the myocardium included changes in staining characteristics, separation of the myocardial fibers, fragmentation, and fibrosis. These were more common in the stimulated animals than in the controls. Frequently there were irregular areas which failed to stain normally in the slides stained with hematoxylin-eosin. They were pale, and it was difficult to discern their cytological detail. Where separation occurred, the myocardial fibers appeared to be shredded, and they were separated along their long axes so that fusiform spaces developed. Such separation was often extensive, covering the width of the myocardium. Fragmentation was characterized by a breaking up of the myocardial fibers at the intercalated discs; six to a dozen would be involved, each breaking up in several places. These fragmented areas were paler, giving the impression that there had been a loss of cytoplasmic staining characteristics.

As time went on, over half the stressed animals showed fibrous tissue which collected around the small vessels and in small, scattered patches throughout the myocardium. In one of ten cases, the process progressed until confluent lesions formed a patchwork of microinfarcts that extended through a considerable portion of the ventricular wall.

Recent studies have demonstrated "contraction band" lesions involving groups of sarcomeres adjacent to the intercalated discs, larger lesions involving hypercontraction and coagulation of contractile proteins throughout entire myocardial cells (Todd, unpublished observations). The majority of stressed animals exhibit these lesions, which Todd regards as catecholamine-induced and corresponding to Baroldi's (1975) coagulative myocytolysis. Baroldi describes the chronic phase of these lesions as involving

> . . . myocytolysis with dissolution of the cells to leave empty sarcolemma spaces. This phase is followed by a mild and diffuse fibrosis. Throughout this process there is little inflammatory cell response, except for a few macrophages and a few fibroblasts.

At least one of these features was found in the hearts of socially stressed mice, and many exhibited two or more. Thus it can be shown that the model of psychosocial stress using mice in population cages induces extensive cardiomyopathy. There is evidence that the accompanying neuroendocrine arousal involving sympathetic adrenal-medullary activation can be associated with arousal of the pituitary adrenal-cortical system (Henry and Stephens, 1977a). Although their roles have not yet been determined, these two systems can be differentiated. For example, animals that retain dominance and control despite challenge display primarily adrenal-medullary and catecholamine arousal. On the other hand, animals that are less dominant but still aggressive experience adrenal-cortical and catecholamine arousal (Ely and Henry 1978; von Holst et al., in press; Sassenrath, in press). Subordinate animals respond predominantly with the adrenal-cortical system only. They can be recognized in a complex population cage by their scarring, lower preputial weight, and by their failure to move out from the subordinate box.

METHODS

We established social groups with equal numbers of mature 4-month-old male and female CBA mice that had been bred in the laboratory and raised as siblings in standard 29 x 18 x 13-cm cages. The animals were fed a commercial diet (Purina Lab Chow) and water *ad libitum*, and their bedding consisted of 5 cm of loose shavings, changed weekly. Stress was induced by placing them in Henry-Stephens complex population cages (Fig. 1). All passageways were so narrow that it was hard for mice to pass each other, forcing repeated confrontations. The multiple entries and exits, the narrow tubes, and the centrally located food and water increased social tension and encouraged the mice to compete vigorously (Henry and Stephens, 1977a). The chronic arousal that ensued could be repeatedly assessed by taking blood samples by orbital puncture. Blood was centrifuged in Natelson pipettes, which provide a hematocrit measure as well as 0.1 ml of plasma. The animals were weighed and scarring was assessed monthly when systolic blood pressure was taken by tail plethysmography without anesthesia. At autopsy the adrenals

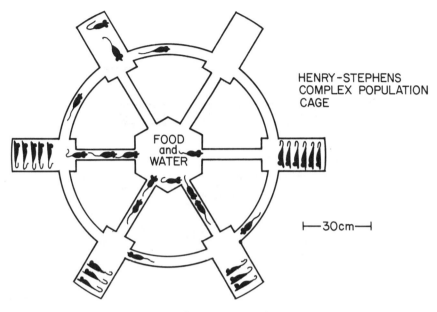

HENRY-STEPHENS
COMPLEX POPULATION
CAGE

FOOD
and
WATER

├──30cm──┤

Fig. 1.　Intercommunicating Henry-Stephens complex population cage used to induce social interaction in mice.　The lucite cages, a standard vivarium shoebox-size of 29 x 18 x 13 cm, are connected into a circle by flexible plastic tubes of 3.8 cm I.D.　The central hexagon holds food and water and is connected to each cage by short tubes of 3.2. cm I.D.　(Henry and Stephens, 1977a.)

were cleaned of fat and weighed to 0.1 mg, while the hearts were weighed to the nearest milligram.　Sibling control animals were maintained 6 to 8 in a cage, and the entire group, both control and stressed animals, were evaluated at autopsy after 6 to 9 months of chronic arousal.

RESULTS

The intense and sustained neuroendocrine stimulation in these socially disordered colonies resulted in a rise in systemic arterial pressure, which could be controlled by a beta blocker such as Metoprolol (Fig. 2) (Henry and Stephens, in press).　The accompanying rise in renin was also controlled by beta blockade, so the combination of catecholamine and renin angiotensin arousal seemed responsible for the chronic hypertension.　Despite the effective beta blockade, when the angiotensin I to II transformation-inhibitor Captopril (SQ 14225) was given to these colonies of mice in the early stages, there was no reduction of arterial pressure.　This indicates that in the early stages hypertension was primarily due to raised catecholamine levels (Fig. 3) (Henry et al., 1979).　After a month or so the mice became sensitive to Captopril, suggesting that renin played a part in the

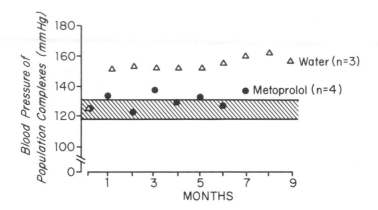

Fig. 2. Mean monthly blood pressure observations of four mouse colonies on 120 mg Metoprolol/kg contrasted with that of three control colonies on water. All were housed in Henry-Stephens complex population cages.

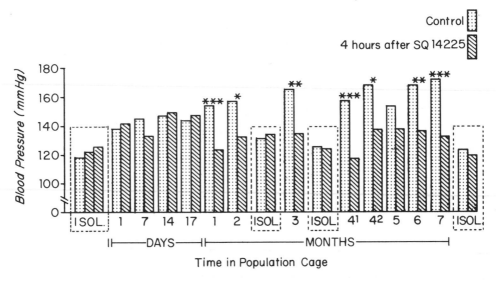

Fig. 3. When exposure to social stress extends beyond one month, the angiotensin enzyme inhibitor Captopril (SQ14225) effectively reduces the blood pressure of male mice exposed to chronic social stress in complex population cages. This reduction persists for at least 4 hr. Controls living in isolation, hence not socially stressed, show no change in blood pressure, regardless of age (Henry et al., 1979).

later stages. After six months of social interaction, heart weights increased uniformly (Fig. 4) (Henry et al., 1975), and histological analysis showed a marked increase of myocardial fibrosis (Fig. 5).

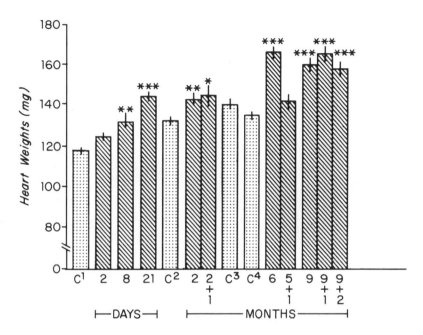

Fig. 4. Average heart weights of male mice in a series of colonies exposed to increasing durations of social stimulation. Dotted columns represent mean heart weight of each colony under study. Hatched columns represent weights of control groups of appropriate age. The significance of the differences between the appropriately aged controls and the various experimental groups was determined by paired Student's t-tests. ** = p<0.01 and *** = p<0.001.

The level of plasma corticosterone was more elevated in the later stages, when the colonies were aging, than during the first weeks (Fig. 6) (Henry and Stephens, 1977b). Thus, after six months, in addition to elevated catecholamines and catecholamine synthesis, these chronically stressed animals also experienced pituitary adrenal-cortical activation. The pathophysiological consequences of the arousal of both the adrenal-medullary and adrenal-cortical systems combined, as opposed to alone, remain to be determined.

DISCUSSION

Catecholamines and Cardiomyopathy

The work of other investigators supports the proposal that although cardiomyopathy is closely related to activation of the sympathetic adrenal-medullary system, adrenal-cortical activation may also play a part.

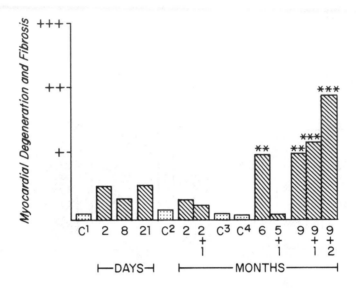

Fig. 5. Incidence of cardiomyopathy and myocardial fibrosis in males of 10 socially disordered colonies of mice. For details see legend to Fig. 4 and Henry and Stephens (1977a). Ordinate: + scattered fibrous tissue between muscle bundles, ++ small scattered patches throughout the myocardium, +++ confluent lesions forming a patchwork of microinfarcts extending a considerable distance in the ventricular wall.

In a recent paper, Tanaka et al. (1980) compared the cardiac lesions induced in rats by isoproterenol with those resulting from the repeated stress of restraint and water immersion. They studied this potent beta agonist with special reference to the etiology of cardiomyopathy, and found myocardial hypertrophy, degeneration, and necrosis replaced by interstitial fibrosis in both sets of animals. They concluded that isoproterenol-induced cardiac lesions can be regarded as analogous to those of stress-induced cardiomyopathy. Also the endogeneously induced beta adrenergic response, produced by 5 hr of restraint and water immersion each day for 30 days, led to cardiac lesions similar to those induced by the drug.

It may be significant that catecholamine-induced arrhythmia can be potentiated by corticoid pretreatment and that the effect of catecholamines cannot be considered alone. If this is so, then a feeling of helplessness in which the pituitary adrenal-cortical axis is strongly stimulated may be more likely to induce cardiac damage than one in which arousal is restricted to the fight-flight response and the sympathetic adrenal-medullary system alone (Guideri et al., 1974).

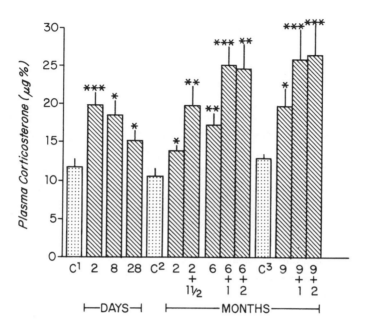

Fig. 6. Plasma corticosterone levels of all males in 11 socially disordered mouse colonies. The general design is the same as described for Fig. 4. There is a trend toward higher values in the older colonies, and the return to isolation is accompanied by even higher values, suggesting that isolation further stimulated the adrenal responses of mice that have experienced a social environment, even a disturbed one.

In their work on the porcine stress syndrome, Johansson and Jonsson (1977) observed that restraint stress induced acute myopathy that involved myofibrillar disintegration and other changes similar to those found in the administration of catecholamines.

In a series of studies on the effects of mental stress on cardiomyopathy, G. Johansson (unpublished observations) found that myofibrillar damage resulting from activation of the fight-flight response in the frightened, immobilized pig was successfully prevented by amygdalectomy. In addition, pulse rate was slower and arrhythmias no longer occurred, suggesting a reduction in catecholamine levels.

Emotionally Arousing States and Cardiomyopathy

Situations in which the individual lacks control and perceives an intense threat are associated with neuroendocrine arousal and cardiomyopathy. Thus, Connor (1969) described the classic focal myocytolysis in a series of victims of spontaneous intracranial hemorrhage. The cause was usually rupture of an aneurysm and it frequently occurred in persons with hypertension. As de Champlain et al. (1981) point out, an important proportion of patients with hypertension have increased sympathoadrenal tone.

In a series of observations on the effects of threatening noises on helpless, wild rats, Raab et al. (1964) found myocardial necrosis in nearly 70 percent of the animals. They suggested that the accompanying adrenal-cortical hypertrophy, due to caging and isolation, may have increased the sensitivity of these rats to cardiotoxic effects of catecholamines.

Spontaneous cardiomyopathy similar to that seen with isoproterenol has been observed in wild baboons exposed to capture, isolation, and surgery (Weber et al., 1973). The adrenals were grossly enlarged, very possibly due to stress. In a follow-up study of social conflict resulting from the intermittent crowding of rabbits, Weber and Van der Walt (1975) showed myocytolysis and eventual myocardial fibrosis in a high percentage of survivors. They concluded that the aggression with fighting and biting, triggered by crowding, may have played a role in cardiomyopathy.

Brain Mechanisms and Cardiomyopathy

Recent observations have established that some of the many descending hypo-thalamo-autonomic pathways pass directly to the preganglionic nuclei of the sympathetic and parasympathetic systems (Saper et al., 1976). In addition, there are direct projections from the nucleus of the solitary tract up to the hypothalamus, amygdala, and other limbic forebrain structures (Ricardo and Koh, 1978). Stock et al. (1978) directly stimulated the basal area of the amygdala to show that a defense or fear response was elicited and that stimulation of the central nucleus aroused fight, and found that typical epinephrine and norepinephrine responses of the peripheral vascular bed were involved. As previously mentioned, Johansson and Jonsson (1977) reported that amygdalectomy interrupts the mediation of the response to threatening immobilization in the pig. They found evidence of diminished catecholamine release and cessation of cardiomyopathy.

The orbital cortex of the frontal lobes has been related to the previously mentioned amygdalar responses. In recent work, Skinner and Reed (1981) showed that cooling of the forebrain, or the posterior hypothalamus, or the fields of Forel of the brain stem will prevent arrhythmias that would otherwise develop after acute coronary occlusion. They cited Johansson's work with immobilization stress and suggested that a central neural projection to the heart must be intact for myocardial ischemia to precipitate lethal arrhythmias. They pointed out that posterior hypothalamic stimulation also induces cardiomyopathy. Melville et al. (1969) suggested that the cardiac damage they occasionally observed after lateral hypothalamic stimulation in the rhesus macaque may relate to the release of catecholamines.

SUMMARY

There is strong evidence linking the development of cardiomyopathy to repeated cognitively mediated arousal of the sympathetic adrenal-medullary system. The possibility exists that pituitary adrenal-cortical mechanisms act in synergism with the catecholamines, increasing the cardiac damage in the later stages of chronic social stimulation.

ACKNOWLEDGMENT

This work was supported by grant HL 25544 from the National Institutes of Health.

REFERENCES

Baroldi, G. (1975) Different types of myocardial necrosis in coronary heart disease: a pathophysiologic review of their functional significance. Amer. Heart J. 89, 742-752.

Champlain, J. de, Cousineau, D., Lapointe, L., Lavallee, M., Nadeau, R. and Denis, G. (1981) Sympathetic abnormalities in human hypertension. Clin. Exp. Hyperten. 3, 417-438.

Connor, R.C.R. (1969) Focal myocytolysis and fuchsinophilic degeneration of the myocardium of patients dying with various brain lesions. Ann. N.Y. Acad. Sci. 156, 261-269.

Ely, D.L. and Henry, J.P. (1978) Neuroendocrine response patterns in dominant and subordinate mice. Horm. Behav. 10, 156-169.

Guideri, G., Barletta, M.A. and Lehr, D. (1974) Extraordinary potentiation of isoproterenol cardiotoxicity by corticoid pretreatment. Cardiovasc. Res. 8, 775-786.

Henry, J.P., Ely, D.L., Stephens, P.M., Ratcliffe, H.L., Santisteban, G.A. and Shapiro, A.J. (1971) The role of psychosocial factors in the development of arteriosclerosis in CBA mice. Observations on the heart, kidney, and aorta. Atherosclerosis 14, 203-218.

Henry, J.P. and Stephens, P.M. (1977a) Stress, Health, and the Social Environment: A Sociobiologic Approach to Medicine. Springer-Verlag, New York.

Henry, J.P. and Stephens, P.M. (1977b) The social environment and essential hypertension in mice: possible role of the innervation of the adrenal cortex. Progr. Brain Res. 47, 263-276.

Henry, J.P. and Stephens, P.M. (in press) Psychosocial stress induces tubulointerstitial nephritis unrelated to hypertension in CBA mice. Clin. Exp. Pharmacol. Physiol.

Henry, J.P., Stephens, P.M. and Santisteban, G.A. (1975) A model of psychosocial hypertension showing reversibiity and progression of cardiovascular complications. Circulat. Res. 36, 156-164.

Henry, J.P., Vander, A.J. and Stephens, P.M. (1979) Effects of an angiotensin converting enzyme inhibitor on psychosocial hypertension in mice. Clin. Sci. Mol. Med. 57, 153-155.

Johansson, G. and Jonsson, L. (1977) Myocardial cell damage in the porcine stress syndrome. J. Comp. Pathol. 87, 67-74.

Melville, K.I., Garvey, H.L., Shister, H.E. and Knaack, J. (1969) Central nervous system stimulation and cardiac ischemic changes in monkeys. Ann. N.Y. Acad. Sci. 156, 241-260.

Raab, W., Chaplin, J.P. and Bajusz, E. (1964) Myocardial necroses produced in domesticated rats and in wild rats by sensory and emotional stresses. Proc. Soc. Exp. Biol. Med. 116, 665-669.

Ricardo, J.A. and Koh, E.T. (1978) Anatomical evidence of direct projections from the nucleus of the solitary tract to the hypothalamus, amygdala, and other forebrain structures in the rat. Brain Res. 153, 1-26.

Saper, C.B., Loewy, A.D., Swanson, L.W. and Cowan, W.M. (1976) Direct hypothalamo-autonomic connections. Brain Res. 117, 305-312.

Sassenrath, E.N. (in press) Studies in adaptability: experiential, environmental, and pharmacological influences; in Hormones, Drugs, and Social Behavior, A. Kling and H.D. Steklis, eds. Spectrum Publications, New York.

Skinner, J.E. and Reed, J.C. (1981) Blockade of frontocortical-brain stem pathway prevents ventricular fibrillation of ischemic heart. Amer. J. Physiol. 240, H156-H163.

Stock, G., Schlör, K.H., Heidt, H. and Buss, J. (1978) Psychomotor behaviour and cardiovascular patterns during stimulation of the amygdala. Pflügers Arch. 376, 177-184.

Tanaka, M., Tsuchihashi, Y., Katsume, H., Ijichi, H. and Ibata, Y. (1980) Comparison of cardiac lesions induced in rats by isoproterenol and by repeated stress of restraint and water immersion with special reference to etiology of cardiomyopathy. Jap. Circulat. J. 44, 971-980.

Vander, A.J., Henry, J.P., Stephens, P.M., Kay, L.L. and Mouw, D.R. (1978) Plasma renin activity in psychosocial hypertension of CBA mice. Circulat. Res. 42, 496-502.

von Holst, D., Fuchs, E. and Stöhr, W. (in press) Physiological changes in male *Tupaia belangeri* under different types of social stress. J. Behav. Med.

Weber, H.W. and Van der Walt, J.J. (1975) Cardiomyopathy in crowded rabbits; in Recent Advances in Studies on Cardiac Structure and Metabolism, Vol. 6, Pathophysiology and Morphology of Myocardial Cell Alteration, A. Fleckenstein and G. Rona eds. University Park Press, Baltimore, pp. 471-477.

Weber, H.W., Van der Walt, J.J. and Greeff, M. (1973) Spontaneous cardiomyopathies in Chacma baboons; in Recent Advances in Studies on Cardiac Structure and Metabolism, Vol. 2, Cardiomyopathies, E. Bajusz and G. Rona, eds. University Park Press, Baltimore, pp. 361-375.

Copyright 1982 by Elsevier Science Publishing Co.,Inc.
Smith, Galosy, and Weiss, editors
CIRCULATION, NEUROBIOLOGY, AND BEHAVIOR

Neurobiology of the Periventricular Tissue Surrounding the Anteroventral Third Ventricle (AV3V) and its Role in Behavior, Fluid Balance, and Cardiovascular Control

ALAN KIM JOHNSON
Department of Psychology and the Cardiovascular Center, University of Iowa, Iowa City, Iowa

INTRODUCTION

Behavioral, hormonal, and cardiovascular (CV) mechanisms function to maintain overall fluid balance as well as regulate distribution of salt and water within the body. These effector systems are controlled by the central nervous system (CNS). In this review of the work in our laboratory, we will (1) describe some of the major effects of lesions of the tissue surrounding the anteroventral third ventricle (AV3V), (2) present some recent findings on the neurobiology of the AV3V region to enhance our understanding of its role, (3) discuss the advantages of the combined study of behavioral and physiological systems that are biologically consistent in their function, and (4) provide a working hypothesis, derived from functional and neuroanatomical studies, on the role of the AV3V in body fluid homeostasis.

BACKGROUND

As depicted in Figure 1, the CNS receives and integrates humoral and neural information reflecting the moment-to-moment hydrational status of the body. Depending on the prevailing conditions, the appropriate effector systems are activated to correct deficits and to retain and optimize the distribution of existing fluid resources. The elucidation of how the brain is informed of derangements in fluid homeostasis, of how such information is processed by the CNS, and of how behavioral, hormonal, and circulatory responses are effected represents a major challenge to scientists fascinated by problems of neural control.

Our studies implicating the AV3V and body fluid homeostasis began with a search for a site of action that would account for the dipsogenic effect of angiotensin II (A II). In early work, we found that intracranially injected A II was most effective in producing thirst when the peptide gained access to the cerebral ventricles (Johnson and Epstein, 1975). We therefore proposed a periventricular site of action for the thirst induced by angiotensin borne via the cerebrospinal fluid (CSF).

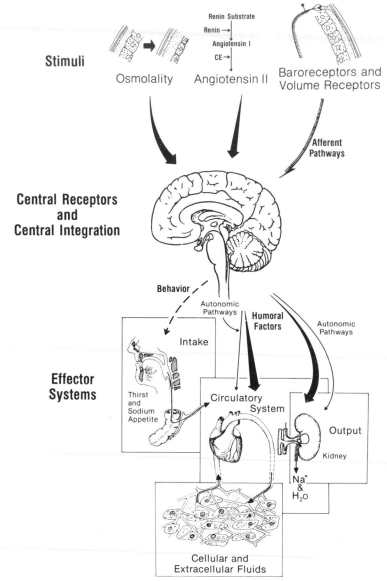

Stimuli

Renin Substrate
Renin →
Angiotensin I
CE →

Osmolality   Angiotensin II   Baroreceptors and
Volume Receptors

Afferent
Pathways

**Central Receptors
and
Central Integration**

Behavior
Autonomic
Pathways   **Humoral
Factors**   Autonomic
Pathways

Intake

**Effector
Systems**

Thirst
and
Sodium
Appetite

Circulatory
System

Output

Kidney

Na⁺
&
H₂O

Cellular and
Extracellular Fluids

Fig. 1. A representation of the major intrinsic stimuli that "inform" the brain of the hydrational and circulatory status of the organism, the site of reception and integration of this information (i.e., the CNS), and the primary effector systems involved in the control of body fluid homeostasis. The control of overall body fluid balance largely depends on water and salt ingestion and excretion by the kidneys. Central systems serve as the neural substrate for thirst and sodium appetite. The excretion of water and salt is largely controlled by the CNS through its influence on the release of antidiuretic hormone and possibly natriuretic hormone. On the background of fluid balance, central systems control CV responses to provide optimal perfusion of body tissues.

Based on the findings of Buggy and colleagues that the periventricular site of action for the dipsogenic response is located in the rostroventral portion of the third ventricle (Buggy, 1974; Buggy et al., 1975; Buggy and Fisher, 1976), we initiated ablation studies to determine whether a more precise determination of the critical periventricular region could be made. To our initial surprise, rats with lesions of the tissue in the most anterior portion of the AV3V virtually ceased water intake (Fig. 2), even though they seemed behaviorally vigorous in other ways (Buggy and Johnson, 1977a,b; Johnson and Buggy, 1977, 1978). The majority of the animals remained adipsic, became moribund, and died of dehydration within a few days.

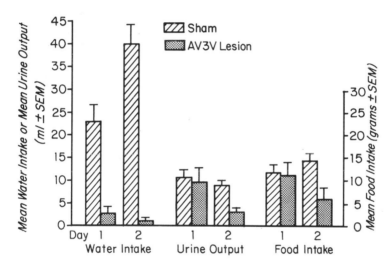

Fig. 2. Food and water intake and urine volume for rats with sham lesions (n = 7) and with AV3V lesions (n = 7) on the first and second days after surgery. (From Buggy and Johnson, 1977a, with permission.)

Histological examination revealed that these rats had sustained damage to the periventricular tissue of the optic recess between the anterior commissure and the optic chiasm. Always included in the lesion were the organum vasculosum of the lamina terminalis, the median preoptic nucleus, and the preoptic-anterior hypothalamic periventricular nuclei. The medial preoptic and anterior hypothalamic nuclei sustained little damage beyond their medial border with the periventricular nuclei.

Because the lesion was not restricted to a single anatomical structure, we decided it would be most appropriate to describe it on the basis of its location in the brain, that is, the AV3V region. Although the lesion is relatively small, destroying only about 1.0 to

1.5 mg of tissue, it destroys several neural structures in this tiny region that are essential for the maintenance of normal body fluid homeostasis.

ACUTE EFFECTS OF AV3V LESIONS
Thirst

The most profound effect of ablation of AV3V periventricular tissue is the immediate and absolute cessation of water intake. This result is all the more remarkable when one sees that the animals exhibit no outstanding behavioral side effects. They show normal neurological signs (e.g., righting reflexes), respond to handling, and continue consuming amounts of food comparable to those consumed by rats deprived of water (Johnson and Buggy, 1977, 1978). The failure to drink water is not due to altered oral motor patterns; animals readily lick and consume large quantities of palatable solutions (saccharin or sucrose) or liquid diet. During this period of acute adipsia, treatments that normally elicit drinking (e.g., systemic injections of hypertonic saline or A II, or hypovolemia produced by polyethylene glycol) have no effect on animals with lesions. Furthermore, the nonregulatory drinking response of schedule-induced polydipsia is attenuated following AV3V lesions (Lind and Johnson, 1978). A rat that has just sustained an AV3V lesion has all the appearances of a normal, intact animal that has been overhydrated and whose further drinking is inhibited by satiety mechanisms.

Vasopressin

The initial studies on rats with AV3V lesions indicated that body weight declined precipitately during the acute postlesion period (Johnson and Buggy, 1978). This weight loss was more severe than that shown by animals deprived of water. These observations suggested that rats with AV3V lesions may have difficulty retaining and concentrating urine because of an impairment in vasopressin release, and subsequent studies showed this indeed to be the case (Johnson et al., 1980a, b). In the face of very severe dehydration (as indicated by an increase in plasma osmolality, plasma sodium concentration, and hematocrit), rats with AV3V lesions do not show an increase in circulating vasopressin. As was the case for drinking during this acute postlesion period, vasopressin cannot be released by even more intense stimuli. For example, intracranial injection of A II is ineffective in rats with lesions, whereas in normal rats it produces an immediate secretion of vasopressin (Bealer et al., 1979b).

The supraoptic nuclei and the posterior pituitary of rats showing postlesion adipsia have been studied with electron microscopy. In contrast to normal rats, which manifest morphological evidence of increased biosynthesis of vasopressin and related precursors, rats with AV3V lesions show no such effects (Carithers et al., 1980). The posterior lobes of affected rats contain an accumulation of secretory material that is not being released from this structure (Carithers et al., 1981). Thus, the acute failure of these rats to release vasopressin is not due to a lack of the peptide in the hypothalamo-hypophyseal system, but apparently is due to the failure of hydration-related stimuli to activate the magnocellular neurons.

CHRONIC EFFECTS OF AV3V LESIONS

As would gladden the heart of any biopsychologist, we especially took note when an animal with an AV3V lesion "spontaneously" recovered water intake after a few days of complete adipsia. Teitelbaum's classic work with Stellar (1954) and Epstein (1962) demonstrated that the terminally adipsic and aphagic rats with lateral hypothalamic lesions would recover if fed and hydrated for a sufficiently long period. We reasoned that it may be possible to enhance survival and promote recovery of water intake by hydrating the rats with AV3V lesions during the postsurgical period. By intubating the animals with water, we could prevent many of them from dying of dehydration. Better yet, the animals did not manifest postlesion motor impairments, and so would hydrate themselves when provided with sweet solutions. They could eventually be "weaned" from sweet solutions to water by having the concentration of sugar or saccharin reduced through successive steps. By 7 to 10 days postlesion, most rats will maintain themselves on water and have average daily water intakes comparable to those of rats with sham lesions. Thus, the rat with a chronic AV3V lesion needs little special attention or maintenance, and can be studied to determine what physiological compromises result from the lesion.

Thirst

Although rats with AV3V lesions can achieve a restored daily fluid intake, they evidence a severely impaired response to all thirst challenges that induce or simulate perturbations in body fluid balance (Table 1). In addition, rats with chronic AV3V lesions show motivational deficits under conditions assessing their drive to acquire water.

We have trained water-deprived rats to press a lever for water on a variable interval schedule in which response rate is an index of motivation (Teitelbaum, 1966). Rats were tested before surgery as well as several weeks after they had recovered from the acute effects of AV3V lesions. As indicated in Figure 3, rats with AV3V and sham lesions consumed comparable amounts of water in a 2-hr free-access drinking test. However, when required to work for water by bar pressing, the rats with AV3V lesions showed a significantly lower response rate (Thunhorst and Johnson, unpublished observations). In other experiments using a nondiscriminated avoidance paradigm, we found that rats with AV3V lesions will lever press to avoid electric foot shock. Therefore, these animals' reduced response rate when responding for water is not due to a nonspecific disruptive effect on lever pressing. In another test of the thirst motivational state, we studied the

TABLE 1

CHRONIC EFFECTS OF AV3V LESIONS ON EXPERIMENTAL THIRST

Challenge	Response
Water deprivation	Attenuated[1]
Cellular thirst	Abolished[1]
Extracellular thirst	
Hormonal	
Angiotensin II	Abolished[1,2]
Hormonal and hypotensive	
Isoproterenol	Attenuated[3]
Caval ligation	Attenuated[4]
Hormonal and hypovolemic	
Polyethylene glycol	Attenuated[5]

[1]Buggy and Johnson, 1977
[2]Buggy and Johnson, 1978
[3]Lind and Johnson, 1981
[4]Shrager and Johnson, 1979
[5]Lind and Johnson, 1982

acceptance of quinine-adulterated water in rats with AV3V and sham lesions (Bealer and Johnson, 1979). The animals with AV3V lesions drank relatively less of each concentration of quinine than did those with sham lesions.

Although, as a group, rats with AV3V lesions show daily intakes at least comparable to those of intact animals, the 24-hr free-access intakes of individual animals over days are highly variable (Lind and Johnson, unpublished results). This variability in drinking is also apparent when the pattern of food and water intake is studied. Although rats with AV3V lesions continue to drink in close temporal proximity with a meal, the correlation between volume drunk and amount of food eaten (relative to that of a normal animal) is abolished (Bealer and Johnson, 1980). Although rats with AV3V lesions apparently can maintain body fluid balance over the long term, they lack the capacity to use thirst mechanisms to achieve fine regulation.

Vasopressin

In the chronic phase, rats with AV3V lesions seem to regain an antidiuretic response because they will reduce urine volume and concentrate urine following water deprivation. However, when they are tested with either intracranial injections of A II (Johnson et al.,

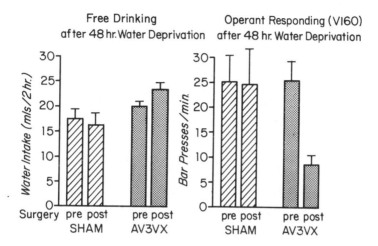

Fig. 3. Water intake in a free-access test and operant response rates for water following 48 hr of water deprivation in rats with sham lesions (n = 4) and AV3V lesions (n = 7). All animals were tested pre- and postsurgery in both the free-access and operant situations. The order of testing was randomized. Although rats with AV3V lesions readily drank in the free-access test, their response rates were significantly lower in the operant test. (Thunhorst and Johnson, unpublished results.)

1978) or systemic hypertonic saline (Johnson et al., 1980a), they show impaired anti-diuretic responses. On the other hand, if extracellular fluid volume is depleted by using subcutaneous polyethylene glycol, vasopressin release can be induced and is comparable to that seen for intact animals (Johnson et al., 1980a). Because extracellular depletion activates not only the renin-angiotensin system but also volume and/or baroreceptor mechanisms, it seems that the latter afferent systems function to mediate the control of vasopressin release in animals with chronic lesions.

Natriuretic Factor

When normal, intact rats are infused with a hypotonic hydrating solution, they show a brisk diuresis and natriuresis; however, when rats with AV3V lesions are treated identically, they exhibit attenuated diuretic and natriuretic responses (Johnson et al., 1978; Bealer et al., 1979a). Recent observations suggest that rats with AV3V lesions are unable to release a natriuretic factor upon volume expansion, which may account for the natriuretic impairment (Bealer et al., 1979a).

Effects on Overall Fluid Balance

One of the manifestations of the AV3V lesion is chronic hypernatremia (Buggy and Johnson, 1977b). Blood samples collected even several months postlesion consistently indicate increased plasma sodium concentration and osmolality. It is of considerable interest that the AV3V preparation parallels almost exactly the frequently reported clinical syndrome of essential hypernatremia (Table 2). Although most of the clinical reports describe the patients as having widespread neurological damage, a commonly affected area seems to be the periventricular zone around the optic recess (Kastin et al., 1965; Lascelles and Lewis, 1972; Skulety and Joynt, 1963; Sridhar et al., 1974).

Our experiments initially began because of an interest in drinking behavior; from this perspective, it is particularly fascinating to note that these patients are uniformly described as having a reduction if not complete absence of the urge to drink. Also, it is especially significant that for the manifestation of essential hypernatremia, impairments in both thirst and antidiuretic mechanisms must exist. A disruption in drinking alone or vasopressin alone will not produce hypernatremia (Ross and Christie, 1969).

TABLE 2

PARALLELS BETWEEN PATIENTS WITH ESSENTIAL HYPERNATREMIA AND RATS WITH AV3V LESIONS

	Patients with essential hypernatremia	Rats with AV3V lesions
Hypothalamic damage	Yes[1]	Yes[2]
Chronically elevated serum sodium	Yes[1]	Yes[2]
Chronically elevated serum osmolarity	Yes[1]	Yes[2]
Reduced or absent thirst	Yes[1]	Yes[2]
Impaired antidiuretic response	Yes[1]	Yes[3]
Elevated plasma renin	Yes[4]	Yes[5]
Reduced pressor response to systemic A II	Yes[6]	Yes[7]
Reduced blood volume	No[1]	No[8]

[1]Ross and Christie, 1969
[2]Buggy and Johnson, 1977b
[3]Johnson et al., 1980b
[4]Wolf et al., 1973
[5]Shrager and Johnson, 1980
[6]Hsieh et al., 1980
[7]Buggy et al., 1977
[8]Unpublished observations

EFFECTS OF AV3V LESIONS ON EXPERIMENTAL HYPERTENSION

Reports from several laboratories (Sweet et al., 1976; Ganten et al., 1976; Phillips and Hoffman, 1977) made it reasonable to hypothesize that the central action of A II was a critical link in the sequence of events leading to some forms of hypertension. If A II did play such a role, it might exert its hypertensive influence through the same target region where it seemed to exert its dipsogenic action, that is, within the AV3V. Working in M.J. Brody's laboratory, we tested this idea by studying the effects of AV3V lesions on experimental hypertension. The first form of hypertension we examined was the one-kidney Grollman model (unilateral nephrectomy plus figure eight ligature). Animals that had previously sustained AV3V lesions were "protected" against the elevated blood pressure produced by this procedure (Buggy et al., 1977). The increased water intake normally associated with this form of renal hypertension was also abolished by the lesion. However, Grollman renal hypertension was not due to increased fluid intake, for when water was restricted to presurgical levels (35 ml/day), the arterial pressure rose to the same level as that of animals with unrestricted access to water.

Since this initial demonstration of the protective effects of AV3V lesions on Grollman renal hypertension, our laboratories extended the evaluation of the effects of this lesion on the development and maintenance of hypertension to several different experimental models (Table 3). The efficacy of AV3V lesions in preventing hypertension was much greater than we had initially envisioned. Two important points related to AV3V lesions and hypertension can be derived from these studies. First, the protective effects of the AV3V lesions must involve mechanisms other than or in addition to disruption of a central action of angiotensin. This is apparent because the lesion is effective in abolishing or aborting not only renin-dependent hypertension but also non-renin-dependent forms such as DOC-salt hypertension (desoxycorticosterone pivalate and saline drinking water) in which the renin-angiotensin system is suppressed. Second, although the AV3V lesion is effective on most forms of experimental hypertension, it is not effective in preventing or reversing the form of genetic hypertension in the spontaneously hyper-tensive rat (SHR) (Buggy et al., 1978; Gordon et al., 1979, in press). Thus, the antihypertensive effects of AV3V lesions are specific in that most but not all forms of high blood pressure are affected by the lesion.

The protective effects of AV3V lesions on experimental hypertension have given rise to several lines of research. Much of this work and its consequences in terms of enhancing our understanding of the neural control of the circulation have been described elsewhere (Brody et al., 1978a, b; Brody and Johnson, 1980, 1981).

STUDIES ON THE NEUROBIOLOGY OF THE AV3V REGION

There are several likely reasons why the AV3V lesion could produce such global effects on body fluid balance and CV function. First, the AV3V region may be a target tissue for circulating humoral factors that mobilize thirst, hormone release from the pituitary, and CV adjustments. Second, the lesion may interrupt fibers that originate from other structures and merely pass through the AV3V enroute to other regions. Third, the AV3V region may act as a focal site receiving afferent information, which is

TABLE 3

EFFECTS OF AV3V LESIONS ON EXPERIMENTAL HYPERTENSION

Model	Prevents or attenuates	Reversed
1 kidney, 1 wrap Grollman hypertension	Yes[1]	Yes (water restricted)[2] No (free access conditions)
2 kidneys, 1 clip Goldblatt hypertension	Yes[3]	Yes[3]
Aortic ligation between the renal arteries	Yes[4]	--
Sinoaortic denervation	Yes[5]	--
Lesions of the nucleus of the solitary tract	Yes[5]	--
DOC-salt hypertension	Yes[6]	--
Dahl S strain rats	Yes[7]	--
Spontaneously hypertensive rats	No*[8]	No[2]
Spontaneously hypertensive, stroke-prone rats	No*[9]	--

*Lesion placed at 4 weeks of age.

[1]Buggy et al., 1977   [4]Hartle et al., 1979   [7]Brody and Johnson, 1980
[2]Buggy et al., 1978   [5]Mow et al., 1978   [8]Gordon et al., in press
[3]Haywood et al., 1978   [6]Fink et al., 1977   [9]Gordon et al., 1979

integrated and relayed to other areas of the nervous system. These three hypotheses are not mutually exclusive, and, given the widespread nature of the effects of the AV3V lesion, more than one of them may be correct. Clearly, our understanding of the function of the AV3V region and of the phenomena associated with AV3V lesions will be enhanced by our understanding of the anatomical organization of this region.

Functional Fractionation of Critical Tissues Within the AV3V Region

While characterizing the physiological effects of AV3V lesions in our earlier experiments, we observed that when the placement or size of the AV3V lesion was varied, the constellation of characteristics associated with the "typical" AV3V lesion could be dissociated from one another. For example, two animals with similar but not identical lesions within the AV3V region might display differences in their response to dipsogenic thirst challenges. In an early report, we described several animals that had drinking deficits to A II but not to hypertonic saline (Buggy and Johnson, 1977b). Such observations emphasized the need to learn much more about the neuroanatomy of the AV3V region in order to substantiate a more precise correlation of structure with function.

By careful reconstruction of lesions and with the aid of lesion overlap analyses, we can describe more fully the tissues within the AV3V that are responsible for specific response deficits. For example, the results of one lesion overlap analysis for drinking deficits to hypertonic saline and to A II are presented in Figure 4 (Lind et al., 1979). Shown is a profile in the midsagittal plane of the area of damage for 12 rats that failed to respond to systemic hypertonic saline and for six rats that failed to respond to A II.

MIDSAGITTAL VIEW OF AN INTACT BRAIN

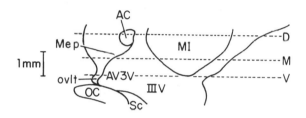

COMMON LESION PROFILE FROM RATS REFRACTORY TO:

HYPERTONIC SALINE   ANGIOTENSIN II

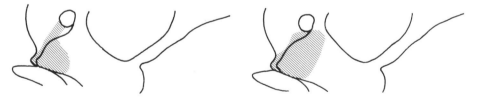

Fig. 4. Above: a midsagittal view of an intact rat brain depicting the AV3V region and major surrounding regions and structures. Also depicted are three planes, dorsal (D), medial (M) and ventral (V), from which horizontal sections were taken for assessment of critical damage. Below: profiles of the area of common overlap (diagonal lines) of lesions in rats in which water intake could not be elicited by a hypertonic saline thirst challenge (left, n = 12) or angiotensin II (right, n = 6). Animals with comparable damage at the ventral level of the lesion but little or no damage at the medial and dorsal levels responded normally to these thirst challenges. Thus, the median preoptic nucleus damage must be critical for the thirst deficits to the challenges studied here (Lind et al., 1979). MI, mass intermedia of the thalamus; AC, anterior commissure; Me p, median preoptic; ovlt, organum vasculosum of the lamina terminalis; OC, optic chiasm; Sc, supra chiasmatic nucleus of the anterior hypothalamus; III V, third ventricle; AV3V, anteroventral third ventricle.

Although a portion of the lesion profile is common to both types of response deficiencies, a distinct region close to the anterior commissure is differentially associated with the two deficits. The results of this analysis support the functional specificity of regions within the AV3V, and have been extended to other response characteristics associated with AV3V lesions.

The AV3V Region as a Target Tissue for the Action of Humoral Substances

Thirst. The experiments by Buggy and colleagues (Buggy, 1974; Buggy et al., 1975; Buggy and Fisher, 1976) demonstrated that CSF-borne A II must have access to the periventricular tissue of the AV3V region in order to be dipsogenic. Similarly, Hoffman and Phillips (1976) demonstrated that angiotensin injected into the lateral ventricles must reach the AV3V to induce a pressor response. For the drinking response to A II, there must be separate sites of action for blood-borne and CSF-borne angiotensin. It is possible, by plugging the AV3V region, to dissociate drinking responses to systemically or intraventricularly applied A II (Buggy and Johnson, 1978). Blood-borne A II still induces thirst after AV3V plugging, but CSF-borne A II does not. Other lesions also make it possible to dissociate the drinking responses to systemic and centrally delivered A II. Ablation of the subfornical organ (SFO) prevents the drinking response to blood-borne A II, but, provided there is access to the AV3V region, drinking to central A II remains intact (Thunhorst et al., 1981). Current data suggest that blood-borne A II acts on the SFO to induce drinking behavior (Simpson et al., 1978) and that CSF-borne A II acts within the AV3V (see Lind and Johnson, 1982, for a review of this problem).

Vasopressin release. As pointed out previously, one of the problems with using lesion techniques in the search for receptors or target tissues is that the lesion may be interrupting fibers of passage. One way to reduce the probability that one is dealing with fibers of passage is to eliminate other regions that are likely to function as target tissues and restrict the analysis to a smaller region.

We recently did some experiments with Celia D. Sladek, who for several years has used a hypothalamic explant preparation that allows her to study the effects of several types of humoral stimuli and their ability to release vasopressin. The explant preparation contains the posterior lobe of the pituitary connected to the basal hypothalamus, which includes the supraoptic nuclei and the ventral portion of the AV3V region. We found that explants from rats with AV3V lesions did not release vasopressin to a hyperosmotic stimulus that was effective in animals with sham lesions (Johnson and Sladek, 1979). On the other hand, acetylcholine, which presumably induces secretion by direct action on the supraoptic magnocellular neurons, was effective in releasing vasopressin in rats with lesions. These results indicate that the AV3V region may contain osmosensitive units, which may have been destroyed by AV3V lesions.

RELATION OF THE AV3V REGION TO OTHER CENTRAL SYSTEMS INVOLVED IN BODY FLUID BALANCE AND CV CONTROL

Since our initial observations on the effect of AV3V lesions, a greater amount of information has accumulated on the anatomical and functional organization of this region. Summarized in Figure 5 are the results from several laboratories, including our own, that have appeared over the past few years. Much of this information was gleaned by use of the new neuroanatomical tract tracing techniques, employing radioactive labeled amino acids and horseradish peroxidase (HRP), as well as by functional studies using electrical stimulation of the AV3V region.

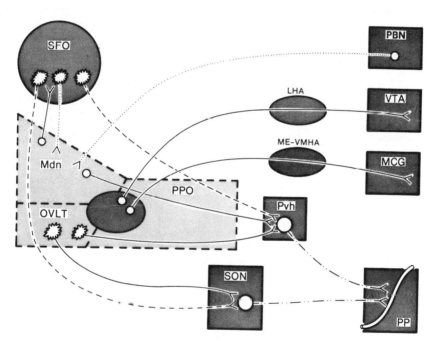

Fig. 5. Afferents, efferents, and fibers of passage associated with the AV3V. The median preoptic (Mdn), the organum vasculosum of the lamina terminalis (OVLT), and the periventricular preoptic (PPO) comprise the major tissue destroyed by the AV3V lesion. The darkened oval within the AV3V depicts the origin of descending projections for which there are functional data but no definitive anatomical evidence. There is good anatomical support for all other projections depicted. The papers from which this summary was constructed are cited in the text. SFO, subfornical organ; SON, supraoptic nucleus; Pvh, paraventricular nucleus; LHA, lateral hypothalamic area; ME-VMHA, median eminence-ventromedial hypothalamic area; PBN, parabrachial nucleus; VTA, ventral tegmental area; MCG, mesencephalic central gray; PP, posterior pituitary.

Two major sources of afferent input into the AV3V arrive from the SFO (Miselis et al., 1979; Miselis, 1980; Grazi and Miselis, 1980; Lind et al., 1981) and from the parabrachial nucleus in the pons (Saper and Loewy, 1980). Currently, excellent evidence supports the observation that the SFO acts as a central target for circulating angiotensin (Simpson et al., 1978). Projections to the nucleus medianus from the parabrachial nucleus may carry pressure/volume information since the parabrachial nucleus receives projections from the nucleus of the solitary tract. There is good anatomical evidence that AV3V efferents project to the supraoptic and paraventricular nuclei (Miselis et al., 1979; Silverman et al., 1981). These projections may influence the secretion of vasopressin. Studies using injections of labeled amino acid into the medial preoptic nuclei and the medial preoptic-periventricular preoptic region describe a medial projection to the mesencephalic central gray and a lateral pathway to the ventral lateral tegmental area (Conrad and Pfaff, 1976; Swanson et al., 1978). Although the injections of labeled tracers in these studies were not confined to just tissues within the AV3V region, some of the labeled descending fibers probably originate from this area. Mogenson and Kucharczyk (1978) have provided functional data suggesting that the projection to the ventral tegmental area is involved in the control of thirst. The medial projection to the central gray is likely to be involved in control of the circulation. Hemodynamic changes produced by electrical stimulation of the AV3V are blocked by an electrolytic ablation of the median eminence-ventromedial hypothalamic region (ME-VMH) (Fink et al., 1978). Also, ME-VMH lesions have been shown to block the development of one-kidney Grollman renal hypertension (Johnson et al., 1981).

Undoubtedly, fibers that course through the AV3V region and are interrupted by the lesion make an important contribution to the phenomena associated with the lesion. Carithers and colleagues (1980) showed that AV3V lesions produced degeneration of nerve terminals ending on supraoptic magnocellular neurons and evidence of degenerating cell bodies in the SFO. Recent studies using HRP, which permitted the point-to-point tracing of fibers, indicate that many of the fibers originating in the SFO and projecting to the supraoptic and paraventricular nuclei course through the AV3V region (Lind et al., 1981).

Taken together, the data obtained from a closer scrutiny of the microstructure of the AV3V region indicate that many aspects of the effects observed after AV3V lesions can be understood on the basis of (1) the sensitivity of the region to humoral substances, (2) the loss of tissue that may integrate information related to humoral and pressure/volume receptors, and (3) removal of efferent output or fibers of passage that project into pathways involved in thirst, vasopressin secretion, and CV control.

ANALYSIS OF THE AV3V REGION: A MODEL FOR THE COMBINED STUDY
OF NEUROBIOLOGY, BEHAVIOR, AND THE CV SYSTEM

In the previous sections, some of the effects of AV3V lesions on behavior and on the circulation have been described as well as recent findings on the neurobiology of the region. Both philosophical and practical reasons support the practice of analyzing the role of the AV3V region by simultaneously studying multiple effector systems. In light of the purpose of this symposium, it seems appropriate to comment on both of these.

Interest in the AV3V region originated because of studies that implicated this area in the neural control of drinking. We have maintained a fundamental concern for the role of this area of the brain in behavior and for the analysis of that behavior.

When only behavioral endpoints have been considered in former analyses, the application of limited experimental approaches (e.g., electrical stimulation of the hypothalamus) has led quickly to a theoretical impasse because of the difficulty involved in demonstrating that the observed behavioral effects were not merely epiphenomena (see Teitelbaum, 1973, for a brief review and statement of theoretical problems of the effects of hypothalamic stimulation on stimulus-bound behavior). One of the major advantages of studying both behavior and related physiological effectors (e.g., in this case, thirst along with hormones and the circulation) is that the "validity" of an observed behavioral effect can be assessed in the other systems.

The analysis of the role of the AV3V region in thirst has been facilitated because it is possible to make logical predictions of what should happen to a complementary physiological response (i.e., the release of vasopressin and sympathetic tone) when a treatment alters drinking in a specific direction. Namely, manipulations that increase water intake are likely to release vasopressin and increase sympathetic tone, or vice versa. If this response constellation is altered, one is compelled to scrutinize the experimental analysis much more carefully for potential methodological flaws.

The second advantage of studying several parallel, complementary systems is that it is sometimes easier, owing to technical limitations, to elucidate a mechanism in one system than in another. For example, it is sometimes easier to measure CV or hormonal endpoints in anesthetized than in unanesthetized animals. After initial observations are established in the anesthetized state, it may be deemed worthwhile and feasible to develop a procedure for studying both the physiological systems and behavior in the unanesthetized state.

WORKING HYPOTHESIS OF THE ROLE OF THE AV3V REGION
IN THE CONTROL OF BODY FLUID BALANCE AND THE CV SYSTEM

The results of functional studies employing electrolytic lesions, knife cuts, and stimulation of the periventricular tissue of the AV3V region clearly implicate the involvement of this area in control of body fluid balance and distribution. As we accumulate experimental data and learn more particularly about the neurobiology of this region, we begin to appreciate why ablation of this tissue has such profound effects on these behavioral and physiological systems. Given the distillate of what is currently known about the effects of AV3V lesions and about the neurobiology of this region, we can adopt a working hypothesis that this region of the brain serves to sense and integrate humoral and neural input, and mobilizes appropriate effector systems to achieve fine regulation of body fluid homeostasis. Further studies designed to test this hypothesis more thoroughly should enrich our understanding of the role of the CNS in the control of behavior and the CV system.

ACKNOWLEDGMENTS

The studies reviewed in this paper involved the collaboration of the many colleagues whose names are presented in the text and in the reference section, and we thank each of them for their extensive contributions. In addition, we are especially grateful to Sarah Bro for her editorial comments and to Becky Rowe for preparation of the manuscript.

Studies from our laboratory were supported in part by USPHS grants HLP14558 and HL24102 and by NIMH grants MH25345 and MH26751. AKJ is the recipient of Research Scientist Development Award MH00064 from NIMH.

REFERENCES

Bealer, S.L., Brody, M.J., Haywood, J.R., Fink, G.D., Gruber, K.A., Buckalew, V.M. and Johnson, A.K. (1979a) Decreased sodium consumption and impaired natriuresis following electrolytic ablation of anteroventral third ventricle (AV3V) periventricular tissue in rats. Soc. Neurosci. Abstr. 5, 430.

Bealer, S.L. and Johnson, A.K. (1979) Preoptic-hypothalamic periventricular lesions: impairment of thirst-motivated behavior. Physiol. Behav. 22, 841-846.

Bealer, S.L. and Johnson, A.K. (1980) Preoptic-hypothalamic periventricular lesions alter food-associated drinking and circadian rhythms. J. Comp. Physiol. Psychol. 94, 547-555.

Bealer, S.L., Phillips, M.I., Johnson, A.K. and Schmid, P.G. (1979b) Effect of anteroventral third ventricular lesions on antidiuretic responses to central angiotensin II. Amer. J. Physiol. 236, E610-E615.

Brody, M.J., Fink, G.D., Buggy, J., Haywood, J.R., Gordon, F.J. and Johnson, A.K. (1978a) The role of the anteroventral third ventricle (AV3V) region in experimental hypertension. Circulat. Res. 43, I2-I13.

Brody, M.J., Fink, G.D., Buggy, J., Haywood, J.R., Gordon, F.J., Kneupfer, M.M., Mow, M., Mahoney, L. and Johnson, A.K. (1978b) Critical role of the anteroventral third ventricle (AV3V) region in development and maintenance of experimental hypertension; in Perspectives in Nephrology and Hypertension, H. Schmitt and P. Meyer, eds. John Wiley & Sons, New York, pp. 76-84.

Brody, M.J. and Johnson, A.K. (1980) Role of the anteroventral third ventricle (AV3V) region in fluid and electrolyte balance, arterial pressure regulation, and hypertension; in Frontiers in Neuroendocrinology (Vol. 6), L. Martini and W.F. Ganong, eds. Raven Press, New York, pp. 249-292.

Brody, M.J. and Johnson, A.K. (1981) Role of forebrain structures in models of experimental hypertension; in Disturbances in the Neurogenic Control of the Circulation. Clinical Physiology Series, American Physiological Society. Williams & Wilkins Co., Baltimore, pp. 105-117.

Buggy, J. (1974) Thirst elicited by intracranial angiotensin: analysis of sensitive sites within the third ventricle. Unpublished doctoral dissertation, University of Pittsburgh.

Buggy, J., Fink, G.D., Haywood, J.R., Johnson, A.K. and Brody, M.J. (1978) Interruption of the maintenance phase of established hypertension by ablation of the anteroventral third ventricle (AV3V) in rats. Clin. Exp. Hypertension 1, 337-353.

Buggy, J., Fink, G.D., Johnson, A.K. and Brody, M.J. (1977) Prevention of the development of renal hypertension by anteroventral third ventricular tissue lesions. Circulat. Res. 40, I110-I117.

Buggy, J. and Fisher, A.E. (1976) Anteroventral third ventricle site of action for angiotensin induced thirst. Pharmacol. Biochem. Behav. 4, 651-660.

Buggy, J., Fisher, A.E., Hoffman, W.E., Johnson, A.K. and Phillips, M.I. (1975) Ventricular obstruction: effects on drinking to intracranial angiotensin. Science 190, 72-74.

Buggy, J. and Johnson, A.K. (1977a) Anteroventral third ventricle periventricular ablation: temporary adipsia and persisting thirst deficits. Neurosci. Lett. 5, 177-182.

Buggy, J. and Johnson, A.K. (1977b) Preoptic-hypothalamic periventricular lesions: thirst deficits and hypernatremia. Amer. J. Physiol. 233, R44-R52.

Buggy, J. and Johnson, A.K. (1978) Angiotensin induced thirst: effects of third ventricle obstruction and periventricular ablation. Brain Res. 149, 117-128.

Carithers, J., Bealer, S.L., Brody, M.J. and Johnson, A.K. (1980) Fine structural evidence of degeneration in supraoptic nucleus and subfornical organ of rats with lesions in the anteroventral third ventricle. Brain Res. 201, 1-12.

Carithers, J.R., Dellmann, H.D., Bealer, S.L., Brody, M.J. and Johnson, A.K. (1981) Ultrastructural effects of anteroventral third ventricle lesions on supraoptic nuclei and neural lobes of rats. Brain Res. 220, 13-29.

Conrad, L.C.A. and Pfaff, D.W. (1976) Efferents from medial basal forebrain and hypothalamus in the rat. J. Comp. Neurol. 169, 185-220.

Fink, G.D., Buggy, J., Haywood, J.R., Johnson, A.K. and Brody, M.J. (1978) Hemodynamic responses to electrical stimulation of areas of rat forebrain containing angiotensin on osmosensitive sites. Amer. J. Physiol. 235, H445-H451.

Fink, G.D., Buggy, J., Johnson, A.K. and Brody, M.J. (1977) Prevention of steroid-salt hypertension in the rat by anterior forebrain lesions. Circulation 56, III-242.

Ganten, D., Hutchinson, J.S., Schelling, P., Ganten, U. and Fischer, H. (1976) The iso-renin angiotensin systems in extrarenal tissue. Clin. Exp. Pharmacol. Physiol. 3, 103-126.

Gordon, F.J., Haywood, J.R., Brody, M.J. and Johnson, A.K. (in press) Effect of ablation of an angiotensin and osmosensitive brain region on the development of hypertension in spontaneously hypertensive rats. Hypertension.

Gordon, F.J., Haywood, J.R., Brody, M.J., Mann, J.F.E., Ganten, D. and Johnson, A.K. (1979) Effect of anteroventral third ventricle (AV3V) lesions on Okamoto strain and stroke prone spontaneously hypertensive rat. Jap. Heart J. 20 (Suppl. I), 116-118.

Grazi, V.M. and Miselis, R.R. (1980) Afferent and efferent projections of the nucleus medianus: an HRP study. Soc. Neurosci. Abstr. 6, 126.

Hartle, D.K., Shaffer, R.A., Johnson, A.K. and Brody, M.J. (1979) The effect of anteroventral third ventricle (AV3V) lesions on aortic coarctation hypertension in the rat. Pharmacologist 21, 254.

Haywood, J.R., Fink, G.D., Buggy, J., Boutelle, S. and Brody, M.J. (1978) Prevention and reversal of two-kidney (2K) renal hypertension in the rat by ablation of anteroventral third ventricle (AV3V) tissue. Fed. Proc. 37, 804.

Hoffman, W.E. and Phillips, M.I. (1976) Regional study of cerebral ventricle sensitive sites to angiotensin II. Brain Res. 110, 313-330.

Hsieh, B., Chen, W., Yen, T. and Tsai, T. (1980) Decreased sensitivity to angiotensin II in chronic sustained hypernatremia. J. Formosan Med. Ass. 79, 370-378.

Johnson, A.K., Bealer, S.L., McNeill, J.R., Schoun, J. and Mohring, J. (1980a) The influence of the periventricular tissue of the anteroventral third ventricle (AV3V) on the release of vasopressin (VP). Soc. Neurosci. Abstr. 6, 696.

Johnson, A.K. and Buggy, J. (1977) A critical analysis of the site of action for the dipsogenic effect of angiotensin II; in International Symposium on the Central Actions of Angiotensin and Related Hormones, J.P. Buckley and C. Ferrario, eds. Pergamon, New York, pp. 357-386.

Johnson, A.K. and Buggy, J. (1978) Periventricular preoptic-hypothalamus is vital for thirst and normal water economy. Amer. J. Physiol. 234, R122-R129.

Johnson, A.K., Buggy, J., Fink, G.D. and Brody, M.J. (1981) Prevention of renal hypertension and of the central pressor effect of angiotensin by ventromedial hypothalamic ablation. Brain Res. 205, 255-264.

Johnson, A.K. and Epstein, A.N. (1975) The cerebral ventricles as the avenue for the dipsogenic action of intracranial angiotensin. Brain Res. 86, 399-418.

Johnson, A.K., Hoffman, W.E. and Buggy, J. (1978) Attenuated pressor responses to intracranially injected stimuli and altered antidiuretic activity following preoptic-hypothalamic periventricular ablation. Brain Res. 157, 161-166.

Johnson, A.K., Schoun, J., McNeill, J.R. and Möhring, J. (1980b) Periventricular tissue of the anteroventral third ventricle: a role for the control of vasopressin (VP) release. Fed. Proc. 39, 986.

Johnson, A.K. and Sladek, C.D. (1979) The effect of anteroventral third ventricle region lesion on osmotic stimulation of vasopressin release by the organ cultured rat hypothalamo-neurohypophyseal system. Soc. Neurosci. Abstr. 5, 448.

Kastin, A.J., Lipsett, M.B., Ommaya, A.K. and Moser, J.M. (1965) Asymptomatic hypernatremia. Amer. J. Med. 38, 306-315.

Lascelles, P.T. and Lewis, P.D. (1972) Hypodipsia and hypernatremia associated with hypothalamic and suprasellar lesions. Brain 95, 249-264.

Lind, H., Lind, R.W., Shrager, E.E., Bealer, S.L. and Johnson, A.K. (1979) Critical tissues within the periventricular region of the anteroventral third ventricle (AV3V) associated with specific thirst deficits. Soc. Neurosci. Abstr. 5, 220.

Lind, R.W. and Johnson, A.K. (1978) Effect of anteroventral third ventricle (AV3V) lesions on schedule-induced polydipsia in the rat. Soc. Neurosci. Abstr. 4, 178.

Lind, R.W. and Johnson, A.K. (1982) Central and peripheral mechanisms mediating angiotensin-induced thirst; in Angiotensin System in the Brain, D. Ganten, M. Printz, M.I. Phillips and B.A. Schölkens, eds. Springer-Verlag, Berlin, pp. 353-364.

Lind, R.W., VanHoeson, G.W. and Johnson, A.K. (1981) Connections of the subfornical organ (SFO). Soc. Neurosci. Abstr. 7, 638.

Miselis, R.R. (1980) New efferents and afferents of the subfornical organ: a strategic neural circuitry for the control of water balance behaviorally and physiologically. Soc. Neurosci. Abstr. 6, 32.

Miselis, R.R., Shapiro, R.E. and Hand, P.J. (1979) Subfornical organ efferents to neural systems for control of body water. Science 205, 1022-1025.

Mogenson, G.J. and Kucharczyk, J. (1978) Central neural pathways for angiotensin-induced thirst. Fed. Proc. 37, 2683-2688.

Mow, M.T., Haywood, J.R., Johnson, A.K. and Brody, M.J. (1978) The role of the anteroventral third ventricle (AV3V) in development of neurogenic hypertension. Soc. Neurosci. Abstr. 4, 23.

Phillips, M.I. and Hoffman, W.E. (1977) Sensitive sites in the brain for the blood pressure and drinking responses to angiotensin II; in Central Actions of Angiotensin and Related Hormones, J.P. Buckley, C.M. Ferrario and M.F. Lokhandwala, eds. Pergamon Press, New York, pp. 325-356.

Ross, E.J. and Christie, S.B.M. (1969) Hypernatremia. Medicine 48, 441-473.

Saper, C.B. and Loewy, A.D. (1980) Efferent connections of the parabrachial nucleus in the rat. Brain Res. 197, 291-317.

Shrager, E.E. and Johnson, A.K. (1980) Anteroventral third ventricle (AV3V) region ablation: chronic elevations of plasma renin concentration. Brain Res. 190, 554-558.

Silverman, A.J., Hoffman, D.L. and Zimmerman, E.A. (1981) The descending afferent connections of the paraventricular nucleus of the hypothalamus (PVN). Brain Res. Bull. 6, 47-61.

Simpson, J.B., Epstein, A.N. and Camardo, J.S., Jr. (1978) Localization of receptors for the dipsogenic action of angiotensin II in the subfornical organ of rat. J. Comp. Physiol. Psychol. 92, 581-601.

Skulety, F.M. and Joynt, R.J. (1963) Clinical implications of adipsia. J. Neurosurg. 20, 793-800.

Sridhar, C.B., Calvert, G.D. and Ibbertson, H.K. (1974) Syndrome of hypernatremia, hypodipsia and partial diabetes insipidus: a new interpretation. J. Clin. Endocrinol. Metab. 38, 890-901.

Swanson, L.W., Kucharczyk, J. and Mogenson, G.J. (1978) Autoradiographic evidence for pathways from the medial preoptic area to the midbrain involved in the drinking response to angiotensin II. J. Comp. Neurol. 178, 645-660.

Sweet, C.S., Columbo, J.M. and Gaul, S.L. (1976) Central antihypertensive effects of inhibitors of the renin-angiotensin system in rats. Amer. J. Physiol. 231, 1794-1799.

Teitelbaum, P. (1966) The use of operant methods in the assessment and control of motivational states; in Operant Behavior: Areas of Research and Application, W.K. Honig, ed. Appleton-Century-Crofts, New York, pp. 565-608.

Teitelbaum, P. (1973) Discussion: on the use of electrical stimulation to study hypothalamic structure and function; in The Neuropsychology of Thirst: New Findings and Advances in Concepts, A.N. Epstein, H.R. Kissileff and E. Stellar, eds. V.H. Winston & Sons, Washington, D.C., pp. 143-154.

Teitelbaum, P. and Epstein, A.N. (1962) The lateral hypothalamic syndrome: recency of feeding and drinking after lateral hypothalamic lesions. Psychol. Rev. 69, 74-90.

Teitelbaum, P. and Stellar, E. (1954) Recovery from the failure to eat produced by hypothalamic lesions. Science 120, 894-895.

Thunhorst, R.L., Lind, R.W. and Johnson, A.K. (1981) Lesions of the subfornical organ (SFO) block drinking to peripheral but not central angiotensin. Soc. Neurosci. Abstr. 7, 638.

Wolf, C.L., Skulety, F.M., Ecklund, R.E. and Gallagher, T.F. (1973) Apparent cerebral hypernatremia secondary to volume regulation of fluid balance. Trans. Amer. Neurol. Ass. 98, 324-325.

Task Force Reports on
Hypertension, Sudden Cardiac Death,
Coronary Artery Disease, and Cardiomyopathy

Task Force Report on Hypertension

Co-Chairmen:

DAVID ANDERSON
Department of Psychiatry, University of South Florida College of Medicine,
Tampa, Florida

ARTHUR J. VANDER
Department of Physiology, University of Michigan, Ann Arbor, Michigan

Three general conclusions have emerged at this conference that have a fundamental bearing on future theory, research and applications in hypertension. First, behavioral and cardiovascular (CV) processes are not separate, independent variables but are integrated at all levels from the periphery to the brain (Calaresu et al., 1975; Cohen and Obrist, 1975; Henry et al., 1967; Hilton and Spyer, 1980; Obrist, 1981; Smith, 1974; Zanchetti et al., 1975). Second, the brain is exquisitely and complexly organized to integrate psychological and neuroendocrine processes, of which the skeletal muscle and CV systems are an important subset (Baccelli et al., 1981; Longhurst and Mitchell, 1979; Obrist, 1981; Peterson et al., 1981). Third, the potential for patterning of CV processes in different behavioral situations is clearly indicated (Herd et al., 1969; Hilton, 1974; Obrist, 1981). A major shift in our thinking is that patterning of biobehavioral processes may be the rule rather than the exception, and that it is organized in a dynamic fashion at both central and peripheral levels.

BASIC STUDIES ON BEHAVIORAL-NEUROENDOCRINE CARDIOVASCULAR INTERACTIONS

Neurophysiology

Although not covered extensively in the conference, there was a feeling that electrophysiological studies have great potential in identifying sites of CV control and integration. Both central and peripheral recording techniques in conscious animals are now available (Lawler et al., 1981).

New information on patterned activity in the nervous system indicates the potential for selective activation of autonomic effectors underlying specific emotional-behavioral states (Brody and Johnson, 1981; Henry and Meehan, 1981; Loewy, this volume). One such example with obvious relations to hypertension would be identification of situations that selectively activate renal sympthetic nerves (Ammons et al., in press; Donald and Shepherd, 1978; Grignolo et al., in press; Weaver, this volume).

Visceral afferents can alter autonomic activity (Schramm, this volume; Thies and Foreman, 1981). The visceral autonomic consequences of behavior might be inhibited or amplified by feedback.

A number of CV reflexes, particularly the baroreflexes, serve to stabilize blood pressure and, to some extent, fix the resting level of blood pressure. These reflexes are generally depressed in established hypertension (Angell-James and George, 1980; Bristow et al., 1969; Gribbin et al., 1971; Jones, 1977; Koushanpour and Kenfield, 1981; Krieger, 1970; Liard, 1980; Mancia et al., 1978; McCubbin et al., 1956; Salgado and Krieger, 1973; Takeshita et al., 1975; Zanchetti et al., 1980). Altered baroreflex function has been attributed to changes in the receptors or effector organs (Andresen et al., 1980; Dworkin et al., 1979; Folkow et al., 1973, 1978; Korner, 1979; Sapru and Krieger, 1979; Sleight et al., 1977; Zucker and Gilmore, 1981). Furthermore, recent research shows a dynamic interplay of the baroreflexes and CV activity associated with various behaviors (Baccelli et al., 1981; Combs, this volume; Goldstein et al., 1977; Guazzi and Zanchetti, 1965; Nathan, 1981; Nathan et al., 1978; Stephenson, this volume; Stephenson et al., 1981; Zanchetti et al., 1975). Studies reviewed at this conference demonstrated that the baroreflexes can modulate CV responses accompanying certain behaviors (Combs, this volume; Djojosugito et al., 1970; Goldstein et al., 1977; Melcher and Donald, in press; Nathan et al., 1978; Stephenson et al., 1981). In turn, areas of the brain that mediate these responses can alter the sensitivity of the baroreflexes (Adair and Manning, 1975; Gebber and Snyder, 1970; Goldstein et al., 1977; Kumada et al., 1975; Laubie and Schmitt, 1979; Nathan and Reis, 1977; Nathan et al., 1978; Stephenson et al., 1981).

A great deal of new information is emerging about the nature of central CV control during exercise. The role of higher brain structures as related to the control of motor behavior in the regulation of associated CV responses is an area of active investigation (Longhurst and Mitchell, 1979; Smith et al., this volume). A question clearly reopened by the conference is whether there are centers that mediate anticipatory CV responses to behavioral stimuli.

Much information has also been forthcoming on the physiological and behavioral interactions of certain peptides with various central loci, particularly within the forebrain proximal to the third ventricle (Brody and Johnson, 1981; Ganten et al., 1981; Swanson, this volume). For example, vasopressin now is suggested to be involved in several forms of hypertension (Brody and Johnson, 1981; Swanson, this volume).

Recommendations

1. Electrophysiological studies need to be applied to the study of conscious, behaving animals.

2. Patterned autonomic responses and visceral sensory mechanisms need to be examined in relation to behavioral-autonomic interactions.

3. The degree of neural integration of autonomic responses that occurs at spinal and ganglionic levels needs emphasis.

4. Studies addressing the interplay of baroreflex regulation of the circulation and CV activity associated with various behaviors should be expanded, especially to conscious, behaving animals and humans.

5. There is a need to identify or define the neuroanatomical pathways and the neurotransmitters used in mediating autonomic responses that accompany emotional-behavioral responses. Similar studies are needed on the autonomic activity that pertains to limbic system behavior patterns of aggression and anxiety.

6. Additional information is needed regarding peptide interactions in the CNS. Further neurochemical, functional, and anatomical studies of known loci of peptide action should be pursued.

Neuropharmacology and Neurochemistry

Techniques are now available for specific immunological and pharmacological intervention into neurophysiological and biosynthetic mechanisms. As described by both Gillis and Swanson (this volume), neurotoxins can locally destroy aminergic projections; specific peptidergic antibodies can be used to antagonize the effects of putative peptide transmitters; antibodies to biosynthetic enzymes can be used to alter the activity of neuronal systems; and pharmacological antagonists can interfere with cerebral neurotransmission at specific loci (see also Anderson, 1981; Anderson and Tosheff, 1973).

Recommendation

1. Specific neuropharmacologic, immunologic, and neurotoxic techniques need to be used to determine whether certain behaviors and their attendant autonomic and CV responses are dependent on particular transmitters and/or sites.

Behavioral Methodology

Although not discussed in any depth in this conference, there are exciting opportunities for the use of recently developed analytical behavioral techniques in studies of the physiological mechanisms involved in CV effects. One example is the use of ethological techniques, including the use of specific postures and facial expressions to produce or identify particular emotional effects (Obrist, this volume; Obrist et al., 1974). Another example is the use of behavioral variables such as active vs. passive avoidance, signaled vs. unsignaled and controllable vs. uncontrollable electric shock, approach-avoidance conflict, and the effects of highly arousing, positively rewarding vs. aversive situations (Anderson, 1981; Anderson and Brady, 1972, 1973; Anderson and Yingling, 1979;

Buchholz et al., 1981; Friedman, 1981; Galosy et al., 1979; Langer et al., 1979; Lawler et al., 1975, 1980a,b, 1981; Light, 1981; Obrist, 1981). Also, social-psychological tasks such as congestion and crowding can be varied systematically (Benson et al., 1969; Campbell and Henry, in press; Galosy et al., 1981; Harris et al., 1973; Henry and Stephens, 1977, 1979; Henry et al., 1975; Miller and Brucker, 1979).

Information on mechanisms whereby learning can influence CV responses is also beginning to emerge (Benson et al., 1969; Harris et al., 1973; Miller and Brucker, 1979). This seems to be an important area, particularly the possibility of developing animal models for using learned reduction in blood pressure to reduce genetic or experimental hypertension in animals. There is need for analysis of the neuroanatomical circuits and neurohumoral mechanisms involved in CV changes induced by learning, as well as for knowledge of the types of hypertension that are subject to reduction by learning.

Recommendations

1. In the types of experiments to be discussed below, the actual stimulus to the animal or person and the behavioral events should be characterized just as carefully as the physiological and pathophysiological responses. The variety available is illustrated in Table 1.

2. Since there is evidence that the effects of such situations are not always monotonic, there is a need for more dose-response and time-response studies (i.e., chronic vs. acute). Closer parallels between intensity of behavioral stimuli and intensity of CV and neurophysiological variations need to be examined. There is also a need to investigate possible critical periods during early stages of development.

TABLE 1

COMMON STRESSES LEADING TO PATHOPHYSIOLOGICAL RESPONSES

Simple Stresses	Social Stresses	Naturally Recurring Life Stresses
Immobilization	Crowding	Death
Deprivation	Separation	War
Aversive stimulation	Competition tasks	Job loss
Electrical	Dominance/aggression	Divorce
Noise	Social anxiety tasks	
Heat/cold	Interviews	**Learning**
Conflict	Speech making	Classical conditioning
	Role playing	Positive
Mental Stress		Negative
Cognitive tasks		Operant
Vigilance		Reward
Reaction time		Avoidance
Discrimination		
Mental arithmetic		

ANIMAL MODELS OF HYPERTENSION

Studies reviewed at the conference showed that emotional conditioning can contribute significantly to the development of sustained hypertension in a variety of animal species (Anderson, 1981; Bianchi et al., 1975; Folkow, 1981; Friedman and Iwai, 1976; Henry, this volume; Henry et al., 1975; Herd et al., 1969; Lawler et al., 1981). In particular, it was shown that prolonged exposure to naturalistic stressors such as psychosocial interactions and auditory stimulation can result in chronic hypertension in rats and monkeys, respectively. It was also reported that specific aversive conditioning procedures can result in sustained hypertension in primates, and that this hypertension can develop rapidly in dogs exposed concurrently to increased salt intake. Moreover, emotional conditioning procedures have been shown to affect the rate of development of hypertension in genetically susceptible rodents. The central role of the brain in experimental hypertension was indicated by experiments showing that lesions of selected CNS sites prevent DOCA-salt hypertension (Cohen and Obrist, 1975; Cowley et al., 1973; Miller, 1981; Nathan and Reis, 1977; Obrist, this volume). Establishment of the hormonal and CV correlates of these kinds of hypertension is necessary so that these models can be compared and contrasted with the various forms of human hypertension. The information may very well be useful not only in determining the etiology of hypertension, but in providing the basic information required for a more rational therapy for the various forms of human hypertension, including combinations of behavioral and pharmacological therapy.

Recommendations

1. Given the advances in basic methods of behavioral science and neurobiological concepts and techniques described above, the Hypertension Task Force gave a very high priority to the full-scale encouragement of research on models of experimental hypertension that focus on environmental-behavioral interactions.

2. Investigators should pursue the potential for using advanced anatomical, physiological and biochemical techniques to study pathophysiological mechanisms of these forms of hypertension.

3. Research efforts should be mounted that include physiological and biochemical observations in the behaving animal. Such efforts, though complex and expensive of time, seem warranted on the basis of recent progress in behavioral hypertension models. There is a need for clarity and precision in the specification of the critical aspects of behavioral factors in experimental hypertension, and for a determination of the extent to which models are applicable across species.

4. Additional information is needed to determine behavioral, neurophysiological and circulatory mechanisms involved in these models. There is an interest in the degree to which psychosocial and conditioning models share basic underlying mechanisms, and studies are needed to characterize variables such as cardiac output, resistances of a

variety of vascular beds, renal and adrenal hormonal changes, and neurobehavioral processes. The technology already exists to measure such variables, thereby facilitating experimental design.

5. There was a general consensus among the Task Force members that the kinds of research on animal models stemming from these recommendations require multi-disciplinary approaches that are particularly difficult to fund, given the structure of present policies. The National Institutes of Health is urged to consider ways in which the establishment of programs to investigate these models could be facilitated. Whether the ideal situation would be in the form of program projects or some other method of combining talents, facilities, and methodologies was felt to be beyond the committee's charge, but there was no doubt that attention to encouraging interdisciplinary studies deserves high priority.

STUDIES ON HUMAN CARDIOVASCULAR FUNCTION

There is emerging evidence that there are individual differences in CV responses to environmental inputs that have emotional connotation (Galosy et al., 1981; Gold and Cohen, 1981; Lawler, 1980; Lawler et al., 1981; Obrist, 1981 and this volume; Smith et al., 1980). There is little information on the mechanisms involved, or the ways in which other environmental factors, such as diet and exercise, interact with behavioral stimuli.

Another area involving humans in which a great deal of new information seems to be emerging is that of the nature of CV control during exercise (Bevegard and Shepherd, 1966; Langer et al., 1979) and other fundamental homeostatic processes such as sodium balance (Grignolo et al., in press; Koepke et al., in preparation), as well as the manner in which "stress" disrupts the efficiency with which these life-sustaining functions are maintained (Gillis, this volume; Obrist et al., in press a, b). There is still a great deal of debate about the role played by various receptors, such as baroreceptors and muscle chemoreceptors, as well as the importance of "central command" (Rowell et al., 1981).

Recommendations

1. There is a need to characterize the various patterns of autonomic responses to different behavioral-emotional stimuli and to determine the mechanisms responsible for these individual differences. One of the aims of this type of research would be to identify those persons at risk from hypertension by delineating the manner in which the myocardium and the vasculature react to environmental demands and the relation of these CV effects to the renal handling of sodium and other electrolytes. Included in these efforts should be an assessment of CV function under naturalistic (field) conditions so as to be able to establish an individual's characteristic means of responding to stress. We are seeking information that goes beyond such established risk factors as parental history,

diet and weight; we need to identify features of the individual-environmental interaction that relate to risk, e.g., life styles or coping strategies.

2. It is important to combine exercise studies with subsequent behavioral paradigms in the same individuals and animals in order to understand the differences and interactions between them. In fact, the use of emotional stimuli introduced during exercise may offer information about additive or conflicting CV outcomes, thus suggesting possible therapeutic outcomes.

3. The studies proposed in this section should be performed on both normotensive and hypertensive persons.

REFERENCES

Adair, R. and Manning, J.W. (1975) Hypothalamic modulation of baroreceptor afferent unit activity. Amer. J. Physiol. 229, 1357-1364.

Ammons, W.S., Koyama, S. and Manning, J.W. (in press) Neural and vascular interaction in renin response to graded renal nerve stimulation. Amer. J. Physiol. (Regulat. Integrat. Comp. Physiol.)

Anderson, D. (1981) Classical conditioning techniques and the induction of experimental hypertension. 3rd Joint U.S.-U.S.S.R. Symposium on Hypertension. National Institutes of Health, Bethesda, Maryland.

Anderson, D.E. and Brady J.V. (1972) Differential preparatory cardiovascular responses to aversive and appetitive conditioning. Condit. Reflex 7, 82-96.

Anderson, D.E. and Brady, J.V. (1973) Prolonged preavoidance effects on blood pressure and heart rate in the dog. Psychosom. Med. 35, 4-12.

Anderson, D.E. and Tosheff, J.G. (1973) Cardiac output and total peripheral resistance changes during preavoidance periods in the dog. J. Appl. Physiol. 34, 650-654.

Anderson, D.E. and Yingling, J.E. (1979) Aversive conditioning of elevations in total peripheral resistance in dogs. Amer. J. Physiol. 236, H880-H887.

Andresen, M.C., Kuraoka, S. and Brown, A.M. (1980) Baroreceptor function and changes in strain sensitivity in normotensive and spontaneously hypertensive rats. Circulat. Res. 47, 821-828.

Angell-James, J.E. and George, M.J. (1980) Carotid sinus baroreceptor reflex control of the circulation in medial sclerotic and renal hypertensive rabbits and its modification by the aortic baroreceptors. Circulat. Res. 47, 890-901.

Baccelli, G., Albertini, R., DelBo, A., Mancia, G. and Zanchetti, A. (1981) Role of sinoaortic reflexes in hemodynamic patterns of natural defense behaviors in the cat. Amer. J. Physiol. 240, H421-H429.

Benson, H., Herd, A.J., Morse, W.H. and Kelleher, R.T. (1969) Behavioral induction of arterial hypertension and its reversal. Amer. J. Physiol. 217, 30-34.

Bevegard, B.S. and Shepherd, J.T. (1966) Circulatory effects of stimulating the carotid stretch receptors in man at rest and during exercise. J. Clin. Invest. 45, 132-142.

Bianchi, G., Baer, P.G., Fox, U., Puzzi, L., Pagetti, D. and Giovonetti, A.M. (1975) Changes in renin, water balance and sodium balance during development of high blood pressure in genetically hypertensive rats. Circulat. Res. Suppl. I, 36-37.

Bristow, J., Hanous, A.J., Pickering, G.W., Sleight, P. and Smyth, H.S. (1969) Diminished baroreflex sensitivity in high blood pressure. Circulation 39, 48-54.

Brody, M.J. and Johnson, A.K. (1981) Role of forebrain structures in models of experimental hypertension; in Disturbances in Neurogenic Control of the Circulation, F.M. Abboud et al., eds. Waverly Press, Baltimore, pp. 105-119.

Buchholz, R.A., Lawler, J.E. and Barker, G.F. (1981) The effects of avoidance and conflict schedules on the blood pressure and heart rate of rats. Physiol. Behav. 26, 853-863.

Calaresu, F.R., Faies, A.A. and Mogenson, G.J. (1975) Central neural regulation of heart and blood vessels in mammals. Progr. Neurobiol. 5, 1-35.

Campbell, R.J. and Henry, J.P. (in press) Animal models of hypertension; in Handbook of Psychology and Health, D.S. Krantz, J.E. Singer and A. Baum, eds. Lawrence J. Erlbaum Ass., Hillsdale, N.J.

Cohen, D.H. and Obrist, P.A. (1975) Interactions between behavior and the cardiovascular system. Circulat. Res. 37, 693-706.

Cowley, A.W., Liard, J.F. and Guyton, A.C. (1973) Role of baroreceptor reflex in daily control of arterial blood pressure and other variables in dogs. Circulat. Res. 32, 564-576.

Djojosugito, A.M., Folkow, B., Kylstra, P., Lisander, B. and Tuttle, R.S. (1970) Interactions between hypothalamic defence reaction and baroreceptor reflexes. Acta Physiol. Scand. 78, 376-385.

Donald, D.E. and Shepherd, J.T. (1978) Reflexes from the heart and lungs: physiological curiosities or important regulatory mechanisms. Cardiovasc. Res. 12, 449-469.

Dworkin, B.R., Filewich, R.J., Miller, N.E., Craigmyle, N. and Pickering, T.G. (1979) Baroreceptor activation reduces reactivity to noxious stimulation: implications for hypertension. Science 205, 1299-1301.

Folkow, B. (1981) Central and peripheral mechanism in spontaneous hypertension in rats. Res. Publ. Ass. Res. Nerv. Ment. Dis. 59, 257-272.

Folkow, B., Hallback, M., Lundgren, Y., Sivertsson, R. and Weiss, L. (1973) Importance of adaptive changes in vascular design for establishment of primary hypertension, studied in man and in spontaneously hypertensive rats. Circulat. Res. 32/33, I2-I16.

Folkow, B., Hallback, M. and Noresson, E. (1978) Vascular resistance and reactivity of the microcirculation in hypertension. Blood Vessels 15, 33-45.

Friedman, R. (1981) Genetic basis for susceptibility for stress-induced hypertension. 3rd Joint U.S.-U.S.S.R. Symposium on Hypertension. National Institutes of Health, Bethesda, Maryland.

Friedman, R. and Dahl, L.K. (1975) The effect of chronic conflict on the blood pressure of rats with a genetic susceptibility to experimental hypertension. Psychosom. Med. 37, 402-416.

Friedman, R. and Iwai, J. (1976) Genetic predisposition and stress-induced hypertension. Science 193, 161-162.

Galosy, R.A., Clarke, L.K. and Mitchell, J.H. (1979) Cardiac changes during behavioral stress in dogs. Amer. J. Physiol. 236, H750-H758.

Galosy, R.A., Clarke, L.K., Vasko, M.R. and Crawford, I.L. (1981) Neurophysiology and neuropharmacology of cardiovascular regulation and stress. Neurosci. Biobehav. Res. 5, 137-175.

Ganten, D., Unger, T., Scholkens, B., Rascher, W., Speck, G. and Stock, G. (1981) Role of neuropeptides in regulation of blood pressure; in Disturbances in Neurogenic Control of the Circulation, F.M. Abboud et al., eds. Waverly Press, Baltimore, pp. 139-152.

Gebber, G.L. and Snyder, D.W. (1970) Hypothalamic control of the baroreflexes. Amer. J. Physiol. 218, 124-131.

Gold, M.R. and Cohen, D.H. (1981) Modification of the discharge of vagal cardiac neurons during learned heart rate change. Science 214, 345-347.

Goldstein, D.S., Harris, A.H. and Brady, J.V. (1977) Baroreflex sensitivity during operant blood pressure conditioning. Biofeedback and Self-Regulation 2, 127-138.

Gribbin, B., Pickering, T.G., Sleight, P. and Peto, R. (1971) Effect of age and high blood pressure on baroreflex sensitivity in man. Circulat. Res. 29, 424-431.

Grignolo, A., Koepke, J.P. and Obrist, P.A. (in press) Renal function, heart rate and blood pressure during exercise and avoidance in dogs. Amer. J. Physiol.

Guazzi, M. and Zanchetti, A. (1965) Blood pressure and heart rate during natural sleep of the cat and their regulation by carotid sinus and aortic reflexes. Arch. Ital. Biol. 103, 789-817.

Harris, A.H., Gilliam, W.J., Findley, J.D. and Brady, J.V. (1973) Instrumental conditioning of large-magnitude, daily, 12-hour blood pressure elevations in the baboon. Science 182, 175-177.

Henry, J.P. and Meehan, J.P. (1981) Psychosocial stimuli, physiological specificity and cardiovascular disease. Res. Publ. Ass. Res. Nerv. Ment. Dis. 59, 305-334.

Henry, J.P., Meehan, J.P. and Stephens, P.M. (1967) The use of psychosocial stimuli to induce prolonged systolic hypertension in mice. Psychosom. Med. 29, 408-432.

Henry, J.P. and Stephens, P.M. (1977) Stress, Health and the Social Environment: A Sociobiologic Approach to Medicine. Springer-Verlag, New York.

Henry, J.P. and Stephens, P.M. (1979) An animal model of neuropsychological factors in hypertension; in Prophylactic Approach to Hypertensive Diseases, Y. Yamori, W. Lovenberg and W. Freis, eds. Raven Press, New York, pp. 299-307.

Henry, J.P., Stephens, P.M. and Santisteban, G.A. (1975) A model of psychosocial hypertension showing reversibility and progression of cardiovascular complications. Circulat. Res. 36, 156-164.

Herd, J.A., Morse, W.H., Kelleher, R.T. and Jones, L.G. (1969) Arterial hypertension in the squirrel monkey during behavioral experiments. Amer. J. Physiol. 217, 24-29.

Hilton, S.M. (1974) The role of the hypothalamus in the organization of patterns of cardiovascular responses; in Recent Studies of Hypothalamic Function, K. Lederis and K.E. Cooper, eds. S. Karger, Basel, pp. 306-314.

Hilton, S.M. and Spyer, K.M. (1980) Central nervous system regulation of vascular resistance. Ann. Rev. Physiol. 42, 399-411.

Jones, J.V. (1977) Time course of carotid sinus baroreceptor threshold resetting in rats with renovascular hypertension. Acta Physiol. Scand. 99, 173-182.

Korner, P.I. (1979) Central nervous control of cardiovascular function; in Handbook of Physiology, Sec. 1, The Cardiovascular System, Vol. 1.

Koushanpour, F. and Kenfield, K.J. (1981) Partition of carotid sinus baroreceptor response in dogs with chronic renal hypertension. Circulat. Res. 48, 267-273.

Krieger, E.M. (1970) Time course of baroreceptor resetting in acute hypertension. Amer. J. Phsyiol. 218, 486-490.

Kumada, M., Schramm, L.P., Altmansberger, R.A. and Sagawa, K. (1975) Modulation of carotid sinus baroreceptor reflex by hypothalamic defense response. Amer. J. Physiol. 228, 34-45.

Langer, A.W., Obrist, P.A. and McCubbin, J.A. (1979) Hemodynamic and metabolic adjustments during exercise and shock avoidance in dogs. Amer. J. Physiol. 236, H225-H230.

Laubie, M. and Schmitt, H. (1979) Destruction of the nucleus tractus solitarii in the dog: comparison with sinoaortic denervation. Amer. J. Physiol. 236, H736-H743.

Lawler, K.A. (1980) Cardiovascular and electrodermal response patterns in heart rate reactive individuals during psychological stress. Psychophysiology 17, 464-470.

Lawler, K.A., Allen, M.T., Critcher, E.C. and Standard, B.A. (1981) The relationship of physiological responses to the coronary-prone behavior pattern in children. J. Behav. Med. 4, 203-216.

Lawler, J.E., Barker, G.F., Hubbard, J.W. and Allen, M.T. (1980a) The effects of conflict on tonic levels of blood pressure in the genetically borderline hypertensive rat. Psychophysiology 17, 363-370.

Lawler, J.E., Barker, G.F., Hubbard, J.W. and Schaub, R.G. (1980b) Pathophysiological changes associated with stress-induced hypertension in the borderline hypertensive rat. Clin. Sci. 59, 307s-310s.

Lawler, J.E., Barker, G.F., Hubbard, J.W. and Schaub, R.G. (1981) Effects of stress on blood pressure and cardiac pathology in rats with borderline hypertension. Hypertension 3, 496-505.

Lawler, J.E., Obrist, P.A. and Lawler, K.A. (1975) Cardiovascular function during pre-avoidance, avoidance and post-avoidance in dogs. Psychophysiology 12, 4-11.

Liard, J.F. (1980) The baroreceptor reflexes in experimental hypertension. Clin. Exp. Hypertens. 2, 479-498.

Light, K.C. (1981) Cardiovascular responses to effortful active coping. Implications for the role of stress in hypertension development. Psychophysiology 18, 216-225.

Longhurst, J.C. and Mitchell, J.H. (1979) Reflex control of the circulation by afferents from skeletal muscle. Int. Rev. Physiol. 18, 125-148.

Mancia, G., Ludbroo, J., Ferrari, A., Gregorini, L. and Zanchetti, A. (1978) Baroreceptor reflexes in human hypertension. Circulat. Res. 43, 170-177.

308

McCubbin, J.W., Green, J.H. and Page, I.H. (1956) Baroreceptor function in chronic renal hypertension. Circulat. Res. 4, 205-210.
Melcher, A. and Donald, D.E. (in press) Maintained ability of carotid baroreflex to regulate arterial pressure during exercise in conscious dogs. Amer. J. Physiol.
Miller, N.E. (1981) Hypertension: effects of learning and stress. 3rd Joint U.S.-U.S.S.R. Symposium on Hypertension. National Institutes of Health, Bethesda, Maryland.
Miller, N.E. and Brucker, B.S. (1979) Learned large increases in blood pressure apparently independent of skeletal responses in patients paralyzed by spinal lesions; in Biofeedback and Self-Regulation, N. Birbaumer and H.D. Kimmel, eds. Lawrence Erlbaum Ass., Hillsdale, N.J., pp. 287-304.
Nathan, M.A. and Reis, D.J. (1977) Chronic labile hypertension produced by lesions of the nucleus tractus solitarii in the cat. Circulat. Res. 40, 72-81.
Nathan, M.A., Tucker, L.W., Severini, W.H. and Reis, D.J. (1978) Enhancement of conditional arterial pressure responses in cats after brainstem lesions. Science 20, 71-73.
Obrist, P.A. (1981) Cardiovascular Psychophysiology: A Perspective. Plenum, New York, p. 236.
Obrist, P.A., Langer, A.W., Light, K.C. and Koepke, J.P. (in press a) A cardiac-behavioral approach in the study of hypertension; in Biological Basis of Coronary-Prone Behavior --Behavioral Approaches to a 20th Century Epidemic.
Obrist, P.A., Lawler, J.E., Howard, J.L., Smithson, K.W., Martin, P.L. and Manning, J. (1974) Sympathetic influences on cardiac rate and contractility during acute stress in humans. Psychophysiol. 11, 405-427.
Obrist, P.A., Light, K.C., Langer, A.W. and Koepke, J.P. (in press b) Psychomatics; in Psychophysiology: Systems, Processes and Applications, M. Coles, E. Donchin and S. Proges, eds. Guilford Press, New York.
Peterson, A. et al. (1981) Noise raises blood pressure without impairing auditory thresholds. Science 211, 1450-1452.
Rowell, L.B., Freund, P.R. and Hobbs, S.F. (1981) Cardiovascular responses to muscle in ischemia in humans. Circulat. Res. 48, 137-147.
Salgado, H.C. and Krieger, E.M. (1973) Reversibility of baroreceptor adaptation in chronic hypertension. Clin. Sci. Mol. Med. 45, 123S-126S.
Sapru, H.N. and Krieger, A.J. (1979) Role of receptor elements in baroreceptor resetting. Amer. J. Physiol. 236, H174-H182.
Sleight, P., Robinson, J.L., Brooks, D.E. and Rees, P.M. (1977) Characteristics of single carotid sinus baroreceptor fibers and whole nerve activity in the normotensive and renal hypertensive dog. Circulat. Res. 41, 750-758.
Smith, O.A. (1974) Reflex and central mechanisms involved in the control of the heart and circulation. Ann. Rev. Physiol. 36, 93-123.
Smith, O.A., Astley, C.A., DeVito, J.L., Stein, J.M. and Walsh, K.E. (1980) Functional analysis of hypothalamic control of cardiovascular responses accompanying emotional behavior. Fed. Proc. 391, 2487-2494.
Stephenson, R.B., Smith, O.A. and Scher, A.M. (1981) Baroreceptor regulation of heart rate in baboons during different behavioral states. Amer. J. Physiol. 241, R277-R285.
Takeshita, A., Tanaka, S., Kuroiwa, A. and Nakamura, M. (1975) Reduced baroreceptor sensitivity in borderline hypertension. Circulation 51, 738-742.
Thies, R. and Foreman, R.D. (1981) Descending inhibition of spinal neurons in the cardiopulmonary region by electrical stimulation of vagal afferent nerves. Brain Res. 207, 178-183.
Zanchetti, A., Baccelli, G. and Mancia, G. (1976) Fighting, emotions and exercise: cardiovascular effects in the cat; in Regulation of Blood Pressure by the Central Nervous System, G. Onesti, M. Fernandes and K.E. Kim, eds. Grune, New York, pp. 87-103.
Zanchetti, A., Mancia, G. and Malliani, A. (1980) Alterations of cardiovascular reflexes in hypertension. Clin. Exp. Hypertens. 2, 451-464.
Zucker, I.H. and Gilmore, J.P. (1981) Atrial receptor modulation of renal function in heart failure; in Disturbances in Neurogenic Control of the Circulation, F.M. Abboud et al., eds. Waverly Press, Baltimore, pp. 1-16.

Published 1982 by Elsevier Science Publishing Co., Inc.
Smith, Galosy, and Weiss, editors
CIRCULATION, NEUROBIOLOGY, AND BEHAVIOR

Task Force Report on Sudden Cardiac Death and Arrhythmias

Co-Chairmen:

JAMES E. SKINNER
Department of Neurology and Neuroscience Program, Baylor College of Medicine, Houston, Texas

RICHARD L. VERRIER
Cardiovascular Research, Department of Nutrition, Harvard School of Public Health, Boston, Massachusetts

SCOPE OF THE PROBLEM

The experience of coronary care units and studies of out-of-hospital resuscitation (Cobb et al., 1975; Friedman et al., 1973) indicate that the main mechanism for sudden death is ventricular fibrillation. In most persons who die suddenly, there is a background of ischemic heart disease. In a large number of cases, the heart disease is no worse than that found at random in persons who died from trauma, and in about 15% of the cases, no underlying pathology is detected (Kuller and Lillenfield, 1966; Moritz and Zamcheck, 1946; Spiekerman et al., 1962; Schwartz and Gerrity, 1975). Undetectable forms of acute ischemia, however, have not been ruled out as underlying causes (e.g., coronary spasm, platelet aggregation, or relative ischemia caused by metabolic overdrive).

In contrast, animal studies suggest that myocardial ischemia alone may not be sufficient to initiate ventricular fibrillation. For example, total cardiac denervation prevents the initiation of ventricular fibrillation following coronary artery occlusion (Ebert et al., 1970; Leriche et al., 1931). Furthermore, coronary artery occlusion in unanesthetized animals does not result in ventricular fibrillation if either psychologic stress is eliminated (Skinner et al., 1975) or a particular descending pathway, arising from the frontal cortex, is physically blocked (Skinner and Reed, 1981). Other investigators have shown that animals adapted to the laboratory do not manifest ventricular fibrillation following coronary artery occlusion (Gregg, 1971; Schaper, 1971), although they did not consider the interpretation of psychologic stress as the explanation of the results. Schaper thought the effect was due to a strain difference in dogs, while Gregg thought it may have been due to previous experience of myocardial ischemia. When these variables are controlled (Skinner et al. 1975), the phenomenon apparently remains.

Animal studies have shown that either exposure to behaviorally defined states of stress (Lown and Verrier, 1976; Skinner et al., 1975; Verrier and Lown, 1981) or electric stimulation of sympathetic neural structures (Corr and Gillis, 1978; Lown and Verrier, 1976; Malliani et al., 1980) will significantly enhance the susceptibility of the heart to ventricular fibrillation. The neural mechanisms that link the environmental stressors to the deleterious autonomic outflow are now beginning to be understood. Electrical stimulation along a frontocortical-hypothalamic-brain stem locus will produce, in the normal heart, both a variety of arrhythmias (Delgado, 1960; Garvey and Melville, 1969; Hockman et al., 1966; Manning and Cotten, 1962; Mauck et al., 1964; Melville et al., 1963; Weinberg and Fuster, 1960; Skinner et al., 1975) and cardiac myopathies (Hall et al., 1974; Hall et al., 1977; Ulyaninsky et al., 1977). The extreme effects include ventricular fibrillation (Garvey and Melville, 1969) and tissue necrosis. The same extreme patterns of lethal arrhythmias and permanent myocardial damage can be produced by external physical and psychological stressors (Corley et al., 1973; Johansson et al., 1974). These same types of external stressors can be shown to evoke specific event-related potentials and chemical perturbations within the frontocortical system (Skinner and Yingling, 1976, 1977; Skinner et al., 1978a,b). Thus, we are beginning to understand how an environmental situation of stress can be translated into specific cerebral events within a specific higher neural system that is known to regulate cardiac vulnerability.

There is now a substantial body of information that shows that psychosocial stressors are statistically significant predictors of sudden cardiac death in human populations (Jenkins, 1976; Parkes, 1967; Rahe et al., 1973; Rees and Lutkins, 1967; Reich et al., 1981; Rissanen et al., 1978; Vikhert et al., 1977; Wolf, 1969). These more recent and well-controlled studies confirm older anecdotal descriptions of the same phenomenon (Burrell, 1963; Cannon, 1942; Wolf, 1967). Although myocardial ischemia is certainly an important factor in sudden cardiac death, the above animal studies strongly suggest that it may not be the single primary cause, but rather is a sensitizing factor that predisposes the heart to ventricular fibrillation. Psychosocial factors may be the precipitating events for persons with ischemic heart disease, and perhaps even causal events in those few cases where pathology is not evident.

RESEARCH STRATEGIES

The objective is to identify the person at risk and then to intervene in the process so that death does not occur. The precipitating environmental stressors must first be perceived and interpreted by the brain before they are converted and delivered to the myocardium as deleterious autonomic outflow. Hence, there are three major points in the process at which potential intervention and containment of sudden cardiac death could occur: stressor source, central nervous system (CNS) transducer, and autonomic effector.

Beginning at the initial point in the process, the source of the environmental stressor could simply be removed. This type of intervention appears to explain why certain rural societies that experience very low incidences of psychosocial stress also manifest low sudden death rates (Vikhert, 1977; Wolf, 1969). However, the moving of participants in modern urban settings to rural surroundings is not only impossible, but the act of moving to a new environment may itself increase risk, as suggested by both human (Rahe et al., 1973) and animal (Skinner et al., 1975) studies.

At the next step, intervention could be sought within the central neural mechanisms that underlie the perception and interpretation of the stressor. Collectively, individuals vary a great deal in their perception of a given stressor, and single individuals can change their reaction to a given stressor over time. This plasticity of cognitive response suggests that a clinically created change in the cerebral interpretation of the environmental stressor, by either a behavioral or pharmacologic means, could minimize the reactive autonomic outflow. Although the results of experiments related to behavioral modification of autonomic outflow have demonstrated the feasibility of this approach, there has been no clear demonstration that such psychological changes have any enduring effects or are of sufficient magnitude to actually achieve intervention in the process of sudden death.

Alternatively, pharmacologic blockade in the higher telencephalic centers could directly and forcefully intervene in the mechanism of sudden death. Three centrally acting drugs have been found to have very significant antiarrhythmic effects in the ischemic hearts of both animals and humans. Imipramine, a tricyclic antidepressant, produces 80% to 90% reduction of premature ventricular beats in depressed patients with chronic arrhythmias (Bigger et al., 1977; Giardina et al., 1979). Diazepam, an antianxiety compound, delays the onset and reduces the severity of ventricular arrhythmias following coronary artery occlusion in stressed dogs (Rosenfeld et al., 1978). Ethmozin, a phenothiazine derivative of the neuroleptic class of drugs, produces almost complete abolition of premature ventricular beats and ventricular tachycardia in patients with chronic arrhythmias (Pratt et al., in press). Both imipramine (Weld and Bigger, 1980) and ethmozin (Hoffman, 1980; Rozenshtraukh et al., 1979) have peripheral quinidine-like properties in the myocardium that could explain their antiarrhythmic effects. Their central action, however, may be the most significant factor. For example, ethmozin at low doses that will block spontaneous arrhythmias of ischemic origin will not affect the induction of arrhythmias produced by electric stimulation of the myocardium in either dogs (Rozenshtraukh et al., 1978) or humans (Mann, personal communication). If the peripheral quinidine-like effects were responsible for reversing the spontaneous arrhythmias, then the threshold for the electric induction of arrhythmias should have been raised.

The third point of intervention in the process by which psychosocial factors increase cardiac vulnerability is in the autonomic pathways between the brain and the heart. Since all autonomic outflow must funnel through the peripheral nerves, total peripheral autonomic blockade by drugs could, logically, have the same beneficial effect as that of total cardiac denervation. Peripheral autonomic blockade by the use of competitive inhibitors, however, is not equal to surgical denervation. There is always a trade-off between the degree of competitive inhibition and its toxicity, and hence, total neural blockade is generally not achievable.

Peripheral adrenergic competitive inhibitors can, however, prevent the increases in some measures of cardiac vulnerability that occur in response to some types of psychologic stressors (Verrier and Lown, in press). For example, tolamolol will prevent the lowering of the repetitive extrasystole threshold in dogs that is produced in the control state by instrumentally conditioned shock-avoidance behavior (Matta et al., 1976). This beta-receptor antagonist will also prevent the shortening of the latency to the first premature ventricular beat after coronary occlusion, which is normally elicited in the control state by an environment unfamiliar to the animal or by cutaneous shocks (Rosenfeld et al., 1978). Beta-receptor inhibition by propranolol, however, will not prevent the onset of ventricular fibrillation following more prolonged coronary artery occlusion when the animal is stressed by an unfamiliar laboratory (Skinner et al., 1975). These findings together suggest that although peripherally acting beta-receptor inhibition may block some measures of cardiac vulnerability in the ischemic heart, it may not prevent the lethal arrhythmia itself.

The use of competitive inhibitors at sites in the CNS may prevent the development of the descending deleterious autonomic outflow. That is, the incomplete blockade in a higher central target may disrupt the functioning of the related system and therefore completely inhibit the deleterious autonomic outflow. This strategy of intervention at the second point in the process has great potential, and is supported by the observation that physical intervention in the brain of a stressed animal does prevent the lethal consequence of coronary artery occlusion (Skinner and Reed, 1981), and by the recent evidence that the centrally acting drugs have striking antiarrhythmic effects (Bigger et al., 1977; Giardina et al., 1979; Pratt et al., in press; Rosenfeld et al., 1978).

RECOMMENDATIONS

1. Because of the great potential for the development of higher central pharmaco logic intervention in the process by which psychosocial stressors trigger sudden cardiac death, this general approach to the problem should receive increased attention. Current methods are available in neuroscience for identifying cerebral structures that impinge upon known autonomic outflow systems. These studies should receive initial support, and then once candidate cerebral systems have been identified anatomically and histo-chemically, specific animal models of psychosocial factors and cardiac vulnerability can be used to determine whether or not the functioning of a specific candidate system is both necessary and sufficient for the occurrence of ventricular fibrillation in the ischemic and/or normal heart. The underlying electrophysiological and neurochemical patterns of

activity within these identified candidate systems can then be sought to provide the rationale for later attempts at pharmacologic intervention. Paralleling these cerebral studies, the development of psychosocial stress tests should be encouraged to enable identification of the patient-at-risk. This will enable the effective application of the pharmacologic interventions that are aimed at the higher cerebral targets.

2. Because myocardial ischemia is the most significant risk factor, research must continue to be directed toward the elimination of ischemic heart diseases. Of particular interest is the effect of stress and catecholamines on platelet aggregation and arterial plaque formation. Also, alpha- and beta-receptor control of coronary vasospasm needs clarification as a possible mechanism that may contribute to sudden cardiac death. Chronic and acute ischemic episodes, and their recovery (e.g., reperfusion), produce electrical instability in the cardiac ventricle. How does this occur and what is the role of the nervous system in this mechanism? The mechanism that relates ischemia to the biobehavioral trigger factors that precipitate ventricular fibrillation is not yet known, and certainly deserves systematic investigation.

3. Since all higher cerebral projections to the heart must funnel through the brain stem, spinal cord, and peripheral nerves, the traditional neurocardiac investigations must continue, but it is now clear that these studies must attend to the idea of powerful descending central neural control, an action that can be observed only in the unanesthetized animal. Evaluations of potential antiarrhythmic therapies must be made in the conscious animal model to determine what the efficacy is, relative to that observed *in situ* or *in vitro*, when the CNS is functionally intact and psychological state is controlled. Promising peripheral therapies include partial surgical sympathectomy, parasympathetic nerve activation, alpha- and beta-receptor inhibition, cholinergic-muscarinic receptor excitation, inward calcium current modulation, cyclic nucleotide regulation, and protein phosphorylation control. Although these therapies show great promise in *in vitro* or *in situ* preparations, they may or may not have a significant impact on models of sudden cardiac death in conscious animals or in human populations suffering from this malady.

4. Other areas of CNS functioning and cardiac vulnerability need to be studied. For example, how behavioral and electric activation of the brain results in cardiac myopathy is not clear. How neural patterns of activity produce arrhythmias in the apparently normal heart requires further investigation. Psychological stressors evoke event-related cerebral potentials; is there a relation between a specific potential and a measure of cardiac vulnerability? Natural sleep stages have an effect on premature ventricular beats of ischemic origin; the central and peripheral mechanisms mediating this phenomenon need to be elucidated.

5. The general conclusion is that there is sufficient evidence to establish that biobehavioral factors have a powerful influence on cardiac vulnerability. The specific

recommendation is that underlying neural mechanisms be sought so that intervention can be made in the process of sudden cardiac death. In view of the fact that no clear reversal of ischemic heart diseases is currently possible, this alternative approach may soon provide a means to prevent the lethal consequences of myocardial ischemia. Even if atherosclerotic heart disease were eliminated completely, evidence indicates that sudden cardiac death might still exist as a major health problem. This means that the pursuit of the neural mechanisms by which psychosocial stressors regulate cardiac vulnerability will have a scientific payoff that is independent of the results obtained from research in the area of ischemic heart disease.

REFERENCES

Bigger, T.J., Giardina, E.G.V., Perel, J.M., Kantor, S.J. and Glassman, A.H. (1977) Cardiac antiarrhythmic effect of imipramine hydrochloride. N. Engl. J. Med. 296, 206-208.

Burrell, R.J.W. (1963) The possible bearing of curse death and other factors in Bantu culture on the etiology of myocardial infarction; in The Etiology of Myocardial Infarction, T.N. James and J.W. Keys, eds. Henry Ford Hospital International Symposium. Little Brown and Co., Boston.

Cannon, W.B. (1942) "Voodoo" death. Amer. Anthropol. 44, 169-181.

Cobb, L.A., Baum, R.S., Alvarez, H. and Schaffer, W.A. (1975) Resuscitation from out-of-hospital ventricular fibrillation: 4 year follow up. Circulation 52, III223-III235.

Corley, K.C., Shiel, F.O'M., Mauck, H.P. and Greenhoot, J. (1973) Electrocardiographic and cardiac morphologic changes associated with environmental stress in squirrel monkeys. Psychosom. Med. 35, 361-364.

Corr, P.B. and Gillis, R.A. (1978) Autonomic neural influences on the dysrhythmias resulting from myocardial infarction. Circulat. Res. 43, 1-9.

Delgado, J.M.R. (1960) Circulatory effects of cortical stimulation. Physiol. Rev. 40, Suppl 4, 146-171.

Ebert, P.A., Vandeerveek, R.B., Allgood, R.J., and Sabiston, D.C., Jr. (1970) Effect of chronic cardiac denervation of arrhythmias after coronary artery ligation. Cardiovasc. Res. 4, 141-147.

Friedman, M., Manwaring, J.H., Rosenman, R.H., Donlon, G., Ortega, P. and Grube, S.M. (1973) Instantaneous and sudden deaths. J. Amer. Med. Ass. 225, 1319-1328.

Garvey, J.L. and Melville, K.I. (1969) Cardiovascular effects of lateral hypothalamic stimulation in normal and coronary-ligated dogs. J. Cardiovasc. Surg. 10, 377-385.

Giardina, E., Bigger, J.T., Glassman, A.H., Perel, J.M. and Kantor, S.J. (1979) The electrocardiographic and antiarrhythmic effects of imipramine hydrochloride at therapeutic plasma concentrations. Circulation 60, 1045-1052.

Gregg, D.E. (1971) Sudden cardiac death; in The Artery and the Process of Arteriosclerosis, S. Wolf, ed. Plenum Press, New York, p. 273.

Hall, R.E., Livingston, R.R. and Bloor, M.D. (1977) Orbital cortical influences on cardiovascular dynamics and myocardial structure in conscious monkeys. J. Neurosurg. 46, 638-647.

Hall, R.E., Sybers, H.D., Greenhoot, J.H. and Bloor, C.M. (1974) Myocardial alterations after hypothalamic stimulation in the intact conscious dog. Amer. Heart J. 88, 770-776.

Hockman, C.H., Mauck, H.P. and Hoff, E.C. (1966) ECG changes resulting from cerebral stimulation. II. A spectrum of ventricular arrhythmias of sympathetic origin. Amer. Heart J. 71, 695-701.

Hoffman, E.G. (1980) Status report of effects of Ethmozin in oral toxicity studies using *Cynomolgus* monkeys. Endo Labs, Garden City, New York.

Jenkins, C.D. (1976) Recent evidence supporting psychosocial risk factors for coronary disease. N. Engl. J. Med. 294, 987 and 1033.

Johansson, G., Johnsson, L., Lannek, N., Blomgren, L., Lindberg, P. and Pouph, O. (1974) Severe stress-cardiopathy in pigs. Amer. Heart J. 87, 451-457.

Kuller, L. and Lillenfield, A. (1966) Epidemiological study of sudden and unexpected death due to arteriosclerotic heart disease. Circulation 34, 1056.

Leriche, R., Herman, L. and Fontaine, R. (1931) Ligature de la coronaire gauche et fonction de colur apres enervation sympathique. C. R. Soc. Biol. (Paris), 107, 547-548.

Lown, B. and Verrier, R.L. (1976) Neural activity and ventricular fibrillation. N. Engl. J. Med. 294, 1165-1170.

Malliani, A., Schwartz, P.J. and Zanchetti, A. (1980) Neural mechanisms in life-threatening arrhythmias. Amer. Heart J. 100, 705-715.

Mann, D. (personal communication) This clinical study is currently in progress in the Methodist Hospital, Houston, Texas. Current results are from 10 patients. Published in abstract form in Houston Electrophysiologic Society Newsletter, 1981.

Manning, J.W. and Cotten, M. de V. (1962) Mechanism of cardiac arrhythmias induced by diencephalic stimulation. Amer. J. Physiol. 203, 1120-1124.

Matta, R.J., Lawler, J.E. and Lown, B. (1976) Ventricular electrical instability in the conscious dog. Effects of psychologic stress and beta adrenergic blockade. Amer. J. Cardiol. 38, 594-598.

Mauck, H.P., Hockman, C.H. and Hoff, E.C. (1964) ECG changes after cerebral stimulation of the mesencephalic reticular formation. Amer. Heart J. 68, 98-101.

Melville, K.I., Blum, B., Shister, H.E. and Silver, M.D. (1963) Cardiac ischemic changes in arrhythmias induced by hypothalamic stimulation. Amer. J. Cardiol. 12, 781-791.

Moritz, A.R. and Zamcheck N. (1946) Sudden and unexpected death of young soldiers. Arch. Pathol. 42, 459-494.

Parkes, C.M. (1967) Bereavement. Brit. Med. J. 4, 13.

Pratt, C.M., Yepsen, S.C., Francis, M.J., Taylor, A.A., Waggoner, A.D., Lewis, R.A. and Miller, R.R. (in press) Ethmozin: a unique antiarrhythmic drug with combined efficacy and excellent tolerance. Circulation.

Rahe, R.H., Bennett, L. Romo, M., Seltanen, P. and Arthur, R.S. (1973) Subjects's recent life changes and coronary heart disease in Finland. Amer. J. Psychiat. 130, 1222-1226.

Rees, W.D. and Lutkins, S.G. (1967) Mortality of bereavement. Brit. Med. J. 4, 13.

Reich, P., DeSilva, R.A., Lown, B. and Murawski, J. (1981) Acute psychological disturbances preceding life-threatening ventricular arrhythmias. J. Amer. Med. Ass. 246, 233-235.

Rissanen, V., Romo, M. and Seltanen, P. (1978) Premonitory symptoms and stress factors preceding sudden death from ischemic heart disease. Acta Med. Scand. 204, 389.

Rosenfeld, J., Rosen, M.R. and Hoffman, B.F. (1978) Pharmacologic and behavioral effects on arrhythmias that immediately follow abrupt coronary occlusion: a canine model of sudden coronary death. Amer. J. Cardiol. 41, 1075-1082.

Rozenshtraukh, L.V., Aniukhovsky, E.P., Beloshapko, G.G., Dremin, S.A., Chikharev, V.N., Lyskovtsev, V.V. and Senova, Z.P. (1979) Decrease in fast inward sodium current as a possible cause of the antiarrhythmic effect of Ethmozin, Mextil, and Lidocaine in the late stage of experimental myocardial infarction; in Sudden Cardiac Death: Second USA-USSR Joint Symposium. DHEW No. (NIH) 81-2101, US Govt. Printing Office, Washington, D.C., pp. 119-138.

Rozenshtraukh, L., Verrier, R.L. and Lown, B. (1978) Effect of Ethmozin in vulnerability to ventricular arrhythmias during the early phases of myocardial infarction. Newslett. Acad. Med. Sci. Soviet Union 10, 52-57.

Schaper, W. (1971) The Collateral Circulation of the Heart. North-Holland, Amsterdam.

Schwartz, C.J. and Gerrity, R.G. (1975) Anatomical pathology of sudden unexpected cardiac death. Circulation 52, 18-26.

Skinner, J.E., Lie, J.T. and Entman, M.L. (1975) Modification of ventricular fibrillation latency following coronary artery occlusion in the conscious pig: the effects of psychological stress and beta-adrenergic blockade. Circulation 51, 656-667.

Skinner, J.E. and Reed, J.C. (1981) Blockade of a frontocortical-brainstem pathway prevents ventricular fibrillation of the ischemic heart in pigs. Amer. J. Physiol. 240, H156-H163.

Skinner, J.E., Reed, J.C., Welch, K.M.A. and Nell, J.H. (1978a) Cutaneous shock produced correlated shifts in slow potential amplitude and cyclic 3', 5'-adenosine monophosphate level in the parietal cortex of the conscious rat. J. Neurochem. 30, 699-704.

Skinner, J.E., Welch, K.M.A., Reed, J.C. and Nell, J.H. (1978b) Psychological stress reduced cyclic 3', 5'-adenosine monophosphate level in the parietal cortex of the conscious rat. J. Neurochem. 30, 691-698.

Skinner, J.E. and Yingling, C.D. (1976) Regulation of slow potential shifts in nucleus reticularis thalami by the mesencephalic reticular formation and the frontal cortex. Electroenceph. Clin. Neurophysiol. 40, 288-296.

Skinner, J.E. and Yingling, C.D. (1977) Central gating mechanisms that regulate event-related potentials and behavior: a neural model for attention; in Progress in Clinical Neurophysiology, Vol. 1, J.E. Desmedt, ed. Karger, Brussels, pp. 70-96.

Spiekerman, R.E., Brandenburg, J.T., Achor, R.W.P. and Edward, J.E. (1962) Spectrum of coronary heart disease in a community of 30,000: clinicopathologic study. Circulation 25, 57.

Ulyaninsky, L.S., Stepanyan, E.P. and Krymsky, I.P. (1977) Cardiac arrhythmias of hypothalamic origin in sudden death; in Proceedings USA-USSR Joint Symposium on Sudden Death. DHEW No. (NIH) 78-1472, US Govt. Printing Office, Wasington, D.C.

Verrier, R.L. and Lown, B. (1981) Autonomic nervous system and malignant cardiac arrhythmias; in Brain, Behavior and Bodily Disease, H. Weiner, M.A. Hofer and A.J. Stunkard, eds. Raven Press, New York. (Ass. Res. Nerv. Ment. Dis., Res. Pub. 59, 273-291).

Verrier, R.L. and Lown, B. (in press) Adrenergic blockade and the prevention of behaviorally induced cardiac arrhythmias. Excerpta Medica.

Vikhert, A.M., Velisheva, L.A. and Matova, E.E. (1977) Geographic distribution and pathology of sudden death in the Soviet Union; in USA-USSR First Symposium on Sudden Death. DHEW No. (NIH) 78-1470, US Govt. Printing Office, Washington D.C., pp. 19-40.

Weinberg, S.J. and Fuster, J.M. (1960) Electrocardiographic changes produced by localized hypothalamic stimulations. Ann. Intern. Med. 53, 332-341.

Weld, F.M. and Bigger, J.T., Jr. (1980) Electrophysiological effects of imipramine on ovine cardiac Purkinje and ventricular muscle fibers. Circulat. Res. 46, 167-175.

Wolf, S. (1967) Neural mechanisms in sudden cardiac death. The Jeremiah Metzger Lecture. Trans. Amer. Clin. Climatol. Ass. 79, 158-176.

Wolf, S. (1969) Psychosocial forces in myocardial infarction and sudden death. Circulation 39/40, IV74-IV81.

Published 1982 by Elsevier Science Publishing Co., Inc.
Smith, Galosy, and Weiss, editors
CIRCULATION, NEUROBIOLOGY, AND BEHAVIOR

Task Force Report on Arteriosclerosis

Co-Chairmen:

DAVID C. RANDALL
Department of Physiology and Biophysics, University of Kentucky, Lexington, Kentucky

J. ALAN HERD
Sid W. Richardson Institute for Preventive Medicine, The Methodist Hospital, Houston, Texas

INTRODUCTION

There is compelling evidence that behaviors that can be objectively defined are reliably associated with characteristic cardiovascular (CV) response patterns. These CV and behavioral patterns are integrated within the central nervous system (CNS) and expressed via classically described neuroendocrine and somatomotor pathways. Such CNS integration of complex response patterns is attracting interest among neurobiologists, particularly as regards the increasingly obvious probability that certain biobehavioral factors may be linked to the development of CV disease including coronary artery disease (CAD) and coronary arteriosclerosis. Much of this evidence was reviewed during the present workshop. The purpose of this report is to summarize (1) the general nature of these behaviorally linked CV response patterns, (2) the evidence linking specific behaviorally coupled risk factors to the development of CAD and/or coronary arteriosclerosis, and (3) recommendations for future research.

Characteristics of Behaviorally Coupled CV Response Patterns

A number of carefully defined behavioral paradigms have been used to study behaviorally coupled CV response patterns. For example, Anderson (this volume) presents data demonstrating that increases in blood pressure (BP) and total peripheral resistance (TPR) with concomitant decreases in heart rate (HR) occur in "anticipation" of shock avoidance sessions in dogs; the avoidance sessions proper result in further elevations in BP and HR, with decreases in TPR (Anderson and Tosheff, 1973). Other examples of such patterns could be cited for classical conditioning in man (Obrist et al., 1974 and this volume), nonhuman primates (Randall et al., 1975, 1976; Smith et al., 1980) and other species (Galosy et al., 1981). Definite links between behavior and CV responses have also been observed in nonaversive situations, including eating, drinking and exercise for food reward (Galosy et al., 1981). Complex social situations involving dominant-subordinate individual interactions or other competitive behaviors are likewise characterized by decided alterations in the CV and neuroendocrine status of the subject (Henry, this volume).

While the ultimate synthesis of the diverse findings reported at this conference will depend on the outcome of much subsequent interdisciplinary research, certain heuristic generalizations regarding these CV response patterns may be made:

(1) Feeding and ingestive behaviors seem to be associated with increases in mesenteric blood flow and cardiac output and with decreases in renal, muscle and skin blood flow.

(2) Classical aversive or avoidance conditioning (also including "defense reactions") elicit increases in cardiac output and muscle blood flow with decreases in renal, mesenteric and skin blood flow; coronary vascular resistance may increase transiently owing to elevated alpha-adrenergic tone.

(3) Diving induces decreases in cardiac output and depression of renal, skin, mesenteric and muscle blood flows.

(4) Preavoidance (Anderson, this volume) and immobile confrontation (Zanchetti, 1976) are characterized by vasoconstriction in skeletal muscle and no change or a decrease in cardiac output.

The nervous system clearly plays a dominant role in overall intergration of these response patterns, and a rather detailed analysis of this neuroendocrine involvement has been possible in a number of cases. With respect to the peripheral autonomic nerves, for example, the vagus plays a predominant role in eliciting the conditional tachycardia during aversive conditioning in healthy college men (Obrist et al., this volume). Increases in sympathetic activity to selected vascular beds and the heart are important in other components of this and similar behaviorally induced CV response patterns (Cohen and Obrist, 1975; Williams et al., 1975; Smith et al., 1979). Other formative experiments have elucidated important aspects regarding the corresponding role of the CNS. For example, stimulation at a specific hypothalamic site gives rise to the same pattern of CV adjustment that is elicited during a behaviorally induced conditioned emotional response (Smith et al., 1979). Placing a bilateral lesion in the brain at this precise location eliminates the CV concomitants of the behaviorally evoked response. In addition, stimulation of the AV3V area of the hypothalamus gives rise to a specific pattern of CV adjustment including changes in hindlimb, renal, and mesenteric blood flow that is reminiscent of some of the flow adjustments enumerated in the previous paragraph (Fink et al., 1978; Brody and Johnson, 1981). For more detailed discussions of the neural involvement in control of these behaviorally mediated CV responses, see Smith (1974) and Randall and Smith (in press).

One particularly important feature of the physiological response to environmental events is that the overall pressure and/or volume load on the heart is often elevated, thereby increasing myocardial metabolic demand. Circulating hormones are often released, including epinephrine, norepinephrine, cortisol, etc., which mobilize the CV and metabolic resources of the organism. Several lines of evidence indicate that certain of these physiological responses influence the basic processes of proliferation of vascular smooth muscle cells, arteriosclerosis and CAD; they may also precipitate vascular spasm, platelet aggregation, lipid mobilization, endocrine hypersecretion, and autonomic dysfunction (Schwartz and Stone, 1980, in press). Furthermore, differences are seen in qualitative and quantitative responses of individuals to environmental and behavioral stress factors and may be predictive of pathological consequences (Williams, 1978, 1981, in press). It is also known that adjustments occur in many of these involuntary as well as voluntary responses since learning of effective coping strategies, classical and operant conditioning, physical conditioning, and adaptations to new situations all affect physiological responses that can predispose to arteriosclerosis and complications of coronary heart disease

BIOBEHAVIORAL RISK FACTORS
IN THE ETIOLOGY OF CAD AND ARTERIOSCLEROSIS
Neural Control of the Coronary Vasculature

Although neural and neuroendocrine factors have long been implicated in the genesis of other CV diseases, notably hypertension, relatively less evidence has been marshaled vis-a-vis CAD and/or coronary arteriosclerosis; this may reflect the traditional viewpoint, which emphasizes the importance of metabolic factors in the control of the coronary circulation while minimizing the role of extrinsic controls. During the course of the conference, in fact, it became apparent that there is still a paucity of data related to neural control of the coronary vasculature. Although some participants suggested possible mechanisms directed to the afferent and efferent interconnections affecting autonomic nervous system and target organs (see chapters by Loewy, Manning, Schramm, Dormer and Stone, Swanson, and Weaver; see also Schwartz and Stone, 1977, 1979; Stone, 1980), the specific effects on the coronary vasculature and myocardium were not addressed. Gillis (this volume) and Segal et al. (in press a) showed that coronary resistance was increased by application of drugs that block GABA in the brain and that sectioning the cardiac sympathetic efferent fibers abolished the increase in coronary resistance. Lesions or electrical stimulation studies of select areas of the CNS, including the AV3V region of the hypothalamus, nucleus tractus solitarius, the A5 catecholamine cell group, and the glycine sensitive area of the medulla, have shown that these loci may (1) serve as target tissue,

(2) contain fibers of passage, or (3) be a source of modulation of fibers controlling CV systems (see chapters by Loewy, Smith et al., Johnson, and Gebber et al.).

Several recent behavioral experiments have indicated that the neural control mechanisms identified above are active in the intact, awake animal. Classical aversive conditioning in dog produces a transient but significant increase in coronary vascular resistance which is mediated by increased alpha-adrenergic tone (Billman and Randall, 1980, 1981). Similar findings have been reported in dogs suspended in a Pavlovian sling in which they had been shocked previously (Verrier and Lown, 1981). Sympathetic vaso-constrictor tone can also limit the increase in coronary blood flow during exercise in dog (Gwirtz and Stone, 1981). Only a few behavioral situations have been studied in this regard, and essentially no work of this nature has been done in animals whose hearts are compromised by existing "disease" states. The effects of long-term exposure to behavioral stress on the coronary vasculature of experimental animals are unknown. Nevertheless, the data do indicate that the autonomic nervous system has the **potential** to modulate coronary vasomotor tone as a component of an ongoing pathological process.

Endocrine Factors Related to Arteriosclerosis and Complications of Coronary Heart Disease

The association between endocrine hypersecretion and coronary arteriosclerosis is most evident with cortisol. Young men with arteriosclerotic lesions of coronary arteries have a reduced rate of decline in plasma cortisol levels during the late morning hours compared with men who have no such lesions (Troxler et al., 1977). Cortisol treatment of patients with lupus erythematosis or rheumatoid arthritis increases the incidence of CAD. Endogenous hypersecretion of cortisol in patients with Cushing's Disease also increases the severity of coronary arteriosclerosis.

Experiments in nonhuman primates support the conclusions from clinical studies that cortisol aggravates arteriosclerosis. Cynomolgus macaques treated with oral cortisol and a high-fat, high-cholesterol diet showed more severe aortic atherosclerosis than animals treated with either the high-fat, high-cholesterol diet or the cortisol alone. Neuro-biological mechanisms whereby cortisol may be secreted in response to psychological or behavioral processes include the simultaneous release of ACTH and beta-endorphin as constituents of the same parent molecule released from the posterior pituitary. Although the mechanism of action for beta-endorphin in peripheral blood is uncertain, both ACTH and beta-endorphin are released into the circulation in response to painful stimuli and during intense physical exertion. ACTH released under such circumstances elicits secretion of cortisol from the adrenal cortex. The neurobiologic mechanisms involved in release of ACTH and beta-endorphin are worthy of further study.

Cortisol secretion influences several metabolic processes, which may influence the development of arteriosclerosis and contribute to complications of CAD. Chronic administration of cortisol enhances lipid mobilization and inhibits glucose transport into cells. Thus, high levels of cortisol elevate the turnover rates of free fatty acids and reduce glucose utilization, thereby potentially enhancing arteriosclerotic processes. Also, the increased myocardial utilization of free fatty acids increases myocardial oxygen requirements and predisposes to dysrhythmias, especially in the presence of inadequate coronary blood flow.

Other endocrines under the influence of pituitary releasing factors include testosterone and thyroid hormone. Both have been shown to influence arteriosclerosis and complications of CAD. Other endocrines under the influence of sympathetic nervous activity include insulin and epinephrine, and both play important roles in lipid metabolism, glucose metabolism, cardiac function, and arteriosclerosis. Finally, manipulations of the CNS, such as placement of lesions (Friedman et al., 1969) or electrical stimulation (Gutstein et al., 1968), have been shown to influence plasma lipid levels; this provides support for elucidating mechanisms associated with coronary heart disease. There are large gaps in our understanding of afferent, integrative and efferent interactions on the coronary vasculature.

Hypertension as a Risk Factor in Atherosclerosis

There is no doubt that elevated arterial pressure, which may occur secondarily to behavioral stress, is a risk factor for atherosclerosis. However, the epidemiologic meaning of a "risk factor" is that these conditions are **correlated** and thus does not imply a causal link. Therefore, although it is widely assumed that hypertension causes atherosclerosis, the epidemiologic data do not allow us to jump directly to this conclusion. In fact, although treatment of hypertension can reduce many of the cardiac sequelae of the disease, it does not actually reduce the risk (i.e., correlation) of atherosclerosis. In fact, one might easily hypothesize that atherosclerosis causes hypertension, through renal disease, through changes in vessel stiffness, through contributions in peripheral resistance, or through other mechanisms. According to this hypothesis, the apparent causal relation that has been widely assumed may simply be an artifact of detectability: the physician can detect hypertension more easily than he can detect hemodynamically insignificant atheromas. Simply because the hypertensive patient has not yet manifested atherosclerotic disease does not rule out the possibility that he may already have such disease. Clearly, a great deal of research remains to be done regarding the role of one of the most cited biobehavioral risk factors in CAD.

Individual Personality Profile and CAD

A great deal of research has been done concerning the hypothesis that individuals with different personalities may have correspondingly different risks for development of CAD (Review Panel on Coronary-Prone Behavior, 1981). As an illustration of such research, we might consider the recent study by Williams et al. (1981). Young men performed a mental arithmetic task (hypothesized to produce a muscle vasodilatation like that seen in defense reaction) and a reaction-time task (hypothesized to produce a muscle vasoconstriction like that seen in immobile confrontation). Responses of several CV parameters to these two tasks were measured and continuous blood samples were obtained during baseline and task periods so that a broad array of neuroendocrine responses could be measured as well. Subjects were characterized as Type A or Type B using the Jenkins Activity Survey (Jenkins et al., 1979). The purpose of the study was to determine whether young male Type A subjects would exhibit CV and/or neuroendocrine hyperresponsivity (relative to the responses of Type B individuals) to either or both behavioral challenges. If so, it might be inferred that hyperresponsivity plays a role in the increased rates of both acute coronary events and coronary atherosclerosis among Type A persons.

In response to mental arithmetic, Type A subjects showed significantly greater muscle vasodilatation as well as larger increases in plasma epinephrine, norepinephrine and cortisol than did Type B subjects, while both types displayed similar increases in plasma prolactin levels. During the reaction-time task, cortisol and prolactin were not increased and there were no differences between Type A and B subjects in CV or neuroendocrine responses. However, there was a larger increase in cortisol during the reaction-time task among Type A men with a family history of CV disease than among Type B men with similar histories. In contrast, among those with no family history of CV disease, Type A men showed a smaller cortisol response to the reaction-time task than did Type B men. As noted in a previous section of this report, cortisol hyperresponsivity could be of particular importance in atherogenesis via effects on both lipid metabolism and sympathetic nervous system function.

Undoubtedly, these CV and neuroendocrine adjustments to the mental arithmetic and reaction-time tasks are mediated in the brain. The hyperresponsivity observed among Type A subjects could help to explain why they are at increased risk of developing coronary atherosclerosis and its complications. Identification of CNS mechanisms responsible for these effects would aid in understanding how they are produced, as well as in formulating means for preventing them.

Reinfarction: Possible Sympathetic Nervous System Involvement

Data presented at these meetings demonstrated that sympathetic outflow can have a target-organ specificity (Weaver, this volume). Thus, it is conceivable that sympathetic vasoconstrictor activity could be directed specifically to the coronary vasculature. Vasospasm is conceivable as a consequence. In light of evidence that a spinal sympathosympathetic reflex, with afferents carried in the cardiac sympathetic nerves, can be triggered by myocardial ischemia or by dyskinetic wall motion (Weaver, this volume), it is possible that the infarcted heart is at greater risk for generating such activity. Because such a reflex may place significant additional metabolic demands on the heart, both through direct inotropic and chronotropic mechanisms and through afterload effects, it may thereby contribute to reinfarction. Elsewhere in this volume, Gillis presents evidence that medullary pathways may stimulate coronary vasoconstriction (Segal et al., in press b), and it now appears that such stimulation can occur owing to a behavioral stressor (Randall, personal communication). Thus, CNS dysfunction or behavioral stressors may further compromise oxygen delivery to the postinfarcted heart. In light of this suggestive evidence, the role that biobehavioral risk factors actually play in reinfarction needs further, careful examination.

RECOMMENDATIONS FOR FURTHER RESEARCH

Additional research is clearly needed to (1) increase our understanding of how the CNS integrates both CV and neuroendocrine adjustments to environmental situations, ranging from psychosocial confrontation (e.g., intraspecific aggression/hostility) to the physical milieu (e.g., sodium content of the diet); and (2) apply such understanding to the problem of elucidating mechansisms of atherogenesis, i.e., predicting who will develop arteriosclerosis and under what circumstances. In this conference we have identified a number of specific phenomena that require additional investigative efforts. Recommendations are given below for general research strategies, rather than for specific experiments. This approach recognizes the nascent status of the field, and emphasizes the broad range of possibilities for development of creative research protocols.

Development of Adequate Experimental Animal Models

It is critically important to use an appropriate model in studying the interaction between behavioral stress and coronary artery disease; in a number of cases such models are lacking or require additional refinement. In recommending animal models for such experiments, we must address several key issues. First, the behavioral stressor should be such that activation of CNS structures subserving CV regulation can be documented. Second, the behavioral stressor must be quantified and reproducible in any given model. Third, CV variables should be recorded that provide a data base adequate to analyze the specific phenomena of interest; this often requires that one measure heart rate, arterial pressure, and a patterned flow response in one or more vascular beds. The endpoints of coronary artery disease/arteriosclerosis may be: (1) alteration in myocardial function, (2) an inappropriate decrease in coronary blood flow/oxygen demand ratio, (3) lactate production by the myocardium, (4) platelet aggregation *in vivo* or *in vitro,* and (5) alteration in the normal electrical properties of the myocardium. The model selected for studies of this nature must, therefore, be appropriately sensitive to these five points as well. An analysis of changes in the normal heart leading to alterations in the above variables is also crucial to our understanding of the interaction between behavior and CV disease. Finally, strategies that could be used to interrupt any synergism between behavioral stress and the disease should be considered where appropriate in model development.

With this background, any animal species in which such measurements and paradigms could be used would be appropriate, although it seems clear that certain animal models are better suited for specific studies. Members of the task force recommend that considerably more attention be given to this important aspect of the overall research problem.

Investigation of Central and Peripheral Autonomic Factors in CAD

A twofold research effort seems warranted in this area. First, continued investigations of the central integration of behavioral and coronary vascular function should be pursued aggressively. Investigators should strive toward clearer definition of the relevant neural pathways by using neuroanatomical techniques, such as autoradiography, horseradish peroxidase and dye transport, immunohistochemistry, and 2-deoxyglucose imaging. Neurophysiological techniques such as extracellular and intracellular recordings and antidromic activation of cells whose axons project to various nuclei should be used to examine the functional nature of these pathways. Microlesions, microstimulations and very small knife cuts in the brain also should be used to examine the control of blood flow in the coronary vascular bed. Central chemical stimulations including iontophoresis, push-pull cannulas, microinjections, local application using perspex rings, and osmotic mini-pumps could also add to our understanding of central integration, as well as efferent outflow. These studies can be done on anesthetized as well as conscious, behaving animals. Neuroendocrine studies of the hypothalamus and the pituitary gland will provide important contributions to our understanding of neural and endocrine interactions. The precise nature of the efferent outflow from the CNS to the coronary vasculature and heart should also be examined. These studies should include efforts to delineate the distribution of afferent and efferent fibers on the coronary vasculature, interactions at the ganglia, parasympathetic and sympathetic interactions, and responsivity of the coronary vasculature to circulating hormones and neurotransmitters.

The second recommended thrust stems from previous observations of behaviorally induced alterations in coronary vascular vasoconstrictor tone. Research should be undertaken to determine what behavioral and physiological manipulations increase the magnitude and/or duration of the potentially deleterious response patterns described earlier. For example, the physiological mechanisms responsible for the large and prolonged increase in coronary vascular resistance demonstrated to result from intra-cerebral infusions of picrotoxin cells (Gillis, this volume) could conceivably be activated during "appropriate" behavioral activities as yet unidentified; if so, the relevance of such situations to the etiology of CAD and arteriosclerosis is immediately obvious. Finally, as a correlated possibility, behavioral and physiological interventions that minimize such responses should be examined as possible preventive measures against coronary disease.

Future Research to Clarify Endocrine Involvement in the Development of CAD

The primary research in this area has focused on the CV components of behaviorally mediated response patterns. Much more work is needed to integrate these findings with concomitant neuroendocrine changes in circulating levels of catecholamines, cortisol, vasopressin, renin/angiotensin, and a myriad of other hormones.

As knowledge increases regarding (1) the specific patterns of CV and neuroendocrine responses that occur in conjunction with specific behaviors, and (2) the CNS mechanisms whereby such somatomotor/CV neuroendocrine response patterns are integrated, this knowledge can be brought to bear on the question of how behavioral factors might play a role in the etiology and pathogenesis of atherosclerosis.

Once again, at least two directions for future research promise to be especially productive at this juncture. The first would focus on explicitly examining the hypothesis that changes in neuroendocrine balances similar to those described during behavioral testing do, in fact, accelerate the development of CAD, arteriosclerosis, and eventual cardiomyopathy. This will require continued, and in some cases accelerated, research at the organ/system and tissue/cellular level.

Second, assuming that such links do exist, the specific humoral stimuli affecting the coronary arteries and other visceral organs need to be examined, including the effects of cortisol, bradykinin, angiotensin, prostaglandins, circulating catecholamines, CO_2, O_2 and hydrogen ion. The afferent, efferent and central pathways controlling these neuro-endocrine systems need to be examined, and their actual involvement during behavioral or environmental challenges documented. That is, to the extent that hemodynamic and neuroendocrine hyperresponsivity might be involved in the putative mechanisms of atherogenesis (endothelial injury, hyperlipidemia, immune function, etc.), a consideration of CNS-mediated, behaviorally induced alterations in these functions may lead to new insights regarding who is at risk to develop arteriosclerosis, and how the disease might be prevented.

Verification of a Causal Role of Hypertension in the Etiology of CAD

Epidemiologic and basic research directed at identifying causality in the relation between risk factors and development of CAD and atherosclerosis is clearly required. At a deeper level, research should be directed towards determining whether various types of hypertension are preferentially coupled with coronary disease, and what mechanisms are responsible for the association.

Strategies for Minimizing Reinfaction

A number of hypotheses regarding the etiology of reinfarction need to be examined critically. For example, it should be determined whether sympathetic hyperreactivity does contribute to the risk of reinfarction. Controlled trials of the CV effects of both alpha- and beta-adrenergic antagonists in at-risk humans are needed. Further research into cardio-coronary sympathetic reflexes and their possible role in the production of vasospasm, atherogenesis and thrombogenesis is warranted. Finally, research involving behavioral stress in postinfarction experimental animals is clearly warranted and may be expected to yield clinically applicable insights.

Further Studies on the Role of Personality in the Etiology of CAD

Epidemiologic studies have demonstrated that a certain type of behavior pattern is associated with an increased incidence in the development of coronary heart disease. This behavior pattern has been well characterized in terms of psychological responses and includes excessive drive, aggressiveness, and self-imposed time restraints (Type A behavior). Individuals with this behavior pattern can be diagnosed and characterized with accepted psychological testing procedures. Less is known, however, concerning the response dynamics of the CV system in these individuals. More studies should be performed to characterize the CV response in these individuals to other conditions such as lower body negative pressure, static exercise, dynamic exercise, pharmacologic activation, and blockade adrenergic receptors. It has also been shown that dynamic exercise training can modify the autonomic neural control of the CV system (Stone, 1977, 1980; Liang and Stone, in press). It would be worth considerable effort to determine whether such exercise-induced changes would alter the CV response of Type A individuals to stress. In addition, dynamic exercise can increase coronary reserve capacity and alter blood coagulation (Foreman et al., 1980; Stone, 1980; Gwirtz and Stone, 1981).

REFERENCES

Abboud, F.M. (1972) Control of various components of the peripheral vasculature. Fed. Proc. 31, 1226-1239.

Anderson, D.E. and Tosheff, J.G. (1973) Cardiac output and total peripheral resistance changes during preavoidance periods in the dog. J. Appl. Physiol. 34, 650-654.

Billman, G.E. and Randall, D.C. (1980) Classic aversive conditioning of coronary blood flow in mongrel dogs. Pavlov. J. Biol. Sci. 15, 93-101.

Billman, G.E. and Randall, D.C. (1981) Mechanisms mediating the coronary vascular response to behavioral stress in the dog. Circulat. Res. 48, 214-233.

Brody, M.J. and Johnson, A.K. (1981) Role of forebrain structures in models of experimental hypertension; in Disturbances in Neurogenic Control of the Circulation. Clinical Physiology Series, American Physiological Society. Williams & Wilkins Co., Baltimore, pp. 105-117.

Cohen, D.H. and Obrist, P.A. (1975) Interactions between behavior and the cardiovascular system. Circulat. Res. 37, 693.

Davis, D.L. and Baker, C.H. (1974) Arterial segment constriction under constant-pressure and constant-inflow perfusion. Amer. J. Physiol. 227, 1149-1157.

Dembroski, T.M., Weiss, S.M., Shields, J.M. et al. (1972) Coronary-Prone Behavior. Springer-Verlag, New York.

Feigl, E.O. (1974) The coronary circulation; in Physiology and Biophysics, T.C. Ruch and H.D. Patton, eds. Saunders, Philadelphia.

Fink, G.D., Buggy, J., Haywood, J.R., Johnson, A.K. and Brody, M.J. (1978) Hemodynamic responses to electrical stimulation of forebrain angiotensin and osmosensitive sites. Amer. J. Physiol. 235, H445-H451.

Foreman, R.D., Dormer, K.J., Ohata, C.A. and Stone, H.J. (1980) Neural control of the heart during arrhythmias and exercise. Fed. Proc. 39, 2519-2525.

Friedman, M., Elek, S. and Byers, S. (1969) Abolition of milieu-induced hyperlipemia in the rat by electrolytic lesion in the anterior hypothalamus. Proc. Soc. Exp. Biol. 131, 288-293.

Galosy, R.A., Clarke, L.K., Vasko, M.R. and Crawford, I.L. (1981) Neurophysiology and neuropharmacology of cardiovascular regulation and stress. Neurosci. Behav. Rev. 5, 137-175.

Gold, M.R. and Cohen, D.H. (1981) Modification of the discharge of vagal cardiac neurons during learned heart rate change. Science 214, 345-347.

Gutstein, W.H., Schneck, D.J. and Appleton, H.D. (1968) Association of increased plasma lipid levels with brain stimulation. Metabolism 17, 535-543.

Gwirtz, P.A. and Stone, H.L. (1981) Coronary blood flow and myocardial oxygen consumption following alpha-adrenergic blockade during submaximal exercise. J. Pharm. Exp. Therapeut. 217, 92-98.

Henry, J.P., Ely, D.L., Stephens, P.M., Ratcliffe, H.L., Santisteban, G.A. and Shapiro, A.P. (1971) The role of psychosocial factors in the development of arterial sclerosis in CBA mice; observations on the heart, kidney, aorta. Atherosclerosis 14, 203-218.

Isselbacher, K.J. et al., eds. (1980) Harrison's Principles of Internal Medicine, 9th edition. McGraw-Hill, New York.

Jenkins, C.D., Rosenman, R.H. and Zyzanski, S.J. (1979) Jenkins Activity Survey. The Psychological Corporation, New York.

Liang, I.Y.S. and Stone, H.L. (in press) Effect of exercise conditioning on coronary resistance. J. Appl. Physiol.

Obrist, P.A., Lawler, J.E., Howard, J.L., Smithson, K.W., Martin, P.L. and Manning, J. (1974) Sympathetic influences on cardiac rate and contractility during acute stress in humans. Psychophysiology 11, 405-427.

Randall, D.C., ed. (1977) Neural Regulation of the Heart. Oxford University Press, New York.

Randall, D.C., Brady, J.V. and Martin, K.H. (1975) Cardiovascular dynamics during classical appetitive and aversive conditioning in laboratory primates. Pavlov. J. Biol. Sci. 10, 66-75.

Randall, D.C., Brady, J.V. and Martin, K.H. (1976) Classical conditioning effects upon left and right ventricular pressures and their derivatives in non-human primates. Pavlov. J. Biol. Sci. 11, 125.

Randall, D.C. and Smith, O.A. (in press) Neural control of the heart in the intact conscious animal; in Nervous Control of the Heart, W.C. Randall, ed. Oxford Univ. Press, New York.

328

Review Panel on Coronary-Prone Behavior and Coronary Heart Disease (1981) Coronary-prone behavior and coronary heart disease: a critical review. Circulation 63, 1199-1215.

Schwartz, P.J. and Stone, H.L. (1977) Tonic influence of the sympathetic nervous system on myocardial reactive hyperemia and on coronary blood flow. Circulat. Res. 41, 51-58.

Schwartz, P.J. and Stone, H.L. (1979) Effects of unilateral stellectomy upon cardiac performance during exercise in dogs. Circulat. Res. 44, 637-645.

Schwartz, P.J. and Stone, H.L. (1980) Left stellectomy in the prevention of ventricular fibrillation due to acute myocardial ischemia in conscious dogs with an anterior myocardial infarction. Circulation 62, 1256-1265.

Schwartz, P.J. and Stone, H.L. (in press) The role of the autonomic nervous system in sudden death. Ann. N.Y. Acad. Sci.

Segal, S.A., Pearle, D.L. and Gillis, R.O. (in press a) Coronary spasm in the cat produced by increasing central sympathetic outflow to the heart. Amer. J. Cardiol.

Segal, S.A., Pearle, D.L. and Gillis, R.O. (in press b) Coronary spasm produced by picrotoxin in cats. Eur. J. Pharmacol.

Smith, O.A. (1974) Reflex and central mechanisms involved in the control of the heart and circulation. Ann. Rev. Physiol. 36, 93-124.

Smith, O.A., Astley, C.A., DeVito, J.L., Stein, J.M. and Walsh, K.E. (1980) Functional analysis of hypothalamic control of the cardiovascular responses accompanying emotional behavior. Fed. Proc. 39, 2487-2494.

Smith, O.A., Hohimer, A.R., Astley, C.A. and Taylor, D.J. (1979) Renal and hind limb vascular control during acute emotion in the baboon. Amer. J. Physiol. 236, R198-R205.

Stone, H.L. (1977) Cardiac function and exercise training in conscious dogs. J. Appl. Physiol. 42, 824-832.

Stone, H.L. (1980) Coronary flow, myocardial oxygen consumption and exercise training in dogs. J. Appl. Physiol. 49, 759-768.

Troxler, R.G., Sprague, E.A., Albanese, R.A., Fuchs, F. and Thompson, A.J. (1977) The association of elevated plasma cortisol and early atherosclerosis as demonstrated by coronary angiography. Atherosclerosis 26, 151-162.

Verrier, R.L. and Lown, B. (1981) Influence of psychologic stress on coronary vascular resistance in the conscious dog. Fed. Proc. 40, 566.

Williams, R.B. (1978) Psychophysiological processes, the coronary-prone behavior pattern, and coronary heart disease; in Coronary-Prone Behavior, T.M. Dembroski, S.M. Weiss, J.M. Shields et al., eds. Springer-Verlag, New York, pp. 141-146.

Williams, R.B. (1981) Behavioral factors in cardiovascular disease: an update; in Update V: The Heart, J.W. Nurst, ed. McGraw Hill, New York, pp. 219-230.

Williams, R.B. (in press) Correlates of angiographic findings; in Biobehavioral Bases of Coronary Heart Disease, T.M. Dembroski and T. Schmidt, eds. Karger, Basel.

Williams, R.B., Bittker, T.E., Bucksbaum, M.S. and Wynne, L.C. (1975) Cardiovascular and neurophysiologic correlates of sensory intake and rejection; I. Effect of cognitive tasks. Psychophysiology 12, 427-432.

Williams, R.B., Eichelman, B.S. and Ng, L.K.Y. (1972) Brain amine depletion reverses the blood pressure response to footshock in the rat. Nature (New Biology) 240, 276-277.

Williams, R.B., Lane, J.D., White, A.D., Kuhn, C.M. and Schonberg, S.M. (1981) Type A behavior pattern and neuroendocrine response during mental work. Paper presented at annual meeting, American Psychosomatic Society, Cambridge, Mass, March 1981.

Williams, R.B., Richardson, J.S. and Eichelman, B.S. (1978) Location of central nervous system neurones mediating blood pressure response of rats to shock-induced fighting. J. Behav. Med. 1, 177-185.

Zanchetti, A. (1976) Hypothalamic control of circulation; in The Nervous System in Arterial Hypertension, S. Julius and M.D. Esler, eds. Thomas, Springfield, Ill.

Task Force Report on Cardiomyopathy

Co-Chairmen:

KARL C. CORLEY, JR.
Department of Physiology, Medical College of Virginia, Richmond, Virginia

NEIL SCHNEIDERMAN
Department of Psychology, University of Miami, Coral Gables, Florida

The task force engaged in the clinical aspects of cardiomyopathy focused on relations among circulation, behavior, neurobiology, and myocardial injury. This report begins with brief descriptions of primary cardiomyopathy and diffuse myocardial injury, and the rationale for studying these pathological changes as a function of neurobiology and behavior. Pathological changes observed in the myocardium in response to behavioral stressors are described. Behavioral conditions leading to diffuse myocardial damage and the manner in which they are investigated are then discussed. Central nervous system (CNS) structures, putative neurotransmitter systems, and neurophysiological mechanisms are implicated in this integration of cardiovascular (CV) and emotional responses. These biological and behavioral mechanisms discussed by the conference participants are suggested as possible contributors to the development of cardiomyopathy. Hypotheses relating cardiac and hemodynamic factors to compromised function resulting from damage to the myocardium are also discussed.

PRIMARY CARDIOMYOPATHY

Primary cardiomyopathy refers to diseases that affect the heart muscle, resulting in hypertrophy or fibrosis, while sparing other cardiac structures. Four major subgroups of primary cardiomyopathy include: (1) left or biventricular hypertrophy, (2) obstructive hypertrophy (idiopathic hypertrophic subaortic stenosis), (3) congestive biventricular dilation, and (4) restrictive cardiomyopathy. In ventricular hypertrophy, the ventricles become enlarged and thickened; in congestive cardiomyopathy, the walls of the heart become enlarged and thinned; and in restrictive cardiomyopathy, the heart wall stiffens owing to amyloid deposits or fibrosis. Although behavioral and autonomic nervous system research has not yet focused on primary cardiomyopathy as an area of study, ventricular arrhythmias (e.g., premature ventricular beats), which have little if any prognostic meaning in overtly normal people, are prognostic of increased mortality in patients with cardiomyopathy (Moss, 1981).

The occurrence of ventricular arrhythmias is common in patients with primary cardiomyopathy, and Holter monitoring seems to be superior to exercise testing for exposing these arrhythmias (e.g., Savage et al., 1979). These arrhythmias, in turn, may play a causal role in the high death rate in such patients. The combination of ischemia promoting vulnerability in cardiomyopathy patients in conjunction with the frequent occurrence of potentially serious arrhythmias suggests that sympathetic nervous system activation occurring in conjunction with emotional behavior could trigger a lethal arrhythmia.

Although some animal research has used coronary artery occlusion to study the role of behavioral factors in precipitating potentially lethal arrhythmias, animal models of hypertrophic or congestive cardiomyopathy have not yet been used in behavioral research. Nor has behavioral or autonomic nervous system research addressed the problems of how hypertrophic or congestive cardiomyopathies develop. Instead, animal behavior models have focused on intense behavioral stressors that lead to scattered foci of coagulation necrosis and/or coagulative myocytolysis. Since some of these behavioral procedures occasionally lead to the production of lethal arrhythmias, it is conceivable that autonomic and behavioral nervous system research using such models might help to provide insight into the causes of some of the 15% of sudden cardiac deaths in which no underlying pathology is apparent (Titus, 1978).

EVALUATION OF DIFFUSE MYOCARDIAL DAMAGE

Pathological changes that are observed in the myocardium in response to intense physical and behavioral stressors develop over time. Within the first 24 hours these changes are best evaluated by electron microscopy (Jonsson and Johansson, 1974), although subtle morphological changes such as eosinophilia and contraction bands at the light microscopy level can be observed as well as indirect histochemical and biochemical changes such as loss of glycogen, loss of cytoplasmic enzymes such as creatine kinase and lactate dehydrogenase, uptake of Ca^{++} complexing radioisotopes, and increased affinity for fuchsin stains (Corley et al., 1977; Miller and Mallov, 1977; Rapundalo et al., 1980). It is not yet known whether all these indirect measures are reliable indicators of reversible myocardial injury. More emphasis needs to be placed on cross-validating all such measures and on quantitative rather than qualitative endpoints. Between 24 and 72 hours, however, myocardial cell damage can be reliably identified in hematoxylin and eosin-stained sections by degenerating myocytes and their replacement by infiltrating cells such as monocytes, lymphocytes, and histocytes (Reichenbach and Benditt, 1970). Most often such changes are observed in scattered foci in subendocardial regions near the apex of the heart. As the healing of these necrotic foci progresses over a week or so, the appearance of fibrosis (acellular collagen formation) can be taken as a long-term indicator of myocardial injury. Such fibrotic changes are easily identified with a variety of staining procedures including Masson's trichrome (Crawford, 1977). With regard to the proximal causes of these pathological phenomena, most attention has been focused on excessive sympathetic and pituitary-adrenal stimulation (Cannon, 1929; Selye, 1950). Continued evaluation of such mechanisms is warranted, but there is a need for more in-depth, interdisciplinary research in which a single phenomenon is evaluated by converging strategies. Moreover, the relation of cardiomyopathy to disorders in other organ systems such as the kidney needs to be considered.

One might question whether the myocardial changes that develop in response to brief experimental stressors are relevant to clinical syndromes that are often chronic in nature. This can be evaluated by examining experimental animals in both short- and long-term studies. It is conceivable that the behavioral conditions producing diffuse myocardial damage may have implications for other CV disorders and should be looked at in relation to and in conjunction with hypertension, arrhythmias, atherosclerosis, myocardial hypertrophy, and congestive cardiomyopathy.

BEHAVIORAL CONDITIONS

The situations that seem likely to be related to diffuse myocardial injury are those in which the organism is subjected to sensory stimuli thought to evoke emotional responses. However, the difficulty of defining the term "emotional" has led investigators to adopt the view that it is best instead to describe the observable stimulus conditions or behavioral responses as the independent variable to be related to cardiomyopathy.

Diffuse myocardial injury has been reported to occur as a function of recordings of a rat-cat fight played to caged wild rats (Raab et al., 1974), shocks delivered by an animal prod in swine restrained by a muscle relaxant (Johansson et al., 1974; Jonsson and Johansson, 1974), the trapping, handling, and transport of baboons (Groover et al., 1963), unsignaled, unpredictable foot-shock in domestic rats (Miller and Mallov, 1977), and avoidance conditioning in squirrel monkeys (Corley et al., 1977). Myocardial degeneration has also been observed as a function of relatively long-term psychosocial interactions in mice (Henry et al., 1971), rabbits (Weber and Van der Walt, 1973), and baboons (Lapin and Cherkovich, 1971). Further behavioral research is needed if we are to specify precisely the stimulus conditions and behavioral responses elicited. Also needed is quantification of myocardial damage as a function of behavioral manipulations. Radionuclide techniques such as those described by Miller and Malov (1977) may be helpful in this regard. Finally, experiments are needed to identify the exact physiopathological mechanisms producing behaviorally induced cardiomyopathy, and a rational means for preventing such myopathy from occurring in aversive situations.

CNS AND DIFFUSE MYOCARDIAL DAMAGE

Various CNS structures have been implicated in the integration of CV and emotional responses. Hess (1957), for instance, provided evidence that the autonomic and behavioral mechanisms involving the cat hypothalamus are organized into an anterior "trophotropic" zone concerned with emergency functions such as defensive threat and escape behavior. These latter behaviors involve the mobilization of the sympathetic nervous system. In work discussed at this conference, Orville Smith showed that bilateral ablation of a region closely corresponding to Hess' ergotropic zone abolished the CV components (increases in heart rate, arterial pressure and terminal aortic flow; decreases in renal artery flow) but not the somatic components of a conditional emotional response in the baboon (Smith et al., 1980).

Similar CV responses associated with emotional behavior have been elicited by stimulating the ventromedial hypothalamus (VMH) in the rabbit (Gellman et al., in press). Of particular relevance to the issue of CV pathology are findings reported by Soviet investigators that intermittent electrical stimulation of VMH in rabbits for up to 2 weeks elicited cardiac arrhythmias including ventricular fibrillation (Ulyaninsky et al., 1978). These were associated with increased catecholamine content in the blood and myocardium. In rabbits in which stimulation of the hypothalamus resulted in pronounced rhythm disorders, the ultrastructure of the myocardial cells exhibited foci of hypercontraction. There was also obvious swelling and destruction of the mitochondria as well as the presence of lipid droplets.

Whereas stimulation of the VMH in the rabbit elicits tachycardia, a pressor response and increased movement, stimulation of a region just lateral to VMH elicits a pronounced pressor response, bradycardia and immobility (Gellman et al., in press). Such findings suggest that relations among sympathetic nervous system specificity, emotional behavior and CNS organization are ready for investigation.

Stimulation of the VMH in rabbits has also been shown to gate vagal preganglionic cardioinhibitory motor neurons in the medulla (Jordan et al., 1979). Similarly, posterior hypothalamic stimulation in the cat can gate baroreceptor neurons in the nucleus of the solitary tract (Adair and Manning, 1975). Interestingly, in the present conference Marc Nathan reviewed some of his work in which aversive Pavlovian conditioning in the rat led to pronounced increases in blood pressure after central deafferentation by lesions of the nucleus of the solitary tract (Nathan et al., 1978).

Smith indicated in his presentation that his group has used horseradish peroxidase (HRP) to trace projections to a posterior hypothalamic site, which, when destroyed, abolishes the CV component of the conditioned emotional responses. In addition, they have used autoradiographic techniques to trace the efferent projections from the hypothalamus (Smith et al., 1980).

Another hypothalamic structure that seems to be involved in sympathetically mediated CV adjustments is the paraventricular nucleus. Electrical stimulation of this nucleus elicits tachycardia and a vasopressor response (Ciriello and Calaresu, 1980). Larry Swanson, in this conference, described the efferent projections of the paraventricular nucleus using both immunohistochemical techniques and double-labeling of cell bodies by retrograde transport of fluorescent dyes (Sawchenko and Swanson, 1981). It is interesting to note that a single paraventricular neuron may send axon collaterals to medullary and spinal areas containing preganglionic parasympathetic and sympathetic neurons. One specific medullary area to which the paraventricular nucleus projects is the ventral medulla. Numerous physiological and pharmacological studies have shown that respiratory, CV and endocrine responses can be elicited from the ventral medulla. Arthur Loewy, in this conference, described the efferent projections of the ventral medulla observed through the use of autoradiographic techniques (Loewy et al., 1981). The descending projections from this area to the ventral horn and intermediolateral cell column may underlie some of the CV responses that can be elicited by chemical or electrical stimulation of the ventral medulla.

Although the central pathways involved in sympathoadrenomedullary function seem to be of considerable importance in the production of cardiomyopathy, other putative pathways also deserve consideration. Jim Henry, in his conference presentation, implicated the hypothalamic-pituitary-adrenocortical axis in the development of CV pathologies, including cardiomyopathy (Henry and Stephens, 1977).

Of particular interest in the conference was the combined use of neurophysiological, neuroanatomical and behavioral procedures by Smith and colleagues, and the combined use of neuropharmacological and neuroanatomical techniques used by Loewy. It should be pointed out, for example, that anatomical connections between structures may be inhibitory or excitatory. It should also be pointed out that while monosynaptic connections between forebrain structures and visceromotor neurons have been reported, electrophysiological studies have invariably shown these connections to be at least oligosynaptic (Kaufman et al., 1979). Therefore, if firm links are to be made among behavioral, CV and neuroanatomical factors as contributions to CV pathologies including cardiomyopathy, programmatic research will have to address itself specifically to this relation.

Abundant experimental evidence reviewed at this conference supports the hypothesis that stress is associated with certain neurochemical changes within the CNS, and that these changes, in turn, may be related to hypertension. A common theme connecting the results presented at this workshop implicated neurotransmitters and modulators with the associated chemistry of their synthesis and action. The relation of central neurochemical and pharmacological factors to myocardial injury is, however, largely unexplained.

Several investigative approaches presented by Reis, Gillis, and Galosy provide examples of avenues that may provide potential direction for research relating pathologic changes in the heart to chemical correlates in the brain (Reis et al., 1979; DiMicco et al., 1979; Galosy et al., 1981). Answers to some of the fundamental molecular mechanisms of neuronal communication could be followed by pharmacologic studies directed at per-fection of new agents with selective action in the CNS.

The multidisciplinary studies presented by Reis illustrate the utility of focusing on a brain region involved in controlling CV function and its relevance to dysfunction in hypertension (Reis et al., 1979). The induction and inhibition of the synthesis of tyrosine hydroxylase and catecholamine transmitters may be useful indices for quantitative studies on cardiomyopathies. The potential role of indoleamines in central CNS pathways is controversial and requires additional studies for resolution. The amino acid transmitters appear to be much more involved in CV function than previously thought. Both Reis and Gillis presented evidence raising the possibility that GABA and glutamic acid are transmitters in neuronal systems subserving the central control of the CNS (Reis et al., 1981; Williford et al., 1981) . These new observations indicate yet another approach to relating chemical changes and drug action in the brain to cardiac pathology. The report by Gillis that the S-T segment is prolonged after central administration of GABA antagonists, biuculline and picrotoxin, is a possible sign precedent to myocardial injury. The specific sites of action for eliciting the change need to be identified.

Many anatomic sites in the CNS, when electrically stimulated, have been related to cardiac ischemic changes (e.g., Melville et al., 1969). The specific chemical changes and transmitter systems related to and interconnecting many of these sites remain to be elucidated. Moreover, use of specific pharmacologic agonists and antagonists is recom-mended to provide molecular explanations in the CNS of the mechanisms linking hypertension and myocardial injury to the CNS.

The parenteral administration of catecholamines and their congeners (Tanaka et al., 1980), and naturally occurring conditions such as pheochromocytoma (Haft, 1974) have been reported to cause cardiac lesions. Such findings suggest a plausible theory that diffuse myocardial damage is mediated by catecholamines or sympathetically mediated events. The blockage of pathologic lesions by drugs such as propranolol has been largely attributed to an effect on the heart (Tanaka et al., 1980). The central action of such agents in preventing stress-related cardiac damage merits study.

The contribution of the autonomic nervous system to the genesis of cardiomyopathy is unknown. Behavioral paradigms that lead to diffuse myocardial damage increase sympatho-adrenal activity, which then may also lead to release of a variety of humoral agents such as vasopressin, angiotensin II, growth hormone, and ACTH. The relative importance of neural and non-neural factors in the etiology of cardiomyopathy must be determined.

If sympathetic neural influences on the heart contribute to the etiology of cardiomyopathy, then the exact nature of disordered neural effects must be determined. The work of Randall and Hasson (1978) indicates complex functional heterogeneity of cardiac innervation. Myocardial injury may be caused by abnormalities among any of the cardiac neural receptors and effectors. This injury may result from aberrant distribution of sympathetic influence on myocardial pacemaker tissues or coronary circulation rather than from generalized increases in cardiac sympathetic activity. Traditional techniques of pharmacological blockade and total cardiac denervation may not be adequate to demonstrate disorders of distribution.

Humoral agents may contribute in an important manner to myocardial injury, either independently or as they potentiate or diminish effects of the nervous system. In addition, neuronal factors may lead to secondary release of humoral agents which could exacerbate pathology.

A flaw in the total integration of neural influences on the viscera may be important to the development of myocardial damage. Manning (1977) stressed the "regulatory" or modulating influence of the sympathetic nervous system on CV function. Disruption of finely balanced input-output relations may lead to many diseases such as hypertension or cardiac arrhythmias. Such imbalances also may lead to cardiomyopathy. There are multiple potential sources of aberrant sympathetic control. Dysfunction of a single "reflex" may be an inappropriately simple view of altered cardiac control. For example, Gebber (1980) demonstrated that neurons within brain stem sympathetic networks are modulated by multiple sources rather than solely by baroreceptor afferents. Perturbations in "spontaneous" discharge of brain stem sympathetic neurons originating from many sources could lead to myocardial damage.

The preganglionic neuron is controlled by brain stem and spinal systems. These multiple sources of input may lead to heterogeneous patterns of outflow as described by Lynne Weaver in this conference (Meckler et al., 1981). The reported differential sympathetic input to the viscera leads to the suggestion that the pacemaker tissue, myocardium, and coronary vasculature may receive a similarly differential input. This again would multiply the potential etiological factors that might lead to diffuse myocardial injury.

Schramm suggested at this conference that total sympathetic activity and patterns of sympathetic activity to the heart may be determined both by descending activity and by afferent input from the heart or other tissues via supraspinal, spinal or ganglionic pathways. Likewise, potentially toxic humoral factors may be released during behaviors either directly or in response to afferent information resulting from the CV or metabolic concomitants of the behavior. In addition to their actions in the myocardium, the effects of these substances may be compounded via their effects on the CNS.

CATECHOLAMINES, MYOCARDIAL LESIONS, AND CARDIOMYOPATHY

Cardiac lesions induced by administration of isoproterenol in rats closely resemble myocardial damage induced by repeated restraint and water immersion (Tanaka et al., 1980). Both sets of animals showed evidence of myocardial hypertrophy, degeneration, and necrosis. Studies such as this suggest that myocardial damage associated with behavior may be due to endogenously induced and adrenergic responses. Potentiation of beta-adrenergic cardiotoxicity may also occur owing to corticoid release (Guideri et al., 1974).

HYPOTHESES

The preceding discussion suggests a number of possible relations that may exist between biobehavioral activity and cardiomyopathy. Sympathetic nervous system activity may change cardiac function in such a way as to generate hypertrophic cardiomyopathy. The adrenal medulla may play an important role in this, since epinephrine is a potent beta-adrenergic agonist. It seems likely that the pituitary adrenal-cortical system acts in synergism with the sympatho-adrenomedullary system. Neural and non-neural factors may contribute to the genesis of cardiomyopathy with increased sympathoadreno-medullary activity leading to the release of humoral agents such as vasopressin, angiotensin II, growth hormone, and adrenocorticotrophin.

The effect of beta-adrenergic sympathetic activity is to increase cardiac contractile activity. At the same time, alpha-adrenergic sympathetic activity may lead to regional vasoconstriction, which in turn leads to increased vasoconstrictor activity. These concomitant increases in sympathetic activity thereby lead to increases in myocardial oxygen consumption and an increase in afterload. The sequelae of increased sympathetic activity with no increased preload may be: (1) increased contractile force, (2) increased systolic emptying with decreased diastolic volume, and (3) endocardial ischemia due to mechanically induced decreases in endocardial perfusion. In addition, increased sympathetic activity may increase coronary arterial resistance despite local vasodilator influence. This neurogenically induced decrease in coronary blood flow can cause a rightward shift in the relation between coronary flow and myocardial oxygen consumption (i.e., lower flow at a given VO_2). Dyskinesia may confound this focal ischemia and lead to regional hypertrophy or to decreased ejection fraction.

RECOMMENDATIONS

1. Specific relations among behavioral contingencies, diffuse myocardial injury and the development of primary cardiomyopathy need to be identified.

2. Quantitative measures of diffuse myocardial injury and cardiomyopathy require further development.

3. Noninvasive measures for assessing myocardial damage should be developed.

4. Animal models should be developed to broaden the basis of cardiomyopathy study. This includes study of chronic behavioral factors that may lead to congestive and left ventricular hypertrophy as well as necrosis. The Syrian hamster may serve as an appropriate model for congestive cardiomyopathy.

5. The mediators of cardiomyopathy, including catecholamines and endocrines, as well as their interaction, should be investigated intensively. There is suggestive evidence that prolonged behavioral stress associated with increased sympathetic nervous system activity can lead to hypertrophic cardiomyopathy. Conceivably, prolonged increases in afterload associated with sympathetic nervous system activity in an otherwise healthy heart and vascular system could lead to hypertrophy. Alternatively, the large release of catecholamines and possibly other substances into the circulation of an organism with poor cardiopulmonary function could make the ventricles thin-walled and dilated owing to the loss of myocardial fiber. In any event, since the etiology of most primary cardiomyopathies is unknown or at least poorly understood, future research should examine the possibilities that (a) increased sympathetic nervous system activity can change cardiac function in such a way as to generate cardiomyopathy; and (b) increased sympathetic nervous system activity associated with different behavioral contingencies, differential release of catecholamines, differential release of other neurohumors, and/or differential cardiopulmonary status among animals lead to hypertrophic versus congestive cardiomyopathies.

6. Interactions among hypertension, atherosclerosis and cardiomyopathy need to be examined.

7. CNS pathways that mediate myocardial lesions require study. This includes looking at specificity of pathology with regard to neurophysiological mechanisms.

An end point of this research should be an evaluation and identification of myocardial lesions and developing cardiomyopathy in patients before the histology is obtained. The results of animal models will identify the constellation of behavioral, physiological and endocrine changes that are associated with myocardial lesions and developing cardiomyopathy, and relate these to other pathophysiological conditions.

REFERENCES

Adair, J.R. and Manning, J.W. (1975) Hypothalamic modulation of baroreceptor afferent unit activity. Amer. J. Physiol. 229, 1357-1364.

Cannon, W.B. (1929) Bodily changes in pain, hunger, fear and rage: an account of recent researches into function of emotional excitements. Appleton, New York.

Ciriello, J. and Calaresu, F.R. (1980) Autoradiographic study of ascending projections from cardiovascular sites in the nucleus tractus solitarii in the cat. Brain Res. 186, 448-453.

Corley, K.C., Shiel, F.O., Mauch, H.P., Clark, L.S. and Barker, J.V. (1977) Myocardial degeneration and cardiac arrest in squirrel monkey: physiological and psychological correlation. Psychophysiology 14, 322-328.

Crawford, T. (1977) Pathology of ischemic heart disease. Butterworths, Boston.

DiMicco, J.A., Gale, K., Hamilton, B. and Gillis, R.A. (1979) GABA receptor control of parasympathetic outflow to heart: characterization and brainstem localization. Science 204, 1106-1109.

Galosy, R.A., Clarke, L.K., Vasko, M.R. and Crawford, I.L. (1981) Neurophysiology and neuropharmacology of cardiovascular regulation and stress. Neurosci. Biobehav. Rev. 5, 137-175, 1981.

Gebber, G.L. (1980) Central oscillators responsible for sympathetic nerve discharge. Amer. J. Physiol. 239, H143-H155.

Gellman, M., Schneiderman, N., Wallach, J. and LeBlanc, W. (in press) Cardiovascular responses elicited by hypothalamic stimulation in rabbits reveal a medio-lateral organization. J. Autonom. Nerv. Syst.

Groover, M.E., Seljeskog, L.L., Haglin, J.J. and Hitchcock, C.R. (1963) Myocardial infarction in the Kenya baboon without demonstrable atherosclerosis. Angiology 14, 409-416.

Guideri, G., Barletta, M.A. and Lehr, D. (1974) Extraordinary potentiation of isoproterenol cardiotoxicity by corticoid pretreatment. Cardiovasc. Res. 8, 775-786.

Haft, J.I. (1974) Cardiovascular injury induced by sympathetic catecholamines. Progr. Cardiovasc. Dis. 17, 73-88.

Henry, J.P., Ely, D.L., Stephens, P.M., Ratcliffe, H.L., Santisteban, G.A. and Shapiro, A.P. (1971) The role of psychosocial factors in the development of arteriosclerosis in CBA mice. Atherosclerosis 14, 203-218.

Henry, J.P. and Stephens, P.M. (1977) Stress, Health and the Social Environment: A Sociobiological Approach to Medicine. Springer-Verlag, New York.

Hess, W.R. (1957) Functional Organization of the Diecephalon. Grune and Stratton, New York.

Johansson, G., Jonsson, L., Lannek, N., Blomgren, L., Lindberg, P. and Poupa, O. (1974) Severe stress-cardiopathy in pigs. Amer. Heart J. 87, 451-457.

Johnsson, L. and Johansson, G. (1974) Cardiac muscle cell damage induced by restraint stress. Virchows Arch. Cell Path. 17, 1-12.

Jordan, D., Khalid, M., Schneiderman, N. and Spyer, K.M. (1979) The inhibitory control of vagal cardiomotor neurons. J. Physiol. (Lond.) 301, 54P.

Kaufman, M., Hamilton, R., Wallach, J., Petrik, G. and Schneiderman, N. (1979) Lateral subthalamic area as mediator of bradycardia responses in rabbits. Amer. J. Physiol. 236, H471-H479.

Lapin, B. and Cherkovich, G.M. (1971) Environmental change causing the development of neuroses and corticovisceral pathology in monkeys; in Society, Stress and Disease: The Psychosocial Environment and Psychosomatic Diseases, L. Levi, ed. London.

Loewy, A.D., Wallach, J.H. and McKellar, S. (1981) Efferent connections of the ventral medulla oblongata in the rat. Brain Res. Rev. 3, 63-80.

Manning, J.W. (1977) Intracranial mechanisms of regulation; in Neural Regulation of the Heart, W.C. Randall, ed. Oxford Univ. Press, New York, pp. 187-210.

Meckler, R., Fry, H. and Weaver, L. (1981) Differential pattern of sympathetic outflow initiated by stimulation of visceral afferent neurones. Neurosci. Abstr. 7, 366.

Melville, K.I., Garvey, H.L., Shister, H.E. and Knaack, J. (1969) Central nervous system stimulation and cardiac ischemic changes in monkeys. Ann. N.Y. Acad. Sci. 156, 241-260.

Miller, D.G. and Mallov, S. (1977) The quantitative determination of stress-induced myocardial damage in rats. Pharmacol. Biochem. Behav. 7, 139-145.

Moss, A.J. (1981) Clinical significance of ventricular arrhythmias in patients with and without coronary artery disease; in Sudden Cardiac Death, E.H. Sonnenblick and M. Lesch, eds. Grune and Stratton, New York.

Nathan, M.A., Tucker, L.W., Severini, W.P. and Reis, D.J. (1978) Enhancement of conditioned arterial pressure responses in cats after brainstem lesions. Science 201, 71-73.

Raab, W., Chaplin, J.P. and Bajusz, E. (1964) Myocardial necroses produced in domesticated rats and in wild rats by sensory and emotional stresses. Proc. Soc. Exp. Biol. Med. 116, 665-669.

Randall, D.C. and Hasson, D.M. (1978) Incidence of cardiac arrhythmias in monkey during classic aversive and appetitive conditioning; in Neural Mechanisms in Cardiac Arrhythmias, P.J. Schwartz, A.M. Brown, A. Malliani and A. Zanchetti, eds. Raven, New York.

Rapundalo, S.T., Persinger, M.A. and Alikhan, M.A. (1980) Cardiohistological changes in rats from single episodes of maintained forced exercise. Physiol. Behav. 25, 433-438.

Reichenbach, D.D. and Benditt, E.T. (1970) Catecholamines and cardiomyopathy: the genesis and potential importance of myofibrillar degeneration. Hum. Path. 1, 125-150.

Reis, D.J., Joh, T.H., Nathan, M.A., Renaud, B., Snyder, D.W. and Talman, W.T. (1979) Nucleus tractus solitarii: catecholaminergic innervation in normal and abnormal control of arterial pressure; in Nervous System and Hypertension, P. Meyer and H. Schmitt, eds. Wiley, New York, pp. 147-164.

Reis, D.J., Perrone, M.H. and Talman, W.T. (1981) Glutamic acid as the neurotransmitter of baroreceptor afferents in the nucleus tractus solitarii: possible relationship to neurogenic hypertension; in Central Nervous System Mechanisms in Hypertension, J.P. Buckley and C.M. Ferrario, eds. Raven, New York, pp. 37-48.

Savage, D.D., Seides, S.F., Maron, B.J. et al. (1979) Prevalence of arrhythmias during 24-hr electrocardiographic monitoring and exercise testing in patients with obstructive and nonobstructive hypertrophic cardiomyopathy. Circulation 59, 866-875.

Sawchenko, P.E. and Swanson, L.W. (1981) Central noradrenergic pathways for the integration of hypothalamic neuroendocrine and autonomic responses. Science 214, 685-687.

Selye, H. (1950) The Physiology and Pathology of Exposure to Stress. Acta, Inc. Publishers, Montreal.

Smith, O.A., Astley, A., DeVito, J.L., Stein, J.M. and Walsh, K.E. (1980) Functional analysis of the cardiovascular responses accompanying emotional behavior. Fed. Proc. 39, 2487-2494.

Tanaka, M., Tsuchihashi, Y., Katsume, H., Ijichi, H. and Ibata, Y. (1980) Comparison of cardiac lesions induced in rats by isoproterenol and by repeated stress of restraint and water immersion with special reference to etiology of cardiomyopathy. Jap. Circulat. J. 44, 971-980.

Titus, J.C. (1978) Pathology of sudden cardiac death; in USA-USSR First Symposium on Sudden Death, Yalta, USSR, 309-318.

Ulyaninsky, L.S., Stepanyan, E.P. and Krymsky, I.P. (1977) Cardiac arrhythmias of hypothalamic origin; Proceedings USA-USSR Joint Symposium on Sudden Death. DHEW No. (NIH) 78-1472, US Govt. Printing Office, Washington, D.C.

Weber, H.W. and Van der Walt, J.J. (1973) Cardiomyopathy in crowded rabbits: a preliminary report. S. Afr. Med. J. 47, 1591-1595.

Williford, D.J., Hamilton, B.L., DiMicco, J.A., Norman, W.P., Yamada, K.A., Quest, J.A., Zauadil, A. and Gillis, R.A. (1981) Central GABAergic mechanisms involved in the control of arterial blood pressure; in Central Nervous System Mechanisms in Hypertension, J.P. Buckley and C.M. Ferrario, eds. Raven, New York.

Index